Practical Pediatric
Gastrointestinal Endoscopy

To my life muse, my wife Irina,
my talented daughter Zhenya,
my precious granddaughter Nikka,
and in memory of my remarkable parents.

George Gershman

Practical Pediatric Gastrointestinal Endoscopy

Second Edition

Edited by

George Gershman

MD, PhD
Professor of Pediatrics
Chief, Division of Pediatric Gastroenterology
Harbor-UCLA Medical Center
Torrance, CA, USA

Mike Thomson

MB ChB, DCH, MRCP(Paeds), FRCPCH, MD, FRCP
Consultant in Paediatric Gastroenterology
Sheffield Childrens NHS Trust;
Honorary Reader
University of Sheffield
Sheffield, UK

With

Marvin Ament

MD
Professor Emeritus of Pediatrics
David Geffen School of Medicine, UCLA;
Medical Director of Pediatric Gastroenterology, Hepatology
and Nutrition at Children's Hospital of Central California
Madera, CA, USA

WILEY-BLACKWELL
A John Wiley & Sons, Ltd., Publication

Library of Congress Cataloging-in-Publication Data
Gershman, George.
  Practical pediatric gastrointestinal endoscopy / George Gershman, Mike Thomson, Marvin Ament. – 2nd ed.
     p. ; cm.
  Includes bibliographical references and index.
  ISBN-13: 978-1-4443-3649-8 (hardcover : alk. paper)
  ISBN-10: 1-4443-3649-5 (hardcover : alk. paper)
  I. Thomson, Mike (Mike Andrew) II. Ament, Marvin Earl, 1938- III. Title.
  [DNLM: 1. Endoscopy, Gastrointestinal. 2. Pediatrics–methods. 3. Child. 4. Infant. WI 141]
  LC classification not assigned
  618.92'3307545–dc23
                              2011029723

A catalogue record for this book is available from the British Library.

Set in 8.5 on 11 pt Utopia by Toppan Best-set Premedia Limited
Printed and bound in Singapore by Markono Print Media Pte Ltd

1   2012

Contents

Contributors

David E. Barlow PhD Vice President, Research and Development, Olympus America, Inc., Center Valley, PA, USA

Luigi Dall'Oglio MD Digestive Endoscopy and Surgery Unit, Ospedale Pediatrico Bambino Gesù – IRCCS, Roma, Italy

Paola De Angelis MD Digestive Endoscopy and Surgery Unit, Ospedale Pediatrico Bambino Gesù – IRCCS, Roma, Italy

Thierry Devreker MD Departments of Pediatric Gastroenterology, Universitair Ziekenhuis, Brussels, Belgium

Francesca Foschia MD Digestive Endoscopy and Surgery Unit, Ospedale Pediatrico Bambino Gesù – IRCCS, Roma, Italy

George Gershman MD, PhD Professor of Pediatrics, Chief, Division of Pediatric Gastroenterology, Harbor-UCLA Medical Center, Torrance, CA, USA

Bruno Hauser MD Departments of Pediatric Gastroenterology, Universitair Ziekenhuis, Brussels, Belgium

David P. Hurlstone FRCP MD (Dist). Consultant Advanced Endoscopist and Gastroenterologist, Barnsley NHS Foundation Trust, Barnsley, UK

Tom Kallay MD Assistant Professor of Pediatrics, Division of Pediatric Critical Care, Harbor-UCLA Medical Center, Torrance, CA, USA

Marsha Kay MD Chair, Department of Pediatric Gastroenterology and Nutrition, Director Pediatric Endoscopy, Children's Hospital, Cleveland Clinic, Cleveland, OH, USA

Antonio Quiros MD Pediatric Inflammatory Bowel Disorders Center, California Pacific Medical Center, San Francisco, CA, USA

Alberto Ravelli MD GI Pathophysiology and Gastroenterology, University Department of Pediatrics, Children's Hospital, Spedali Civili, Brescia, Italy

Hendrik Reynaert MD, PhD Department of Gastroenterology, Universitair Ziekenhuis, Brussels, Belgium

Mike Thomson MB ChB, DCH, MRCP(Paeds), FRCPCH, MD, FRCP Consultant in Paediatric Gastroenterology, Sheffield Childrens NHS Trust; Honorary Reader, University of Sheffield, Sheffield, UK

Daniel Urbain MD Department of Gastroenterology, Universitair Ziekenhuis, Brussels, Belgium

Yvan Vandenplas MD, PhD Professor of Pediatrics, Chief Division of Pediatric Gastroenterology, Chair, Department of Pediatrics, Universitair Ziekenhuis, Brussels, Belgium

Jorge H. Vargas MD Professor of Pediatrics, Division of Gastroenterology, Hepatology and Nutrition, Mattel-Children's Hospital, Geffen-UCLA School of Medicine, Los Angeles, CA, USA

Krishnappa Venkatesh MD Sheffield Childrens NHS Trust; Honorary Reader, University of Sheffield, Sheffield, UK

Robert Wyllie MD Chief Medical Officer, Cleveland Clinic Professor, Lerner College of Medicine Vice Chair, Office of Professional Staff Affairs Cleveland Clinic Department of Pediatric Gastroenterology and Nutrition Children's Hospital, Cleveland Clinic, Cleveland, OH, USA

Part One

Pediatric Endoscopy Setting

Introduction

George Gershman

Esophagogastroduodenoscopy (EGD) was an exotic procedure in children until the mid-70s when prototypes of pediatric flexible gastro- and panendoscopes became commercially available. Within the next few years, hundreds of pediatric EGDs were performed in Europe and the US leaving no doubts about safety, high-efficacy and cost-effectiveness of upper gastrointestinal (GI) endoscopy in children.

Over the next ten years, EGD and ileocolonoscopy became routine diagnostic and therapeutic procedures for pediatric gastroenterologists around the world.

Flexible gastrointestinal endoscopy is a unique method of investigation of the GI tract. It combines direct visualization of the GI tract with a target biopsy, application of different dyes, endoluminal ultrasound, injection of contrast materials with various therapeutic procedures. By definition, it is an invasive procedure. When applied to pediatric patients, safety becomes the major priority. In order to minimize morbidity associated with pediatric GI endoscopy, the endoscopist, especially the beginner, should familiarize themselves with all technical aspects of the procedure including:

- Endoscopic equipment: endoscopes, light sources, biopsy forceps, snares, graspers, needles, electrosurgical devices and all other accessories

- Appropriate setting for the endoscopic equipment and doses of commonly used medications and solutions such as epinephrine, glucagon and sclerosing agents.
- Proper techniques of basic diagnostic and therapeutic procedures.

In addition, a pediatric gastroenterologist should also become familiar with age-related characteristics of the esophagus, stomach, duodenum, and common adoptive reactions induced by intubations of the esophagus and insufflation and stretching of the stomach and the colon.

The evolution of the equipment and technological innovations of the last decade opened the door to the new diagnostic and therapeutic procedures in pediatrics such as double-balloon enteroscopy, confocal laser endomicroscopy, removable and biodegradable stents for treatment of refractory esophageal strictures, and endoscopic treatment of gastroesophageal reflux disease.

We believe that the second edition of Practical Pediatrics Gastrointestinal Endoscopy will serve as a perfect guide to trainees, simplifying the learning process of basic endoscopic techniques and highlighting the important background data, technical aspects and outcomes of new endoscopic procedures in children to both pediatric and adult gastroenterologists.

Practical Pediatric Gastrointestinal Endoscopy, Second Edition. George Gershman, Mike Thomson, Marvin Ament.
© 2012 Blackwell Publishing Ltd. Published 2012 by Blackwell Publishing Ltd.

2

Settings and staff

George Gershman

 KEY POINTS

- Endoscopy is complex procedure.
- A proper setting of the endoscopy unit is essential for provision of the optimal working environment and maximal patient flow.
- Meticulous preparation of endoscopic equipment is necessary for a "smooth" operation during endoscopy.

- A well-trained endoscopy nurse is an important key for safety and quality provision of the endoscopic procedure.
- High-quality disinfection of the instruments is a vital component of patient safety.
- Accurate paper type and electronic documentation of information related to the endoscopic procedure is vital for immediate and follow-up treatment.

Pediatric GI endoscopy can be performed in three different settings: an endoscopy unit, the patient's bedside, and the operating room. The endoscopy unit is designated for elective procedures. Typically, it has five functional areas:

- A pre-procedure area consisting of a reception lobby and admitting room dedicated for parental consent, patient dressing, triage, and the establishment of an intravenous access;
- A procedure area with examination rooms;
- A recovery area;
- A medical staff area with a working station for units with more than three procedure rooms;
- A storage space and a section dedicated for cleaning and disinfection of endoscopes.

The average volume of pediatric GI endoscopic procedures is usually not high enough to run a separate pediatric endoscopic GI unit. Typically, pediatric and adult gastroenterologists share the same endoscopy units, either in the hospital or the outpatient surgical center.

Such units must have a nursing and ancillary support staff trained to work with both children and adults. Although some units designate a special room for pediatric patients, it is more con-

venient if pediatric procedures can be performed in all examination rooms.

Most bedside endoscopies for infants and children are done in pediatric and neonatal intensive care units.

Bedside pediatric endoscopy is typically limited to children with acute GI bleeding or complicated recovery following bone-marrow or solid organ transplantation. It is usually a complex and labor-intensive procedure in critically ill patients, which requires:

1. Full cooperation between a skillful endoscopist, a resident, an endoscopy nurse and an attending physician;
2. Proper function of all endoscopic equipment;
3. A well-organized and appropriately equipped mobile endoscopy station.

The mobile station should be loaded with age-appropriate endoscopes and bite-guards, a light source, electrosurgical unit, biopsy forceps, retractable needles, polypectomy snares, graspers, hemostatic clips, rubber bands, epinephrine, biopsy mounting sets, fixatives, culture medias, cytology brushes and slides. The bedside area should be large enough to accommodate the

Practical Pediatric Gastrointestinal Endoscopy, Second Edition. George Gershman, Mike Thomson, Marvin Ament.
© 2012 Blackwell Publishing Ltd. Published 2012 by Blackwell Publishing Ltd.

endoscopic station, a portable monitor and equipment for general anesthesia. Two separate suction canisters should be available for endoscopy and oral or tracheal aspiration.

The position of the bed should be adjusted to the height of the endoscopist and any specific indications for the procedure. For example, reverse Trendelenburg position reduces the risk of aspiration and improves visibility of lesions (acute ulcers or gastric varices) in the gastric cardia and subcardia.

Endoscopic procedures in the neonatal intensive care unit should be performed under the warmer.

Pediatric GI endoscopy in the operating room is restricted to children with obscure or occult GI bleeding, Peutz–Jeghers syndrome, or other conditions which require intraoperative enteroscopy. The needs for such procedures have been recently reduced due to the availability of capsule or double-balloon enteroscopy. The endoscopy team should be familiar with the operating room environment and regulations.

Pediatric endoscopy nurse

A well-trained nurse is the key to a successful pediatric endoscopy team. This individual should be skilled in many areas such as:

1. Communication with the parents and the child targeting the level of stress and anxiety before the procedure;
2. Establishing and securing intravenous (IV) access;
3. Preparing all monitoring devices including EKG leads, pulse oximeter sensors, blood pressure cuffs appropriate for the child's size and life-support equipment such as nasal cannulas, correct size of oxygen masks, ambu-bags, and intubation trays;
4. Selecting and preparing appropriate endoscopic equipment for the procedure;
5. Monitoring patients during sedation, procedure and recovery;
6. Proper mounting of the biopsy specimens and preparation of the cytological slides;
7. Mechanical and chemical cleaning of the equipment and disinfection of the working space;
8. Quality control maintenance.

It is very convenient having an endoscopy nurse on-call for urgent procedures which occur after hours.

Disinfections of the endoscopes and accessories

Thorough mechanical cleaning of the endoscope and any non-disposable instruments is an essential part of any procedure especially a bedside endoscopy. It is an important initial phase of disinfection and is also an effective preventive measure against the clogging of the air-water channel and future mechanical failure of very expensive devices. The final cleaning of the endoscopic equipment is usually performed with glutaraldehyde, which destroys viruses and bacteria within a few minutes. Typically, endoscopes soak for a 20 minute period, although high-risk situations including known or suspected mycobacterial infections may require longer chemical exposure.

Glutaraldehyde can exacerbate reactive airway disease, asthma or dermatitis in sensitive patients or staff. For this reason, instruments are thoroughly rinsed in water and allowed to dry prior to their next use. Air-water and suction channels are further rinsed in a solution containing 70% alcohol and also require compressed air-drying to prevent bacterial growth. Instruments should be hung and stored in a vertical position in a well-ventilated cupboard to ensure dryness and minimize any opportunity for bacterial growth.

A more detailed description of disinfection technique is presented in Chapter 3.

Documentation

Different types of photo-documentation are available during endoscopy. Polaroid photographs and real-time videotaping have been replaced by digital photo printers since the early 1990s. Currently, digitized endoscopic images can be stored on a computer hard-drive or external device. The snapshots of the procedure can be printed on paper or recorded on DVD in real-time. Images can be e-mailed through a secure website for a second opinion or on-line discussion.

FURTHER READING

Association of periOperative Registered Nurses. (2002) Recommended practices for managing the patient receiving moderate sedation/analgesia. *Association of Operating Room Nurses Journal*, **75**, 649–652.

Association of periOperative Registered Nurses. (2005) Guidance Statement: preoperative patient care in the ambulatory surgery setting. *Association of Operating Room Nurses Journal*, **81**, 871–888.

Association of periOperative Registered Nurses. (2005) Guidance Statement: postoperative patient care in the ambulatory surgery setting. *Association of Operating Room Nurses Journal*, **81**, 881–888.

AGA. (2001) The American Gastroenterological Association Standards for Office-Based Gastrointestinal Endoscopy Services. *Gastroenterology*, **121**, 440–443.

ASGE. (2007) Informed consent for GI endoscopy. *Gastrointestinal Endoscopy*, **2**, 626–629.

Berg JW, Appelbaum PS, Lidz CW, *et al.* (2001) *Informed consent: Legal Theory and Clinical Practice.* Oxford: Oxford University Press.

Braddock CH, Fihn SD, Levinson W, *et al.* (1997) How doctors and patients discuss routine clinical decisions: informed decision making in the outpatient setting. *Journal of General Internal Medicine*, **12**, 339–45.

Foote MA. (1994) The role of gastrointestinal assistant. In: Sivak MV (Ed), *Gastrointestinal Endoscopy Clinics of North America*, 523–39. Philadelphia: WB Saunders.

Guidelines for documentations in the gastrointestinal endoscopy setting. (1999) Soc Gastroenterol Nurses Associates Inc. *Gastroenterology Nurse*, **22**, 69–97.

Kowalski T, Edmundowicz S, Vacante N. (2004) Endoscopy unit form and function. *Gastrointestinal Endoscopy Clinics of North America*, **14**(4), 657–666.

Marasco JH, Marasco RF. (2002) Designing the ambulatory endoscopy center. *Gastrointestinal Endoscopy Clinics of North America*, **12**(2), 185–204.

Role delineation of the registered nurse in a staff position in gastroenterology. Position statement. (2001) Soc. Gastroenterol Nurses Assistants. *Gastroenterology Nurse*, **24**, 202–3.

Society of Gastroenterology Nurses and Associates Inc. Guidelines for documentation in the gastrointestinal endoscopy setting. http://www.sgna.org/Resources/guidelines/guideline7.cfm [accessed on 22 October]

Video endoscope: how does it work?

David E. Barlow

 KEY POINTS

- The modern flexible endoscope is a complex, highly-engineered medical instrument. Systems for air, water, suction, tip angulation and the endoscope's basic controls are common across manufacturers and models. Differentiation is often in subtle areas such as handling characteristics, breadth of product line, image quality, and the manufacturer's special features (insertion tube flexibility adjustment, options for image enhancement, image documentation options, etc.).

- RGB sequential endoscopes offer incrementally superior color accuracy but suffer from motion artifacts and a strobed image. Color-chip endoscopes are more popular due to good color reproduction and a natural view of moving objects (e.g. mucosa).

- Recent advancements in imaging include high-definition imaging, narrow-band imaging and wide-angle, close-focusing optics.

- An understanding of the basic components of the endoscope and how they interrelate will help the endoscopist troubleshoot many equipment problems.

- Specific background information on the safe use of chemicals, personal protective equipment and all applicable regulations, plus thorough training on the specific steps of instrument reprocessing are necessary to clean and disinfect an endoscope safely and effectively. Reprocessing errors can lead to instrument damage, costly repairs and an infection control risk.

Overview

The modern video endoscope is the result of more than 25 years of refinements in solid-state imaging technology and improved mechanical design. The basic shape, controls and method of use are relatively unchanged from fiberoptic endoscopes used in the mid-1970s. Although alternative designs for the control section have been proposed (e.g. "pistol-grip" controls), the basic layout of GI endoscopes is similar across all models (gastroscopes, colonoscopes, etc.) and all manufacturers. The basic components and con-

trols of the video endoscope are illustrated in Figure 3.1. The instrument is designed to be held and operated by the endoscopist's left hand, while the endoscopist's right hand primarily controls the insertion tube.

Insertion tube

Figure 3.2 illustrates the internal components of a typical videoscope insertion tube. Both gastroscopes and colonoscopes employ similar components. While its outer appearance is

Practical Pediatric Gastrointestinal Endoscopy, Second Edition. George Gershman, Mike Thomson, Marvin Ament.
© 2012 Blackwell Publishing Ltd. Published 2012 by Blackwell Publishing Ltd.

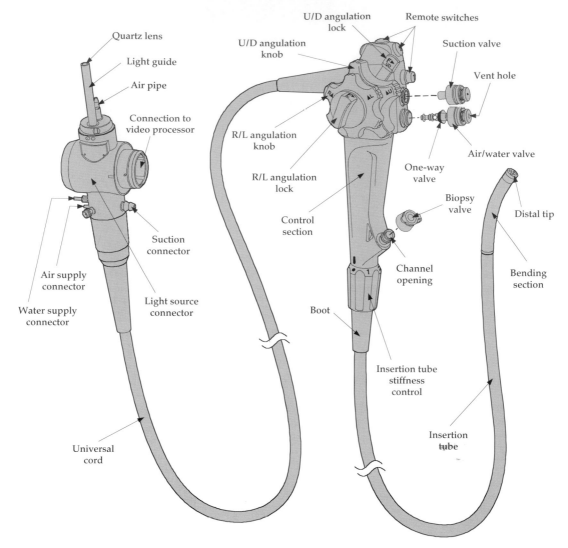

Figure 3.1 Colonoscope – Components and controls. Gastroscopes have a similar construction.

deceptively plain, internally, the insertion tube is filled with a collection of lumens, control wires, electrical wires, glass fibers and other components. The largest tube housed in the insertion tube is typically the instrument "channel" and is used for suctioning fluid and taking biopsies. Smaller internal tubes are used to convey air and water for insufflation and lens washing, respectively. Some models, more often colonoscopes, have an additional forward water-jet tube for washing the mucosa. Four angulation control wires run the length of the insertion tube and control the deflection of the distal tip. A group of

very fine electrical wires connect the CCD (charge-coupled device) image sensor at the distal tip of the endoscope to the video processor. These wires are housed in a protective sheath to prevent them from being damaged as the instrument is manipulated. One or two bundles of delicate glass fibers convey light from the light source to the distal end of the endoscope. These fragile fiberoptic bundles also require protection, and are enclosed in a soft protective sheath. Colonoscopes with adjustable insertion tube flexibility have an additional component – a tensioning wire to control insertion tube stiffness.

The endoscope designer packs these individual components into the smallest possible cross-sectional area in order to minimize the outer diameter of the insertion tube. A small diameter insertion tube is especially important in instruments used in pediatric endoscopy, but the components cannot be packed too tightly. The designer must plan for enough free space to permit the components to move about without damaging the more fragile components (CCD wires, fiberoptic strands) as the instrument is torqued and flexed during use. A dry-powdered lubricant is applied to the internal components to reduce the frictional stress they place on each other during insertion tube manipulation.

Insertion tube flexibility

The handling characteristics of the endoscope's insertion tube are extremely important. For ease of insertion, any rotation applied by the endoscopist to the proximal shaft must be transferred to the distal tip in a 1:1 ratio. In order to transmit this torque and prevent the instrument shaft from simply twisting up, the insertion tube is built around several flat, spiral metal bands that run just under the skin of the insertion tube (*see* Figure 3.2). Because these helical bands are wound in opposite directions, they lock against one another as the tube is torqued, accurately transmitting rotation of the proximal end to the distal end of the tube. At the same time, the gaps in the helical bands allow the shaft to flex freely. These metal bands also give the insertion tube its round shape

and help prevent the internal components of the insertion tube from being crushed by external forces.

The helical bands are covered by a layer of stainless steel mesh. This thin wire mesh creates a metal, fabric-like layer, which covers the sharp edges of the spiral bands, and creates a continuous surface upon which the outer layer of the tube can be applied. The external layer (observable to the user) is composed of a plastic polymer, typically black or dark green, which is extruded over the wire mesh to create a smooth outer surface. This polymer layer provides an atraumatic, biocompatible, watertight exterior for the insertion tube. It is typically marked with a scale to allow the endoscopist to gauge depth of insertion. While each component of the insertion tube has some effect on the overall flexibility of the tube, the endoscope designer most often adjusts the construction of the wire mesh and the outer polymer layer to fine-tune the handling characteristics of the instrument.

Years of experience have shown that a more rigid insertion tube is optimal for examining the fixed anatomy of the upper GI tract. On the one hand, the colon, with its tortuosity and freely moving loops, is best examined by a more flexible instrument. The ideal colonoscope insertion tube must be flexible, yet highly elastic, and sufficiently floppy (non-rigid) to conform easily to the tortuous anatomy of the patient. It should not exert undue force on the colon or its attached mesentery. On the other hand, the instrument must have sufficient column strength to prevent buckling when the proximal end of the instrument is pushed. (In contrast, a wet noodle is extremely flexible but lacks column strength and collapses when pushed). In addition to its flexibility, the colonoscope must have sufficient elasticity to pop back into a straightened condition whenever it is pulled back. This aids the endoscopist in removing colon loops. The goal in designing the proximal portion of the insertion tube, therefore, is to prevent the reformation of bowel loops as the instrument is advanced. Obtaining the ideal combination of flexibility, elasticity, column strength and torqueability is the art and science of insertion tube design. Often, improvements in one of these characteristics negatively impacts one or more of the others. The final design is usually a compromise of these ideal characteristics, confirmed by months of clinical testing.

For ease of insertion, both gastroscopes and colonoscopes vary in flexibility from end to end.

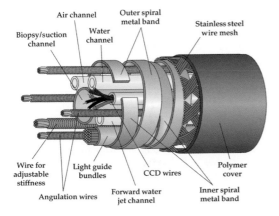

Figure 3.2 Insertion tube – Internal components and construction.

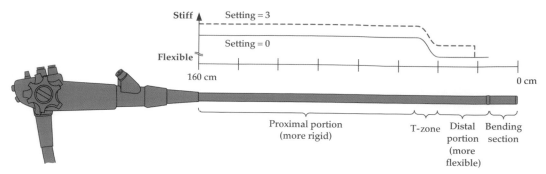

Figure 3.3 The flexibility of the colonoscope insertion tube varies over its length. On some models, it can be further stiffened by changing the setting on the adjustable stiffness control.

As Figure 3.3 illustrates, the distal 40 cm of the colonoscope insertion tube is significantly more flexible than the proximal portion of the tube. This variation in flexibility is achieved by changing the formulation of the tube's outer polymer layer as it is extruded over the underlying wire mesh during the manufacturing process. The extrusion machine that manufactures the outer coating of the insertion tube contains two types of plastic resins, one significantly harder than the other. Initially, as the distal end of the insertion tube passes through the machine, a layer of soft resin is applied to the first 40 cm. This soft resin is gradually replaced by the harder resin within a transition zone (T-Zone in Figure 3.3) near the middle of the tube. The remaining proximal portion of the insertion tube (50 cm to 160 cm) is constructed totally from the hard resin (Moriyama 2000). The end result is a colonoscope insertion tube that has a soft distal portion for atraumatically snaking through a tortuous colon, with a stiffer proximal portion that is effective at preventing the reformation of loops in those portions of the colon that have already been straightened. The flexibility of a gastroscope's insertion tube varies in a similar manner – being more flexible at the distal end and stiffer at the proximal end.

Due to differences in training, insertion technique and personal preference, endoscopists often disagree over what are the "ideal" characteristics for a particular insertion tube. In addition, some endoscopists have expressed a desire to change the characteristics of the insertion tube during the procedure itself, based on insertion depth or the patient's anatomy. This has led to the development of an insertion tube with adjustable stiffness (Moriyama 2001). Colonoscopes with adjustable-stiffness have a tensioning wire that

runs the length of the insertion tube (*see* Figure 3.2). The amount of tension in this wire is controlled by rotating a ring at the proximal end of the insertion tube, just below the control section (*see* Figure 3.1). When the inner wire in the stiffening system is in the "soft" position, the stiffening system provides no additional stiffness to the insertion tube beyond that provided by the wire mesh and polymer coat. When the control ring is rotated to one of the "hard" positions, the pull wire is retracted and placed under heavy tension. This stiffens the coil wire surrounding the pull wire and adds significant rigidity to the insertion tube. As Figure 3.3 summarizes, the base stiffness of the insertion tube (Setting = 0) is established by varying the mixture of hard and soft resins in the outer polymer coat of the insertion tube. This base stiffness however, can be further enhanced by increasing the tension in the variable-stiffness pull wire (Setting = 3).

Distal tip

The distal tip of all forward viewing endoscopes (e.g. gastroscopes, colonoscopes) is constructed of the components illustrated in Figure 3.4. Light to illuminate the interior of the body is carried through the instrument via a bundle(s) of delicate fiberoptic illumination fibers. Each of these glass fibers is approximately 30 microns in diameter. A lens at the tip of this fiberoptic bundle evenly disperses the transmitted light across the endoscope's field of view. It is important to achieve even and balanced illumination across the entire field. Some endoscopes have a single illumination bundle. Larger diameter models may have two or three fiberoptic bundles and matching light guide lens systems to improve illumination on both

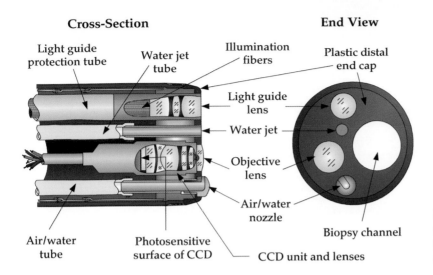

Cross-Section

Light guide protection tube
Water jet tube
Illumination fibers
Light guide lens
Water jet
Objective lens
Air/water nozzle
Air/water tube
Photosensitive surface of CCD
CCD unit and lenses

End View

Plastic distal end cap
Biopsy channel

Figure 3.4 Endoscope distal tip – Typical components and construction.

sides of the biopsy forceps (snare, etc.), and to facilitate the packing of components within the insertion tube.

The objective lens is typically the largest lens on the tip of the instrument. The CCD unit, the solid-state image sensor that creates the endoscopic image, is located in the distal tip just behind the objective lens. The CCD image sensor captures and sends a continuous stream of images back to the video processor for display on the video monitor. The objective lens and CCD unit must be completely sealed to prevent condensation from fogging the image, and to protect the imaging system from damage, if fluid were to accidentally enter the endoscope. Care should be taken in handling the endoscope to prevent the distal tip from hitting the floor, the equipment cart or any other hard object. If the objective lens is cracked, fluid can invade the CCD unit, requiring an expensive repair.

The channel used for biopsy and suction exits the distal tip close to the objective lens. The relative position of the biopsy channel with respect to the objective lens determines how accessories will appear in the endoscopic image as they enter the visual field. On some model endoscopes, the accessory (e.g. biopsy forceps) appears to emerge from the lower right corner of the image. On other models, accessories will enter from the lower left corner, and so forth, depending on the relationship of the channel to the viewing optics.

Air for insufflation, and water for lens washing, travel through the insertion tube in separate small tubes. However, to conserve space and exit

through a single nozzle, these tubes typically merge into a single tube just prior to the bending section of the instrument (*see* Figure 3.6). This combined air/water tube then connects to the air/water nozzle on the tip of the instrument (*see* Figure 3.4). The endoscopist feeds water across the objective lens to clean it, or air from the same nozzle for insufflation. Some endoscopes (more commonly colonoscopes) have an additional water tube and water-jet nozzle on their distal tip for washing the lumen wall (*see* Figure 3.4). In earlier years, pediatric colonoscopes often eliminated some of the functions of standard colonoscopes in order to minimize their size. Improvements in technology have allowed many pediatric colonoscopes to now have functions such as water-jet nozzles, adjustable stiffness controls, and high density CCDs just like their standard sized counterparts.

Bending section and angulation system

The distal-most 7–9 cm of the insertion tube can be angulated under the control of the endoscopist to look around corners or view lesions *en face*. This deflectable portion of the instrument is referred to as the bending section. As Figure 3.5 illustrates, the bending section is able to bend freely because it is composed of a series of metal rings, each one connected to the ring immediately preceding and following it via a freely moving joint. These joints consist of a series of pivot pins, each one displaced from its neighbors by 90°. This construction allows

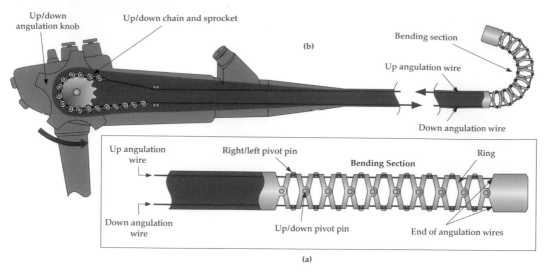

Figure 3.5 Construction of bending section and angulation system.

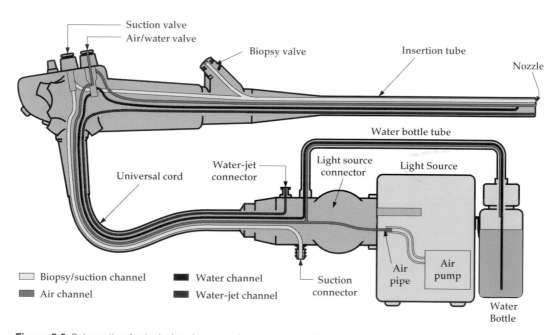

Figure 3.6 Schematic of a typical endoscope air, water and suction system.

the bending section of the endoscope to curl in any direction, often up to a maximum of 180 degrees to 210 degrees. The direction of the curl is controlled by four angulation wires that run the length of the insertion tube (*see* Figure 3.2). These four wires are firmly attached to the distal end of the bending section in the 3, 6, 9 and 12 o'clock positions, respectively. Pulling on the wire attached at the 12 o'clock position will cause the bending section to curl in the UP direction. Pulling on the wire attached at the 3 o'clock position will cause the tip to deflect to the RIGHT. Pulling the other two wires will cause DOWN and LEFT deflections, respectively.

These wires are pulled by rotating either the up/down, or right/left angulation knobs. (For simplicity, Figure 3.5 illustrates only the up/down angulation system.) Rotating both knobs together will produce a combined tip movement (e.g. upward and to the right). Colonoscopes typically have 180 degrees of deflection in the up and down directions. Deflections to the right and left are typically limited to 160 degrees to avoid over-stressing the internal components. Gastroscopes typically have a much tighter bending radius and can achieve a full 210 degree deflection of the tip in the UP direction – ideal for examining the gastro-esophageal junction from a retroflexed position.

Air, water & suction systems

A schematic of the typical system used for air, water and suction is shown in Figure 3.6. Air under mild pressure is supplied by a pump in the light source to a pipe protruding from the endoscope's connector. This air is directed via the air channel tube to the air/water valve on the control section. If this valve is not covered, the air simply exits from a hole in the top of the valve (*see* Figure 3.1). Continuously venting the system via this hole reduces wear and tear on the pump. To insufflate the patient, the endoscopist places a fingertip over the vent hole. This obstructs the vent and forces air down the air channel until it exits the endoscope through a nozzle on the distal tip. The maximum flow out of the tip of the instrument is typically around $30\,cm^3/sec$.

A one-way valve incorporated into the removable air/water valve (*see* Figure 3.1) prevents air which has been insufflated into the patient from flowing backwards, and from exiting out of the hole in the air/water valve whenever the operator lifts his finger off the valve's vent hole.

Water used to clean the objective lens of the endoscope is stored in a water bottle attached to the light source or cart (*see* Figure 3.6). In addition to feeding air for insufflation, the air pump within the light source also pressurizes this water container. This forces water out of the bottle and up the universal cord to the air/water valve. When the endoscopist depresses the air/water valve, it allows the water to continue down the water channel in the insertion tube, and out of the nozzle on the distal tip. The nozzle then directs this water across the surface of the objective lens to clean the lens.

In a similar manner, suction is also controlled by a valve. A suction line from a portable suction pump or wall suction outlet is connected to the endoscope. When the endoscopist depresses the suction valve, any fluid (or air) present at the distal tip of the endoscope will be drawn into the suction collection system. The proximal opening of the biopsy channel must be capped off by a biopsy valve to prevent room air from being drawn into the suction collection system.

There are several inherent safety features in the design of the air, water and suction system shown in Figure 3.6, including the following: (i) There is no air valve in the system which could stick in the "on" position – resulting in accidental over-insufflation of the patient. Rather, the air simply exits the vent hole in the valve unless the physician has his or her finger over the opening. (ii) In the event that the suction system becomes obstructed and the endoscopist has difficulty with possible over-insufflation, he or she can simply quickly remove all valves from the endoscope. This will stop all supply of air and water, and will allow the patient's GI tract to depressurize through the open valve cylinders.

Illumination system

Video endoscopes bring light into the interior of the body via an incoherent fiberoptic bundle. This fiberbundle is composed of thousands of hair-like glass fibers, each one only $30\,\mu m$ in diameter. Each fiber is optically coated to trap light within the fiber. Light rays entering one end of the fiber travel through the fiber's core by reflecting off of the walls of the fiber many thousands of times by means of a phenomenon referred to as *total internal reflection*. The type and thickness of glass used to make the core and cladding of the fiber are all carefully selected to enable the fiberbundle to carry as much light as possible (*see* Kawahara 2000 for a more complete discussion of fiberoptics).

Modern endoscopic light sources typically employ 300 watt xenon arc lamps to produce the bright, white light required for video imaging. A burn-resistant quartz lens at the tip of the endoscope's light guide bundle (*see* Figure 3.1) collects light from the light source lamp and directs it into the endoscope. At the other end of the endoscope, the light guide lens at the distal tip of the instrument spreads this light uniformly over the visual field (*see* Figure 3.4). An automatically controlled aperture (iris) in the light source controls the intensity of the light emitted from the endoscope. When the endoscope is in the body of the stomach and significant light is required to produce a bright image, the aperture in the light source opens up, allowing the endoscope to transmit maximum light. Conversely, when the endoscope tip is very close to the mucosa and illumination will therefore be very bright, the aperture automatically closes down to reduce the amount of light exiting the light source. If illumination of the tissue is too low, the image on the monitor will be dark and grainy. On the other hand, if the illumination is too strong, the image on the monitor will be washed out (i.e., "bloom"). The light source and video processor work together to automatically maintain the illumination at an ideal level for the CCD image sensor.

Video image capture

The image sensors used in video endoscopes are typically referred to as CCDs (charge-coupled devices). These sensors are solid-state electronic imaging devices made of silicon semiconductor material. The silicon on the surface of the sensor responds to light and exhibits a phenomenon called the *photoelectric effect*. When a photon of light strikes the photosensitive surface of the CCD, it displaces an electron from a silicon atom

in the material. This produces a free, negatively charged electron and a corresponding positively charged "hole" in the crystalline structure of the silicon at the location where the electron was previously bound. As photons hit the surface of the sensor, free electrons and corresponding positively charged holes are generated. The minute charges being built up on the surface of the sensor are directly proportional to the amount of light falling on the CCD.

To reproduce an image, the brightness of every point in the image must be measured. Therefore, the photosensitive surface of the image sensor must be divided up into a matrix of thousands of small, independent brightness-measuring photosites. Knowing the brightness of every point in the image allows the image processing system to subsequently recreate the image on a viewing monitor.

All CCD sensors have a rectangular array of discrete photosites on the imaging surface. These photosites individually correspond to the *picture elements*, or *pixels* which make up the final digital image.

Figure 3.7 illustrates a sensor with such an array of photosites. For simplicity this array contains an 8 by 8 matrix of photosites, for a total of 64 pixels. GI endoscopes typically contain CCDs with several hundred thousand to more than a million pixels.

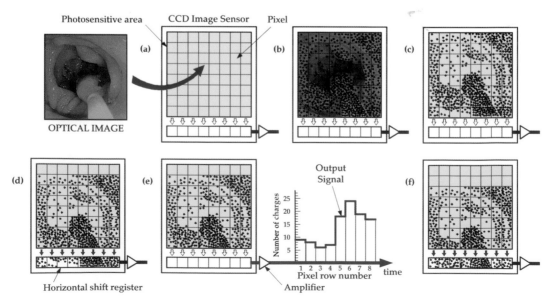

Figure 3.7 Schematic representation of how a line-transfer CCD captures an optical image. The "electrical representation" of the image is then read off in an orderly manner.

The higher the number of pixels in the image sensor, the greater the resolution in the reproduced image.

As illustrated in Figure 3.4, the CCD is located in the distal tip of the endoscope directly behind the objective lens. The objective lens focuses a miniature image of the observed mucosa directly on the surface of this sensor (*see* Figure 3.11). The pattern of light falling on the CCD (that is, the image) is instantly converted into an array of stored electrical charges, as a result of the previously described photoelectric effect. Because the charges stored in each of the individual pixels are isolated from neighboring pixels, the sensor faithfully transforms the optical image into an electrical replica of the image. This electrical representation of the image is then processed and sent to a video monitor for reproduction.

As Figure 3.7 illustrates, pixels in darker areas of the image develop a low voltage, due to the generation of fewer charges. Pixels in brighter areas of the image develop a proportionately higher voltage. The photoelectric process is linear. Doubling the number of photons falling on a pixel doubles the number of charges generated at that photosite.

"Reading" the image created on the CCD

The first step in the imaging process is to measure the brightness of each point in the image by systematically quantifying the number of charges generated in each photosite. After the CCD is exposed to the image, the charges developed in the CCD must be "read out" in an orderly manner, and then processed to create the dataset necessary to reproduce the original image. The steps required to create and then read the charges are schematically illustrated in Figure 3.7.

As shown in Figure 3.7a, the first step is the projection of an optical image of the mucosa onto the photosensitive surface of the CCD. Electrical charges are instantly developed at each photosite within the array based on the brightness of the light falling on each individual photosite (*see* Figure 3.7b–3.7c). (For simplicity, Figure 3.7 illustrates an array with only a very few pixels and only a very few stored charges. The charges are represented by small dots within the photosites.)

The charges within each pixel are then controlled and shifted over the surface of the CCD via electrodes (not shown) located adjacent to each photosite. By varying the voltages applied to these electrodes, the electrons within individual photosites are transferred as "charge packets" from one pixel to another. Sequential voltage changes on these electrodes march the charges across the matrix toward the bottom edge of the CCD and then into a horizontal shift register (*see* Figure 3.7d). The charges in the horizontal shift register are then passed through an output amplifier and are converted into an output electrical signal. The output signal fluctuates in direct proportion to the number of charges stored in each pixel. The processing of the image replica continues, in a step-by-step fashion, until all of the stored charges have been transferred down to the horizontal shift register and counted, pixel by pixel. Once the CCD is read and cleared, it is ready for another exposure. In current video endoscopes, the CCD is exposed, read out, and re-exposed 60 to 90 times each second.

The CCD illustrated in Figure 3.7 is representative of a line transfer CCD. One characteristic of a line transfer CCD is that the photosensitive area of the CCD (the photosite array) must be shielded from light during the entire time that the image is being moved through the matrix and read out. If the CCD is exposed to additional light during the reading process, new charges generated at the photosites by the continuing illumination will mix with the charges generated by the previous image as they are being transferred through the photosite array. To preserve the original image, the photosites must be completely dark while the image replica is being transferred. One method of doing this, in endoscopic applications, is to strobe, or momentarily interrupt the light emitted by the endoscope as the CCD is being read out. Strobing the light source creates a momentary burst of light to expose the image sensor, followed by momentary darkness as the CCD is read out and cleared. Endoscopists who have used an RGB sequential endoscopy system (typically called a "black & white" CCD system) are very familiar with the concept of strobed endoscopic light sources.

The line transfer CCD is just one type of CCD. There are, in fact, several different types of CCDs used in endoscopes today. The manner in which the charges are moved about within the CCD as they are read out depends upon the configuration (type) of CCD employed. The three most common types of CCDs are the Line Transfer CCD, the Frame Transfer CCD, and the Interline Transfer CCD. Each type has specific advantages and disadvantages in terms of the CCDs sensitivity to light (and in turn, the brightness required of the endoscope's illumination system), the type of light source required (strobed versus non-strobed), the physical size of the CCD (which, in turn, affects the diameter of the distal tip of the endoscope), and the speed at which the charges can be transferred out of the CCD. While strobed endoscopic video systems use line transfer CCDs as described above, so-called "color-chip" endoscopy systems typically employ interline transfer CCDs because they do not require strobing of the light source. (See Barlow 2000 for additional information regarding the various types of CCDs used in endoscopy.)

Resolution, magnification & angle of view

The resolution of the endoscope is largely a function of the number of pixels on the surface of the CCD. The greater the number of pixels, the greater the amount of information contained in the image. Large diameter video endoscopes currently contain more than a million pixels. In recent years, the increasing resolution obtained by video endoscopes finally exceeded the display capability of standard video monitors. Monitors for Standard Definition Television (SDTV) typi-cally have 480 horizontal scan lines to display their image. Images which exceed this level of resolution require the use of a High Resolution Television (HDTV) monitor which has 1080 horizontal scan lines, more than twice as many as SDTV.

While there are several different display formats within the digital SDTV and HDTV standards, the best SDTV displays will have a screen composed of 704 columns of pixels by 480 rows of pixels – creating a matrix with a total of 337,920 pixels. The highest resolution digital HDTV monitors, on the other hand, will have a matrix of 1920 columns by 1080 rows – for a total of 2,073,600 pixels. It should be pointed out that high definition CCDs used in endoscopes do not yet use the full display capability of HDTV (there is room for further improvement as CCD technology advances). Furthermore, an endoscopic HDTV system requires an endoscope, video processor and flat panel display, all having HDTV capability. And finally, displaying an endoscope with SDTV-level resolution on an HDTV display does not increase its resolution.

The endoscope's resolving power is a measure of the smallest object detail that an endoscope can capture and display. It is typically measured by a placing a standard optical test chart at a specified distance from the tip of the endoscope and observing sets of line pairs that are increasingly spaced closer and closer together (*see* Figure 3.8b). The spacing between closest line pairs that can be discerned before blending together is the resolving power of the endoscope at that particular distance from the object (Figure 3.8c). High definition endo-

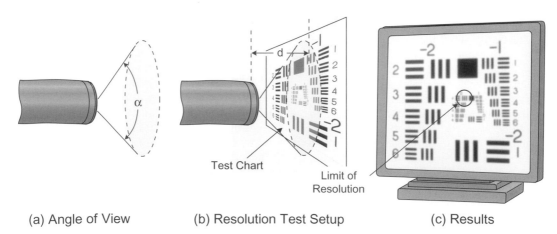

Test Chart

Limit of Resolution

(a) Angle of View (b) Resolution Test Setup (c) Results

Figure 3.8 Specifications of the endoscopic image. (a) endoscope's angle of view, (b) test setup for measuring the endoscope's resolving power, and (c) the image resolution limit can be observed on the video monitor.

scopes obviously have greater resolving power than standard definition endoscopes.

It is also obvious that, as the endoscope is moved closer to the test chart (or the mucosa), it will be able to see finer and finer detail due to an increase in the magnification of the object. However, when the endoscope reaches its close focus point, moving the endoscope closer to the subject will actually begin to deteriorate the image as the image gets increasingly out of focus. On older model endoscopes, this limit of close focus was approximately 6–8 mm from the tissue. Newer endoscopes have advanced optics which not only employ high definition CCDs for greater resolution, but also have a close focus point of 3 mm from the tissue which greatly increases image magnification as well. As a result, an HDTV endoscope with close focus capability can see line pairs on the test chart that are approximately three times closer together than a standard SDTV endoscope.

All video endoscopes offer an electronic magnification feature. However, this feature does not actually improve the resolving power of the endoscope. The image may appear larger (more magnified), as if you moved the endoscope closer to the mucosa, but this is an illusion. The video processor has simply discarded the pixels on the periphery of the image, separated the central pixels to expand the image, interpolated image information in the spaces between the separated pixels, and displayed an electronically "zoomed" imaged. However, there is no real gain in resolving power when using electronic magnification. Real increases in resolving power are only obtained by: (1) Switching to an endoscope with an increased number of pixels, such as an HDTV endoscope. (2) Switching to an endoscope with close-focus capability. Or (3), Switching to an endoscope that has true "optical zoom" as opposed to "electronic zoom". Endoscopes with optical zoom have a control that allows the user to physically move the distal lens of the endoscope to provide a view of the tissue with extreme close focus.

Along with improvements in resolution, with advancing technology endoscope manufacturers have typically been able to increase the angle of view of the endoscope (α in Figure 3.8a) with each successive generation. Standard gastroscopes and colonoscopes now have an angle of view of 120–140 degrees, while new wide-angle colonoscopes have an impressive 170 degree angle of view. The increase in field of view allows the endoscope to see further around the backsides of mucosal folds and to observe a greater area of tissue at any one time.

Reproduction of color

All solid-state image sensors are inherently monochromatic devices. As monochromatic devices, they can produce only a black-and-white image of the mucosa under observation. The silicon photosites employed on the surface of the CCD develop charges in proportion only to the intensity (brightness) of the light falling on the array. The color of the light is not captured and is not known. However, color is extremely important in endoscopic diagnosis. For an endoscope to reproduce the necessary attribute of color, the imaging system must have some additional means to analyze the color (wavelength) of the light falling on the sensor.

To understand color reproduction, it is helpful to first understand how humans perceive color – because all photographic and electronic imaging systems attempt to mimic the manner in which the human eye and brain respond to color. As Figure 3.9 illustrates, the sensitivity of the human eye to light varies with the wavelength or color of the light. The CCD has a similar, but broader sensitivity to light as the eye, ranging from the infrared (wavelengths greater than 780 nm), through the visible spectrum, and into the ultraviolet spectrum (wavelengths less than 380 nm).

Any artist who mixes paints knows that two or more colors mixed together produces a single, newly created color. When observing a mixture of

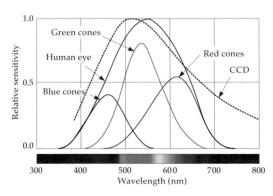

Figure 3.9 Light sensitivity of CCDs compared to the human eye.

colors, the human eye is non-analytical and cannot distinguish the original component colors. The perceived hue of this newly created color is determined by a phenomenon that scientists refer to as *trichromatic vision*.

Trichromatic vision

Nearly any color, to which the human eye is sensitive, can be simulated by mixing light of only three special colors – red, green and blue (RGB). If three light projectors were fitted with proper red, green and blue filters, and the projected light were overlapped, we would obtain an image similar to that shown in Figure 3.10. The color resulting from the overlap of the red and green projectors would be indistinguishable from monochromatic yellow light. Likewise, light from the overlapping green and blue projectors would produce the mental sensation of cyan. And the overlap of red and blue light produces magenta. It is somewhat amazing that where all three of the projectors overlap in the center, the observer will see an area of pure white, with no evidence of the three component colors. If the intensities of each of the three projectors were accurately controlled and varied, it would be possible to reproduce essentially any spectral color in the central area of the overlap. It is upon this phenomenon that all video imaging is based.

In the early 1800s, Thomas Young performed such experiments with projectors and was the first to propose the theory that humans possess trichromatic vision. His experiments, and those of his successors, have caused scientists to postulate that humans perceive color through the stimulation of three different types of neural cells (*cones*) located in the retina of the eye. These cells are presumed to have the approximate sensitivity curves depicted for the red, green and blue cones

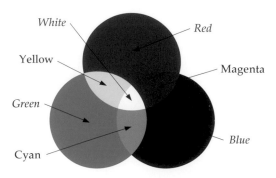

Figure 3.10 Color theory – Additive primary colors.

illustrated in Figure 3.9. The concept of trichromatic vision serves as the foundation for all color reproduction.

Theory of color video

Because red, green and blue (RGB) can be additively combined to mimic all other spectral colors, they are commonly referred to as the *additive primary colors*. It is these three colors (RGB) that are, in fact, the colors used to create the full color images we see on every color video monitor (*see* Figure 3.11) or flat panel video screen.

There are currently two very different types of color imaging systems used in commercial video endoscopes. The first commercial video image endoscope system, the VideoEndoscope™ introduced by Welch Allyn in 1983, was based on an *RGB Sequential Imaging System*. Many current instruments continue to use this system. The second system, the so-called "color-chip" endoscope, despite being developed later, has now become the predominant system worldwide. Each of these systems has specific advantages and disadvantages, as explained below.

RGB sequential imaging

The components of an RGB sequential video endoscope system are schematically shown in Figure 3.11. The endoscope has a monochromatic (black & white) CCD mounted in its distal tip. The objective lens at the tip of the endoscope focuses a miniature image of endoscope's field of view on the photosensitive surface of this CCD. The endoscope's field of view is illuminated via a fiberoptic bundle that runs through the length of the endoscope carrying light from a lamp within the light source to the distal tip of the endoscope. Unlike the light used for fiberoptic endoscopes or color-chip videoscopes, this light is not continuous, but is strobed or pulsed. It is not only strobed, but it is variously colored.

The high-intensity xenon lamp within the light source produces a continuous white light with the approximate color temperature of sunlight. A rotating filter wheel with three colored segments (red, green, and blue) is placed between this lamp and the endoscope's light guide bundle. This filter wheel chops and colors the light falling on the endoscope's light guide bundle into sequential bursts of red, green and blue illumination. The purpose of this unique illumination is to produce three separate monochromatic images,

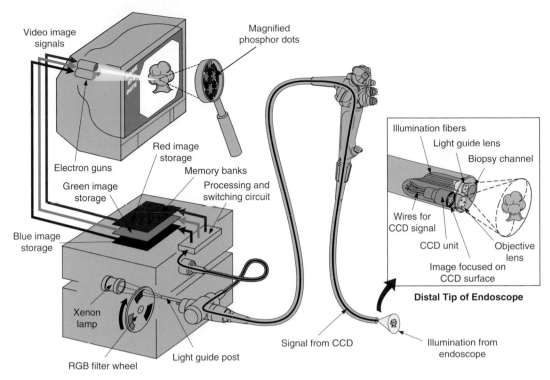

Figure 3.11 Schematic of an RGB sequential endoscope imaging system.

each obtained when the field of view is sequentially illuminated by the three primary colors in turn. During the fraction of a second when the red filter is in the light path, the GI mucosa is illuminated by red light only. The CCD image sensor instantly captures a monochromatic (black & white) image of the mucosa as it appears under this red illumination (*see* Figure 3.12). Tissue that is naturally reddish in color reflects heavily under red light and appears to be bright. Areas of the tissue with less red reflect red light weakly and appear dark under red illumination.

After an image is obtained under red illumination, the filter wheel rotates to the adjacent opaque portion of the wheel. At this point the endoscopic illumination goes momentarily dark and the image on the CCD is read out, directed through a processing and switching circuit, and stored in the "red image" memory bank of the video processor (*see* Figure 3.11).

After the red image is stored, the filter wheel rotates to place the green filter in the light path. A monochromatic image of the tissue as it appears under green illumination is captured and sent for storage in the "green image" memory bank. In a similar manner, a third image under blue illumination is captured and stored. This sequence of capturing a set of images for each of the three primary colors is repeated 20–30 times each second, the exact rate being determined by the video processor.

Color image display

The steps just described, explain the process used to capture images with an RGB sequential imaging endoscope. The technology used to display the resulting image, however, is common to all video systems. The face of the video monitor or flat panel display is actually composed of a repeating pattern of hundreds of thousands of red, green and blue rectangles or dots (*see* Figure 3.11). By feeding the signal from the red memory bank to the monitor's circuit for controlling the red dots, the monitor will reproduce an image of the GI mucosa as it appears under red illumination. This is illustrated by the red component image depicted in Figure 3.12. Likewise, feeding the images from

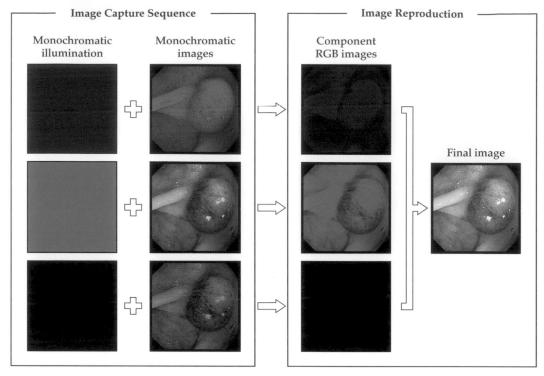

Figure 3.12 RGB sequential imaging system – The tissue is sequentially illuminated by red, green and blue light while monochromatic (B&W) images are captured in sequence. These component images are then fed to a video monitor that generates RGB component images that the observer's eye then fuses into a full-color image.

the green and blue memory banks to the green and blue monitor circuits, respectively, will reproduce the green and blue components of the original image.

It is a phenomenon of human vision that when two or more sources of color are placed close together, but not overlapping, and are viewed from a sufficient distance, the colors will blend together to form a third color. This third color is the color predicted by the theory of trichromatic vision. This fusion of color sources is referred to as the *juxtaposition of color sources*. Because of this phenomenon of vision, the three co-mingled red, green and blue images on the video monitor appear to blend together into a single, full-colored, natural-appearing image – rather than remaining as a confusing collection of intermixed colored dots. The RGB sequential imaging process just described is summarized in Figure 3.12.

Color-chip video imaging

A "color-chip" CCD is essentially a black and white image sensor with a custom-fabricated,

miniaturized, multicolored filter bonded to its photosensitive surface. This filter allows the CCD to directly and simultaneously resolve the component colors of the image.

Although color-chip endoscopes can theoretically use any combination of filter colors, the filter colors shown in Figure 3.13 (yellow – Ye, cyan – Cy, magenta – Mg, and green – G) are a typical choice. These segments are arranged in a 2 × 2 pixel box pattern that regularly repeats over the face of the CCD. Since the final output signals to be sent to the observation monitor must be the standard red, green, and blue component images, the image produced behind this color mosaic filter must first be converted into its primary red, green and blue components prior to display.

From Figure 3.10 it can be determined that a yellow filter will pass both red and green light. A cyan filter will pass both green and blue light; and a magenta filter will pass both red and blue light. As Figure 3.13b illustrates, image brightness information from the pixels located behind the yellow and magenta filter segments is used to create the red component image. Brightness information from

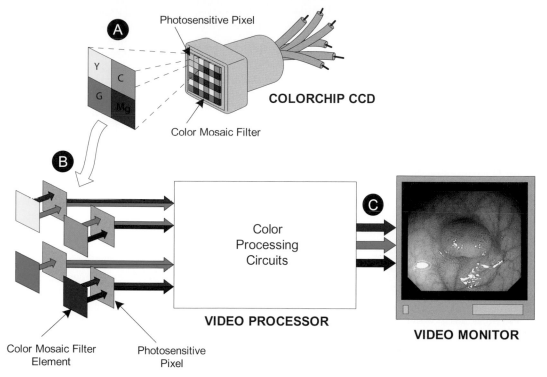

Figure 3.13 Schematic of how a color-chip endoscope captures and reproduces color images. (A) A color mosaic filter element precisely covers each pixel of the CCD. (B) Individual filter segments pass red, green and blue image information to the CCD pixels located behind them, dependent upon the color of the filter segment. (C) Circuitry in the video processor receives color information from the CCD and creates the RGB component signals necessary to reproduce a color image on the video monitor.

the cyan and magenta pixels is used to create the blue component image. And the green component image is created from brightness information obtained from the yellow, cyan and green filtered pixels. All of this information from the CCD is sent to the video processor which then creates the standard RGB (red/green/blue) video signals required by the video monitor.

It may be asked why a CCD would be designed with a color mosaic filter using yellow, cyan and magenta elements, if using red, green and blue filter segments would yield the RGB component values directly, without calculation. The answer lies in the fact that the mosaic filter shown in Figure 3.13 has a significant advantage in terms of brightness. When red, green, and blue filter segments are used, each pixel is filtered to receive only one of the three primary colors. A cyan-filtered pixel, on the other hand, is exposed to both blue and green light. It is, therefore, more heavily illuminated than a pure blue or a pure green pixel. Likewise, pixels behind a yellow

filter (red + green) or a magenta filter (red + blue) receive more photons (light) than pixels behind a pure red, a pure green or pure blue filter.

Because of the increased light intensity passing through a mosaic filter such as that shown in Figure 3.13, a CCD with this construction exhibits far greater light sensitivity. The improved light sensitivity allows the video endoscope designer to construct an endoscope with a smaller illumination bundle, to maximize the endoscope's angle of view, and to increase the endoscope's depth of field. All of these features improve the instrument's optical performance, but require additional light.

Reproduction of motion

The color-chip video endoscope has an inherent advantage over the RGB sequential endoscope in reproducing motion. The filter wheel in current

RGB sequential video processors typically rotates at 20 to 30 rps. Since all the color component images are captured individually in sequence, it takes 1/30 sec (with a 30 rps filter wheel) to capture the three component images that make up a single video image. If there is any relative motion during this time between the endoscope and the object being viewed, as often occurs during endoscopy, the three component images may differ with respect to object size and position. When these three RGB images are subsequently superimposed on the video monitor, they will be misaligned. This misalignment will be clearly visible if the endoscopist happens to freeze the image while it is moving rapidly. This color separation is present, to a greater or lesser extent, continuously throughout the entire examination. However, it gives the images an unnatural, highly colorful, stroboscopic appearance whenever there is rapid motion of the endoscope, the object being viewed, or both. This color separation is especially apparent when the endoscopist feeds water to clean the objective lens.

Second generation RGB sequential video processors are engineered to reduce the problem of color separation on captured images. These processors incorporate an anti-color-slip circuit to analyze the video signal in real time and to freeze the image at the moment when color separation is at a minimum (see Barlow 2005). This circuit is remarkably effective in reducing color separation within captured still images. However, this system does not reduce the strobing, color separation, and water-droplet flicker observed during real-time endoscopy.

The color-chip videoscope, on the other hand, has no problem imaging moving tissue. Because a color-chip endoscope captures all three color components of the image simultaneously, there is never any color separation with either moving or "frozen" images. Since the color-chip endoscope's illumination is continuous and unstrobed, and the frame rate is matched to contemporary TV standards, the reproduction of moving images is always smooth and natural.

Narrow-band imaging

Observation of the tissue's microvascular structure and the interpretation of recognizable "pit patterns" on the surface of the mucosa is often key to endoscopic diagnosis. Pit patterns can be enhanced via chromoendoscopy, however, this is time consuming and messy. In recent years, Olympus (Tokyo, Japan) has developed a new technology called *narrow-band imaging* (NBI) to aid in the observation of surface detail and to add image contrast to microvascular structures.

NBI is based on oxyhemoglobin's highly selective absorption of light at 415 and 540 nm, as shown in Figure 3.14a. Because oxyhemoglobin is highly absorptive of these wavelengths, if light containing only wavelengths around 415 and 540 nm were used as the source of endoscopic illumination, structures which contained high concentrations of hemoglobin (e.g. capillaries) would heavily absorb this light and appear much darker than the surrounding tissue. In addition, if the reflected light were artificially assigned a different color, rather than producing the typical red vessels surrounded by pink tissue, as normally seen in endoscopic images, it would add additional visual contrast to the microvasculature. This is the goal of NBI – to optically enhance the observation of the tissue's surface by identifying structures rich in hemoglobin and increase their visual contrast against the background tissue.

NBI requires the insertion of a special filter in the light path of the endoscopic light source. The NBI filter prevents the light source from emitting its normal "white light" covering the entire visual spectrum as shown in Figure 3.14 (1), to emitting only two narrow bands of light, one with wavelengths centered at 415 nm (blue), the other centered at 540 nm (green), as shown in Figure 3.14 (2).

In color-chip videoscopes, this special light is emitted continuously from the tip of the endoscope when operated in the NBI mode. The color-chip CCD images the tissue as it appears under this special narrow-band illumination. The resulting image information is sent back to the video processor. Note that there are no red wavelengths in the NBI illumination. Therefore, the CCD detects no red in the image that it captures from the tissue. However, it does capture information on how the tissue reflects blue and green light. Note that as shown in Figure 3.14, instead of sending the green image information to the green input of the video monitor, the video processor intentionally reassigns the green image information to the red channel of the monitor. The video processor sends the blue image information to the blue input of the video monitor, but it also sends the same blue image information to the green input of the video monitor as well. The end result is an NBI image such as that shown in

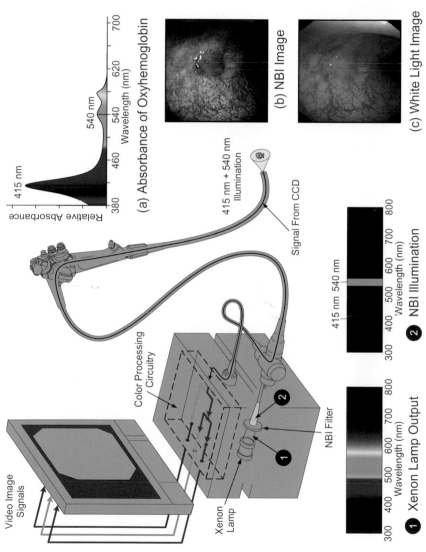

Figure 3.14 Schematic of narrow-band imaging. (a) NBI imaging is based on oxyhemoglobin's high absorbance of light at 415 nm and 540 nm. (b) The full spectrum white light emitted by the xenon lamp (1) is filtered to create the characteristic blue/green narrow-band illumination (2) required for NBI imaging. The colors of the captured image are intentionally reassigned by circuitry in the video processor to create an NBI image for display on the video monitor. (c) A white light image of the same tissue is shown for comparison.

Figure 3.14b. Note the reassignment of colors as well as the enhancement of both the blood vessels and the lesion. For comparison, a standard white light image of the same lesion is shown in Figure 3.14c.

Digital imaging post-processing

When the image from the CCD is transferred to the video processor, it is typically converted into a digital format. This allows the endoscopist to "freeze" the image on the monitor, and also allows the image to be manipulated in real-time by various image-processing algorithms. These algorithms can be used for various purposes such as producing edge enhancement or texture enhancement of the image. Emphasizing the edges of small structures within the image gives the impression of "sharpening" the image.

Recently Fujinon (Saitama, Japan) introduced a feature called FICE (Fuji Intelligent Color Enhancement). Pentax (Montvale, NJ) has introduced a similar feature called i-Scan. These algorithms allow the user to manipulate endoscopic images obtained under normal white light imaging by exaggerating, diminishing and reassigning colors within the endoscopic image. The FICE system, for example, allows the user to select specific colors of interest and to assign these to any of the RGB channels of the monitor. There are ten factory-determined color presets, however, the presets can also be customized by the user. Research is on-going to identify clinically valuable algorithms.

Color chip versus RGB sequential video endoscopes

The advantages and disadvantages of the two basic endoscopic imaging systems described above are summarized in Table 3.1.

Troubleshooting

Many problems encountered during endoscopy can be corrected instantly given a little knowledge of how the equipment works. Endoscopes must be handled with care, thoroughly cleaned to remove all debris which could comprise performance (and present an infection control risk) and stored in a protected environment to prevent damage. Routine leak testing is essential to prevent the

Table 3.1

Feature	RGB Sequential Video Endoscopes	Color-Chip Video Endoscopes
Image Resolution	Have a theoretical advantage because each pixel has unique, image intensity information. The advantage is primarily seen only in the very smallest of endoscopes.	Have a slight disadvantage because information from multiple pixels must be combined together.
Color Accuracy	Have a theoretical advantage because each pixel measures RGB intensity values directly. Ideal for research based on spectroscopy and color-analysis algorithms.	Have a slight disadvantage because color at each point in the image is calculated from information obtained from adjacent pixels.
Reproduction of Motion	Stroboscopic illumination creates problems with rapid motion. Motion produces color slip and brightly colored artifacts. Newer generation systems have advanced image capture algorithms to reduce the color-slip problem.	Smooth, natural reproduction of motion. No stroboscopic effect. No color artifacts. A "fast shutter" mode reduces blurring of quickly moving objects.
Abdominal Transillumination	Strobed illumination produces very weak transillumination. "Transillumination Mode" results in good transillumination but normal imaging is impossible.	The system's bright, continuous, white light illumination is ideal for transillumination.

invasion of fluid into the instrument. Fluid invasion will necessitate extensive and expensive repairs to the instrument.

As endoscopes have become more complex, and have become increasingly integrated with computerized image management systems, the steps required to troubleshoot problems have also become more complex. Table 3.2 contains general troubleshooting information for selected problems. Confirm the details of how to troubleshoot

Table 3.2	
Problem	**Troubleshooting**
Poor air or water feeding	1) Check the air pump is turned on. 2) Check the water bottle contains sufficient water, the lid is screwed on tightly, and that the water bottle tube is connected to the endoscope. **Note**: If the nozzle on the tip of the endoscope Is obstructed by debris, air and water feeding will be compromised Thoroughly clean all internal channels each time the instrument is reprocessed. Some manufacturers supply special adapters for bedside precleaning of the air/water system.
Image is not clear	1) Feed water and then air to wash debris off distal objective lens. 2) If permanently obscured, clean the objective lens by carefully rubbing with gauze moistened with alcohol. 3) Repair the endoscope if the distal lens is damaged or has moisture trapped behind it. **Note**: A cracked or badly scratched lens cannot produce sharp images. Never let the tip of the endoscope contact the floor or other hard surface. Protect the distal tip from damage. Have the endoscope repaired if moisture is trapped behind the lens.
Image color is not correct	1) "White balance" the image while pointing the endoscope at a manufacturer-supplied test fixture or a piece of white gauze. 2) Make sure all color adjustment controls on both the video processor and the video monitor are set in a neutral position. 3) Check for loose or broken video cables. **Note**: If the endoscope is "white balanced" while pointing at a non-white surface, distorted color will result. Many video systems use separate wires for transmitting the red, green and blue component images. If one of these wires is disconnected or broken, the color of the image on the monitor will be severely distorted.
Image is permanently frozen or completely absent	1) Turn both the light source and video processor on and off again. This may correct the problem if it is microprocessor related. 2) Check all wires for accidental disconnection. 3) Check the input selector on the video monitor to ensure that it is set to display the input with the endoscopic image. 4) Press the "Reset" button on the video processor, if one is available. This will return the video processor settings back to its factory defaults.
The image cannot be restored and the endoscope must be withdrawn from the patient	1) Close and remove all accessories from the endoscope channel. 2) If using a colonoscope with adjustable stiffness, set the stiffness control to the most flexible setting. 3) Make sure that the angulation locks are off. 4) Return both angulation knobs to their neutral position in order to straighten the distal tip. 5) Carefully withdraw the endoscope. **Note**: If the endoscope cannot be withdrawn easily, stop and contact the endoscope manufacturer's service center for additional instructions.
The endoscope is damaged	If the endoscope insertion tube is damaged by a patient bite, by accidental closure in the carrying case hinge, or by other means, do not continue to use the endoscope. Further use of the endoscope could cause additional damage to internal components of the instrument, adding to the repair cost.

your particular equipment via your manufacturer-supplied user manuals.

Endoscope reprocessing

After each patient use the endoscope must be reprocessed prior to reuse or storage. The person(s) responsible for reprocessing endoscopes must be thoroughly trained in: 1) Standard Precautions, 2) Occupational Safety and Health Administration (OSHA) rules on exposure to blood borne pathogens, 3) procedures for the safe handling of reprocessing chemicals, 4) professional society guidelines (e.g. those promulgated by ASGE, SGNA, APIC, etc.), and 5) the manufacturer's specific instructions. Reprocessing personnel must also be adequately outfitted with appropriate personal protective equipment for protection against splattering of microorganisms, organic matter, and reprocessing chemicals. Adequate personal protective equipment includes: 1) long-sleeved gowns that are impervious to fluid, 2) gloves that are long enough to extend up the arms to protect the forearms, and 3) eye or face protection.

Cleaning

Following patient use, the endoscope should be immediately precleaned at the bedside by flushing the internal channels and wiping down the insertion tube. Following bedside precleaning, the endoscope is brought to the reprocessing room for manual cleaning. Thorough manual cleaning is often described as being "the most important step" of the entire reprocessing procedure. Cleaning removes gross debris and organic matter that can dry on the instrumentation and hinder future performance (e.g. flow through the air/water nozzle). Studies have shown that cleaning alone can reduce the number of microorganisms and the organic load on the instrument by 4 logs, or 99.99%. This significantly reduces the organic and microbial challenge to the high-level disinfectant or sterilant. Furthermore, residual debris may inhibit germicide penetration and shield microorganisms from contact with the germicide. The recommended channel cleaning brushes and any special brushes (e.g. channel opening cleaning brush) supplied by the manufacturer must be used to mechanically abrade all lumens while they are filled with detergent. After manual cleaning is complete there should be no visible debris left on the instrument.

When cleaning and disinfecting the endoscope, the cleaning tubes and attachments recommended by the endoscope manufacturer for flushing the internal lumens of the endoscope must be used. This ensures that the required volume of fluid for cleaning, disinfection/sterilization, and rinsing passes through the internal channels. Figure 3.15 illustrates one such manufacturer's range of cleaning attachments. The Food and Drug Administration (FDA) requires that the endoscope manufacturer validate the steps listed in each instrument's instruction manual. These instructions must be followed explicitly. Shortcutting the prescribed procedure may result in an inadequately reprocessed instrument that presents an infection control risk to medical personnel and the next patient.

Leak testing

Routine leak testing is an essential part of the reprocessing procedure. Leak testing the endoscope ensures that the seals, lumens and external surface of the endoscope are fluid tight and will not allow reprocessing fluids to enter the interior of the endoscope. If a leak is detected, have the endoscope repaired immediately. Fluid invasion of the endoscope can cause extensive and expensive damage. Furthermore, a breach in the surface integrity of the endoscope can allow microorganisms to enter the endoscope body, where they can reside and later emerge, creating an infection control risk.

High-level disinfection

In 1968, Dr Earle H Spaulding devised a classification system that divided medical devices into three categories (critical, semi-critical, and non-critical) based on the risk of infection involved with their use. Based on the Spaulding classification system, gastrointestinal endoscopes are considered by FDA to be *semi-critical medical devices*. Semi-critical medical devices are instruments that do not enter sterile areas of the body and are generally in contact with intact mucous membranes. As such, both high-level disinfection and sterilization are acceptable methods for reprocessing GI endoscopes.

High-level disinfection is most commonly used. High-level disinfection destroys all vegetative

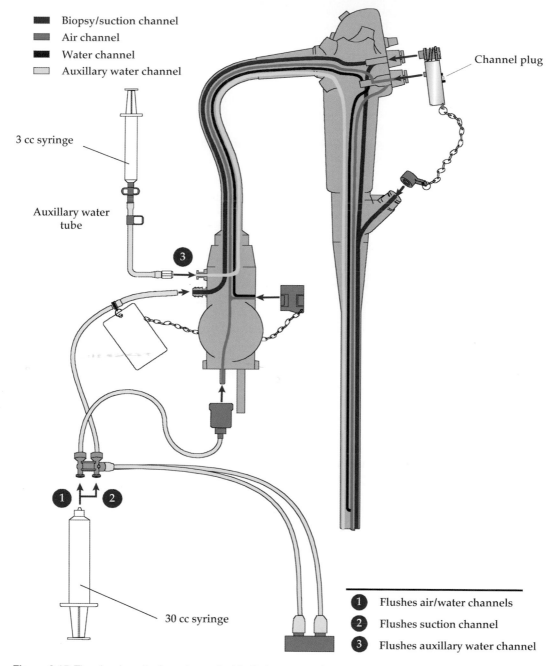

Biopsy/suction channel
Air channel
Water channel
Auxillary water channel

Channel plug

3 cc syringe

Auxillary water tube

3

1 **2**

30 cc syringe

1 Flushes air/water channels
2 Flushes suction channel
3 Flushes auxillary water channel

Figure 3.15 The cleaning attachments required to flush reprocessing chemicals through the lumens of a typical Olympus 160/180-series video endoscope.

organisms, but not necessarily all bacterial endospores. FDA has approved several high-level disinfectants for use on medical devices, including 2.0–3.4% glutaraldehydes, 7.5% hydrogen peroxide, 0.2% peracetic acid, 0.08% peracetic acid/1% hydrogen peroxide, and 0.55% orthophthalaldehyde. Each of these germicides has advantages and disadvantages in terms of cost, contact time, temperature and fume control requirements. However, it is important to note that not all of these products are compatible with all endoscopes. Always check with the endoscope manufacturer regarding chemical compatibility. Some germicides can be used at room temperature for manual reprocessing. Others require heating and are only approved for use in automated reprocessors.

The efficacy of any chemical germicide is dependent upon the manufacturer's instructions for use. The label instructions regarding activation (if required), reuse life, and shelf-life must be followed explicitly. All reusable germicides should be tested regularly, as recommended by the manufacturer, to ensure that they exceed the *minimum effective concentration* (MEC) of the active ingredient. The addition of significant quantities of microbes and organic matter, dilution by rinse water, and aging of the chemical solution will all result in a gradual reduction in the effectiveness of reusable germicides.

Alcohol flush

While many automated reprocessors use 0.2 micron microbial retention filters to produce "sterile" water for the final rinse following disinfection, other endoscopy units rinse their endoscopes in tap water. Irrespective of the quality of the final water rinse (tap water, "bacteria-free" water, and "sterile" water), the entire endoscope should be dried and each of its channels flushed with 70% alcohol followed by an air purge prior to reuse or storage. Alcohol aids in the drying process and inhibits the recontamination of the internal channels with water-borne organisms.

Special channels

Some endoscopes have special channels, such as an auxiliary water or water-jet channel. These channels must be fully reprocessed after each patient use, regardless of whether the channel was used during the preceding patient examination. Patient debris and microorganisms can enter these channels even if they are not used during the endoscopy exam. Reprocessing of these channels often requires additional steps and the use of special attachments (*see* Figure 3.15).

Automated reprocessors

Automated reprocessors standardize the disinfection process and decrease the exposure of personnel to reprocessing chemicals. If an automated endoscope reprocessor is used, the endoscope must be connected to the reprocessor using the correct set of connecting tubes. Some endoscope models, particularly those with special channels, may require a different set of connecting tubes from those used on standard instruments. Failing to connect a specific channel opening or port to the reprocessor may result in patient debris and infectious material remaining in the channel.

Rinsing & disposal

Whether reprocessing manually or with an automated machine, all disinfectant must be flushed from the endoscope's internal lumens during the rinse process. There are published reports of patients receiving chemical burns and/or chemical colitis when disinfectant solution which was retained in the endoscope was expelled from the endoscope's channels during a subsequent patient exam.

Some germicides may require neutralization prior to disposal. State or local ordinances may prohibit the dumping of certain germicides into the city waste water system. Check with the germicide manufacturer and with state and local authorities regarding disposal requirements.

Accessories

Many endoscopic accessories are deemed to be *critical medical devices* by the Spaulding classification system, since they either penetrate mucous membranes (e.g. endoscopic biopsy devices) or enter normally sterile areas of the body (e.g. biliary ducts). As such, they should be sterilized prior to reuse. Steam sterilization is the preferred method of sterilizing any reusable endoscopic accessory that is autoclavable.

Storage

Store reprocessed endoscopes in a well-ventilated area where they are protected from damage and contamination. To facilitate drying, endoscopes should be stored with all valves and removable parts detached. The endoscope carrying case should never be used for the storage of patient-ready endoscopes. Carrying cases are not ventilated, easily contaminated, cannot be reprocessed, and are intended for shipping and long-term storage only. Never put an endoscope that has not been completely reprocessed into its carrying case. In addition, reprocess any endoscope that is removed from a carrying case prior to subsequent patient use.

📖 FURTHER READING

Alvarado CJ, Mark R. (2000) APIC guidelines for infection prevention and control in flexible endoscopy. *American Journal of Infection Control*, **28**, 38–55.

Barlow DE. (2000) Flexible Endoscope Technology: The Video Image Endoscope. In: Sivak MV Jr, (Ed). *Gastroenterologic Endoscopy* (2nd edn, Vol 1) pp. 29–49, WB Saunders Company, Philadelphia.

Barlow DE. (2005) How Endoscopes Work. In: Ginsberg GG, Kochman ML, Norton I, Gostout CJ (Eds). *Clinical Gastrointestinal Endoscopy*, pp. 29–47, Elsevier Saunders, Philadelphia.

Food and Drug Administration. FDA-Cleared Sterilants and High Level Disinfectants With General Claims for Processing Reusable Medical and Dental Devices – (March 2009). Available at http://www.fda.gov/MedicalDevices/ DeviceRegulationandGuidance/ ReprocessingofSingle-UseDevices/ UCM133514. [accessed April 27, 2010.]

Gono K. (2007) An introduction to high-resolution endoscopy and narrowband imaging. In: Cohen J (ed). *Advanced Digestive Endoscopy: Comprehensive Atlas of High Resolution Endoscopy and Narrowband Imaging*. pp. 9–22, Blackwell Publishing, Oxford.

Gono K, Obi T, Ohyama N, *et al.* (2004) Appearance of enhanced tissue features in narrow-band endoscopic imaging. *Journal of Biomedical Optics*, **9**, 568–577.

Kawahara I, Ichikawa H. (2000) Flexible Endoscope Technology: The Fiberoptic Endoscope. In: Sivak MV Jr (ed). *Gastroenterologic Endoscopy* (2nd edn, Vol 1). pp. 16–28, WB Saunders Company, Philadelphia.

Knyrim K, Seidlitz H, Vakil N, *et al.* (1989) Optical performance of electronic imaging systems for the colon. *Gastroenterology*, **96**, 776–782.

Kodashima S, Fujishiro M. (2010) Novel image-enhanced endoscopy with i-scan technology. *World Journal of Gastroenterology*, **16**, 1043–1049.

Kwon RS, Adler DG, Chand B, *et al.* (2009) Prepared by: ASGE Technology Committee. High-resolution and high-magnification endoscopes. *Gastrointestinal Endoscopy*, **69**, 399–407.

Moriyama H. (2000) Engineering characteristics and improvement of colonoscope for insertion. *Early Colorectal Cancer*, **4**, 57–62.

Moriyama H. (2001) Variable Stiffness Colonoscope – Structure and Handling. *Clinical Gastroenterology*, **16**, 167–172.

Nelson DB, Jarvis WR, Rutala WA, *et al.* (2003) Multi-society guideline for reprocessing flexible gastrointestinal endoscopes. *Gastrointestinal Endoscopy*, **58**, 1–8.

Nelson DB, Barkun AN, Block KP, *et al.* (2001) Transmission of infection by gastrointestinal endoscopy. *Gastrointestinal Endoscopy*, **54**, 824–828.

Osawa H, Yoshizawa M, Yamamoto H, *et al.* (2008) Optimal band imaging system can facilitate detection of changes in depressed-type early gastric cancer. *Gastrointestinal Endoscopy*, **67**, 226–234.

Recommended practice for cleaning and processing endoscopes and endoscopic accessories. (2003) *Association of Operating Room Nurses Journal*, **77**, 434–442.

Rutala WA. (1996) APIC guideline for selection and use of disinfectants. *American Journal of Infection Control*, **24**, 313–342.

SGNA Guidelines: Guidelines for the Use of High-Level Disinfectants and Sterilants for Reprocessing of Flexible Gastrointestinal Endoscopes. (2004) *Gastroenterology Nursing*, **27**, 198–206.

Sivak MV Jr, Fleischer DE. (1984) Colonoscopy with a video endoscope. Preliminary experience. *Gastrointestinal Endoscopy*, **30**, 1–5.

Togashi K, Osawa H, Koinuma K, *et al.* (2009) A comparison of conventional endoscopy, chromoendoscopy, and the optimal-band imaging system for the differentiation of neoplastic and non-neoplastic colonic polyps. *Gastrointestinal Endoscopy*, **69**, 734–741.

Wong Kee Song LM, Adler DG, *et al.* (2008) Narrow band imaging and multiband imaging, Prepared by: ASGE Technology Committee. *Gastrointestinal Endoscopy*, **67**, 581–589.

4

Pediatric procedural sedation for gastrointestinal endoscopy

Tom Kallay

 KEY POINTS

- Uniform sedation guidelines should be in place when performing any level of procedural sedation for children.

- The sedation practitioner must be able to recognize the various levels of sedation in children of different ages.

- Children often require deep sedation for optimal procedural conditions.

- Many risks can be avoided by proper presedation assessment and monitoring, as

well as having personnel with adequate knowledge and skills regarding medications and rescue techniques.

- Open communication between the gastroenterologist and monitor provides an environment which allows for timely adjustments in medication titration or endoscopic technique.

Definitions/levels of sedation

There are four levels of sedation defined by the American Society of Anesthesiologists (ASA), and these may be thought of as a continuum. These are minimal sedation (anxiolysis), moderate sedation and analgesia (conscious sedation), deep sedation (unconscious), and general anesthesia.

Anxiolysis is a drug-induced state where motor and cognitive functions may be impaired, but the patient responds to verbal commands. Ventilatory

and cardiovascular functions are largely unaffected with anxiolysis.

During moderate sedation, also known as conscious sedation, the child may respond purposefully to verbal commands (e.g. "open your eyes,") with or without light tactile stimulation. Older patients generally will be interactive, and younger ones will cry appropriately, for example. Airway and cardiovascular function are unaffected; however, endoscopy presents a unique challenge as the tools employed for the procedure can predispose some patients to airway obstruction. This is especially relevant in the smaller children, where the trachea is smaller and with soft cartilagi-

Practical Pediatric Gastrointestinal Endoscopy, Second Edition. George Gershman, Mike Thomson, Marvin Ament.
© 2012 Blackwell Publishing Ltd. Published 2012 by Blackwell Publishing Ltd.

nous rings, and more prone to obstruction than that of an older child with a larger, more rigid airway. In some cases, where there is considerable risk of airway obstruction with endoscopy, intubation may be indicated. Due to the relative size of the endoscope and discomfort involved in its placement, moderate sedation is rarely successful in children when performing this procedure, unless the patient is old enough to cooperate.

Deep sedation refers to a state in which the children respond only to deep or repeated stimulation, and ventilation may be impaired. Patients may require assistance with ventilation or maintaining an airway, but cardiovascular function is usually maintained. One can anticipate a partial or complete loss of airway protective reflexes in this state, and preparations must in place to accommodate for this.

General anesthesia describes a state in which there is no response to painful stimuli, and ventilation assistance is usually required due to depressed consciousness and neuromuscular function. Hemodynamic function may be compromised as well.

An inherent difficulty in childhood sedation is interpreting the physical responses while gauging the level of sedation, usually between conscious and deep sedation. A child who responds by saying "ouch" or purposefully pushes a hand away is consciously sedated. Reflex withdrawal from pain by itself is not considered a sign of conscious sedation, unless it is accompanied by some purposeful activity. This would be consistent with deep sedation.

Sedation and analgesia for diagnostic and therapeutic endoscopy in children carries a number of considerations dependent on differences in age, developmental status, and presence of comorbidities. Sedating a child is different from the sedation of an adult. One of the goals in sedating children is to control behavior, which is entirely dependent on their chronological and developmental age. Children younger than 6 or 7 years often require a deep level of sedation in order to safely complete an uncomfortable procedure, where respiratory drive, airway patency and protective reflexes may be compromised. Studies have shown that it is common for children to pass from the intended level of sedation into a deeper state in an effort to control their behavior, where physiologic compromise may occur. In order to provide the safest conditions for a child undergoing sedation, it is important to understand the definitions pertaining to level of consciousness, as well as having the ability to rescue a child from a deeper level of sedation than was intended.

Goals of sedation

The goals of procedural sedation are to

1. Guard the patient's safety and welfare.
2. Minimize physical discomfort and pain.
3. Control anxiety; minimize psychological trauma (in the child and parents).
4. Control behavior and/or movement to allow the safe completion of the procedure.
5. Return the patient to a state in which safe discharge from medical supervision is possible.

When choosing sedation medications for pediatric gastrointestinal endoscopy, an analysis of the procedure itself is helpful. The placement of an endoscope into the esophagus of a child can be painful, uncomfortable and frightening, therefore, medications must be chosen with these considerations in mind. As previously discussed, due to the instrumentation used in an area adjacent to the airway, compromise of airflow can occur. Proper sedative/hypnotics and analgesic medications must be employed together and carefully titrated in order to maintain the delicate balance of sedation/analgesia and spontaneous, adequate ventilation. Certain patients may benefit from a regimen which includes anxiolytic or amnestic medications prior to procedure, which may reduce the amount of sedatives or analgesics needed for the procedure. Knowledge of the medication onset, peak effect and duration are crucial for making good decisions when titrating, and gauging when it is appropriate to administer another dose of medication. This is particularly relevant when considering discharging toddlers or infants in car seats, where there is a risk of airway obstruction, due to prolonged residual effects of certain longer-acting medications.

Risks and complications associated with monitored sedation

There are two reports on the frequency of complications related to sedations in pediatric endoscopy. A cross-sectional review was published reviewing all complications and risk factors associated with endoscopy in children looking at 10 236 procedures at 13 centers that take part in the Pediatric Endoscopy Database System Clinical Outcomes Research Initiative (PEDS-CORI). The overall complication rate was 2.3%, the most common being hypoxemia. None of the adverse reactions were fatal. Younger age, higher ASA class, female sex, and intravenous administration of medication were noted to be risk factors for developing complications in this study.

Another group published data on performing endoscopy in the endoscopy suite with a pediatric sedation team present; 296 patients with predetermined ASA physical status levels of I-III were examined for complications. Transient desaturation was the only adverse event reported, and occurred in 21 patients (7%). The authors concluded that sedation for pediatric endoscopy could be safely carried out outside the operating room area, provided that adequate monitoring and staff (in this case, a dedicated pediatric sedation team) were present.

Looking beyond endoscopy, a large review of pediatric sedation events for any procedure was performed by the Pediatric Sedation Research Consortium, an international collaborative group involving 35 institutions dedicated to improving pediatric sedation. A total of 30 037 sedation encounters were reviewed, and the overall complication rate was found to be 3.4%. There were no deaths, although cardiopulmonary resuscitation was required in one case where the patient had significant co-morbidities. The most common adverse event was hypoxemia (defined as oxygen saturation <90% for greater than 30 seconds), which occurred at a rate of 157 per 10 000 sedations (1.6% of all cases). Vomiting, apnea, and excessive secretions occurred at rates of 47.2, 24, and 41.6 per 10 000 encounters, respectively. Stridor and laryngospasm both occurred at a rate of 4.3 per 10 000. The incidence of procedures requiring timely rescue interventions was 1 in 89.

Another report published data specifically on adverse events which occurred during pediatric procedural sedations for any procedure. This was a systematic investigation of medications associated with adverse events; a critical analysis of 118 case reports involving complications were reviewed. These cases included procedures in a hospital setting as well as dental offices. Overall, the outcomes of these cases involved death or permanent neurologic disability in 63% of cases. The authors found that adverse events evenly distributed across all classes of drugs (sedative/hypnotics, opioids, benzodiazepines, and barbiturates), and across all routes of administration (intravenous, intramuscular, oral, subcutaneous, rectal, or intranasal). It is important to note that adverse events occurred even when recommended doses were delivered. Factors associated with negative outcome were: inadequate monitoring, a lack of knowledge or skill of the practitioner providing sedation, inadequate presedation evaluation, drug errors or overdose, premature discharge, and the use of 3 or more sedating medications. Most of these adverse events were avoidable, and highlights the fact that uniform guidelines are necessary when any level of sedation is employed. This demonstrates the high risk nature of pediatric sedation, and the need for pediatric sedation practitioners to be knowledgeable of the medications employed, as well as skilled at rescue methods which include airway management and resuscitation.

Before sedation

There are a number of precautions which must be considered when sedating a child for endoscopy. Adequate support staff in pharmacy and nursing is necessary. It must be ensured that equipment and medications are immediately available and routinely maintained. A crash cart or kit should include age and size-appropriate equipment and medications necessary to resuscitate a child who is unconscious and not breathing. Airway equipment must include size-appropriate bag-valve-mask, airway delivery devices (nasal cannula, face mask), and intubating equipment with age-appropriate endotracheal tube sizes and laryngoscope blades. Some institutions employ the use of laryngeal mask airways (LMAs), which are considered acceptable by the American Heart Association guidelines for pediatric advanced life support (PALS). Cardiorespiratory monitoring should include electrocardiography, respiratory tracing, pulse oximetry, capnography if available, and non-invasive blood pressure monitoring with size-appropriate cuffs. An oxygen source and suction with catheters must be available. A defibrillator, with pediatric paddles and adhesive pads, should be accessible. There should be a protocol for accessing a higher level of care such as a pediatric intensive care or step-down unit, and in non-hospital environments, a system for accessing ambulance services must be in place.

A thorough presedation assessment is crucial in order to identify patients at risk for adverse events. Sedation for endoscopy must be tailored for each individual, yet preparations should be approached in the same stepwise fashion for every patient. The components of a presedation evaluation should include:

1. Informed consent.
2. Verbal and written instructions.
3. The child's medical history.
4. Physical exam.
5. A risk assessment.

Informed consent specific to the procedural sedation must be obtained and documented in accordance with institutional guidelines. Verbal and written instructions to the parent or guardian should include the objectives of the sedation, as well as anticipated effects during, and after the procedure. Special instructions should be given to those transporting children in a car seat, especially pertaining to head position and the potential for airway obstruction. A 24-hour phone number should be provided for follow-up, as well as dietary instructions.

The issue of fasting intervals before an elective procedure generally follows those for elective anesthesia. Children should follow the general guidelines set forth by the ASA. *Nil per os* (NPO) status for 6 hours is considered sufficient time for most foods, including infant formula; 8 hours for a full meal. Four to six hours is considered safe for breast milk and clear liquids. For emergent procedures, the risks of sedation and possible aspiration must be weighed against the need for the procedure. The use of the lightest effective sedation may be employed, or if deep sedation is required, intubation may be indicated to protect the airway.

The medical history should focus on any current or past medical illnesses affecting the cardiovascular, respiratory, hepatic or renal systems, which may affect the child's response to the medications chosen. Current home medications should be determined; it is generally acceptable for routine medications to be taken with a sip of water on the day of procedure. Certain medications can affect the metabolism and pharmacodynamics of sedative medications through inhibition of the cytochrome P450 system, and cause unwanted prolonged effects. Erythromycin, cimetidine, some HIV medications, anticonvulsants and psychotropic medications can cause clinically relevant side-effects when sedatives or analgesics are given concomitantly. Consultation with a pharmacist may be necessary when there is a concern for drug interaction. A thorough history of allergies to any medications or foods is important. As an example, propofol is manufactured in an oil-in-water base with egg and soybean oil, and, therefore, is absolutely contraindicated for use in a patient with egg or soybean allergy.

Past medical history should elicit previous experiences with procedures in order to uncover events that the child may be predisposed to, and a family history regarding anesthesia should be obtained. A history of obstructive sleep apnea or snoring could increase the risk for airway obstruction. Other key points to bring forth are recent colds or croup, poorly controlled asthma, and presence of a seizure or other neurologic disorder. Patients with complex congenital heart disease should have an evaluation by a pediatric cardiologist prior to the procedure to determine candidacy for deep sedation. Children with complex anatomy or pulmonary hypertension are usually considered high risk, and consultation with an anesthesiologist is recommended for these cases.

The physical exam must include a complete set of vital signs, which includes temperature, heart and respiratory rate, blood pressure, and pulse oximetry. A current weight is needed for appropriate medication dosing. Particular attention must be paid to the oropharynx for findings such as micrognathia, facial dysmorphism, loose teeth, tonsillar hypertrophy, or any other condition which could affect the airway. Heart exam should focus on the presence of murmurs or gallops which could indicate anatomical or functional issues. The airway exam should focus on the presence of stridor or wheezing.

Risk assessment includes assigning an ASA physical status classification level (Appendix 4.1). Children who are Class I and II are considered appropriate candidates for minimal, moderate, and deep sedation. Situations which would indicate consultation with an anesthesiologist would be ASA class III or IV, children with congenital heart disease, significant upper or lower airway obstruction (such as tonsillar hypertrophy or poorly controlled asthma), or morbid obesity. Neurologic conditions such as poorly controlled seizures, central apnea, or severe developmental delay are also considered high risk, and warrant consultation with appropriate specialty services.

During sedation

At a minimum, the number of staff required for pediatric endoscopy with procedural sedation consists of three individuals. In addition to the gastroenterologist and circulating nurse, there must be another practitioner dedicated to monitoring the patient, whose sole responsibility is to continually observe and respond to the patient's vital signs, physiologic status, and level of sedation. The practitioner should be skilled in assessment of cardiopulmonary function: respiratory rate and depth, early recognition of cyanosis, perfusion and pulse assessment. Optimally, this individual would have a dedicated sedation nurse; however, this may not be possible at some institutions. Whether the sedation practitioner is a physician, physician assistant or nurse practitioner, they should be PALS certified and have adequate specialized training in pediatric procedural sedation and rescue techniques. Regular maintenance of these skills is recommended.

Before the administration of medications, a baseline set of vital signs should be documented. The name, route, site, time, and dosage of all drugs administered should be documented. Once medication administration has begun, level of consciousness and vital signs should be documented on a time-based flow sheet every 5 minutes. The vital signs documented should include heart and respiratory rate, oxygen saturation, and blood pressure. Once the procedure is complete, and no more medications are to be administered, vital signs should be documented every 15 minutes until the child awakens.

Whether administration of medications is performed by the gastroenterologist or the sedation practitioner, good communication is crucial in order to provide optimal procedural sedation. It is important in order to anticipate physiologic changes or the conclusion of the procedure, which could affect a decision to administer a dose of medication or not. Timing of medication administration should be predicated on anticipating patient responses, which is best performed by maintaining an awareness of the procedure through observation and communication. It is the responsibility of the individual monitoring the patient to alert the gastroenterologist of physiologic deterioration, and to temporarily stop the procedure if rescue measures are required.

The nature of gastrointestinal endoscopy mandates a discussion of the specific physiological considerations inherent to the procedure. For example, esophageal intubation can induce apnea and bradycardia due to stimulation of the laryngeal branch of the vagus nerve. Infants or children with spastic neuromuscular disorders are especially prone to this, due to their small size and high cricopharyngeal tone, respectively. When air is insufflated into the gastrointestinal tract, it has the potential to cause respiratory insufficiency. Excess air in the stomach can elevate the left hemidiaphragm, impeding respiratory excursion and subsequently tidal volumes, which can be deleterious for ventilation and oxygenation. The loss of functional residual capacity can subsequently cause hypoxemia from loss of alveolar recruitment, and positive pressure ventilation, along with gastric decompression, may be necessary to recover adequate oxygen saturation.

Mesenteric stretch can cause various degrees of abdominal discomfort in some individuals, and adequate analgesia is needed to blunt this response. Intense pain during a colonoscopy, for example, is a sign of excessive mesenteric stretching and requires not only adequate analgesia but immediate adjustment of endoscopic technique. This situation highlights the need for constant communication between the gastroenterologist and monitor, as adjustments must be made by both individuals for the best procedural conditions.

The issue of standard supplemental oxygen use is controversial. Due to the nature of the procedure, supplemental oxygen is often needed to maintain adequate oxygen saturations. It must be kept in mind that failure in ventilation may be masked by supplemental oxygen, due to the law of partial pressures in the alveoli. End-tidal CO_2 monitoring by a nasal cannula-type device may be employed which can provide objective evidence of ventilatory function, if utilized properly. This does not, however, obviate the need for continued close observation of respiratory function at all times.

Postsedation care

The child who has received moderate or deep sedation must be monitored in an appropriate environment which includes ECG monitoring and pulse oximetry until they are awake. The period of wakefulness should be sustainable, as children emerging from sedation often drift between states of sleep and consciousness as the drugs are metabolized. The recovery area should include qualified staff to continuously record vital signs every 15 minutes, suction apparatus, and oxygen delivery devices including bag-valve-mask. Patients, who have received medications with a long half-life, or reversal agents such as naloxone or flumazenil, should be monitored for a longer period of time due to the risk of resedation.

The following are recommended discharge criteria:

1. Cardiovascular function and airway patency are adequate and stable.
2. The patient is easily arousable and protective reflexes are intact.
3. The patient can talk (if age appropriate).
4. The patient can sit up without assistance (if age appropriate).
5. For patients who are very young, or developmentally delayed, the presedation level of responsiveness or a level as close as possible for that child should be achieved.
6. The state of hydration is adequate.

Specific sedation techniques

Watching preparations to begin the procedure and administer medications is an anxiety provoking time for most children. There are many factors which determine how easy or difficult it is to achieve a desired level of sedation in children. Patient-to-patient variability in drug pharmacodynamics, medication choice, level of distress and anxiety before the procedure, previous hospital experiences, age and developmental stage of the child are all considerations that must be taken into account when preparing to sedate a child. Parental presence and a quiet, calm environment are helpful in reducing the patient's stress and may decrease the amount of medications needed. Any means to distract the child from what is about to happen should be sought by asking the parents what might work, and attempts should be made to perform them. For certain children, techniques such as parental presence for induction, distraction, hypnosis, and use of local anesthetics may reduce the amount of medication needed to complete the procedure.

For IV insertion, EMLA cream®, a topical mixture of 2.5% lidocaine and 2.5% prilocaine, is helpful, if applied locally to the skin 1 hour before the IV is placed. Side-effects of EMLA include local skin reactions: rash, blanching, erythema, edema, and alterations in temperature sensations. Systemic or anaphylactic reactions are rare due to the small amount absorbed. EMLA is contraindicated in children with known hypersensitivity to local anesthetics. Also, children with rare congenital or idiopathic methemoglobinemia, or under 12 months and receiving treatment with methemoglobin inducing agents (phenytoin, phenobarbital, sulfonamides, acetaminophen), should not receive EMLA. For children less than 3 months, EMLA application time should not exceed 1 hour; for all other children maximum contact time is 4 hours.

When considering medications for a child undergoing endoscopy outside of the operating room, the two main components that should be considered are: anxiolysis/sedation and analgesia. Nausea and vomiting are potential side-effects which are universal to all sedatives and analgesics; specific adverse reactions to the following medications are addressed individually.

Anxiolysis and sedation

For anxiolysis and sedation, the most commonly employed medications are the benzodiazepines. Midazolam is an intravenous short-acting agent which also causes retrograde amnesia, which is beneficial in reducing disturbing memories of the procedure. It is usually administered intravenously for procedures. For the particularly anxious child, it can be administered as a pre-treatment by mouth or intranasally, although mucosal pain and discomfort is a significant side-effect associated with the nasal route. For intravenous use, the usual intermittent dosage is 0.05–0.1 mg/kg, and the maximum cumulative total should not exceed 10 mg. Contraindications to its use would be patients with marginal hemodynamic status, as one of the common side-effects is hypotension. Other side-effects include apnea and the phenomenon of paradoxical excitement. Paradoxical reactions are impossible to predict, and occur when the disinhibition has an agitating effect on the child. Increasing or repeating the dose will further increase the agitation, and predispose the child to eventual unconsciousness and respiratory compromise. Once a paradoxical reaction is recognized, an immediate change in the medication strategy is warranted.

The reversal agent for benzodiazepines is fluma-zenil, and will reverse both the sedative and respi-ratory depression effects. The usual initial dose is 0.01 mg/kg (maximum 0.2–0.5 mg depending on age), with repeat doses of 0.005–0.01 mg/kg given every minute for 5 minutes.

Etomidate is an intravenous sedative hypnotic that has less hemodynamic or respiratory effects when compared with midazolam, although apnea has been reported with its use. Usual dosage is 0.1–0.3 mg/kg. Etomidate has no analgesic effects or a reversal agent. A known side-effect of etomi-date is adrenal suppression by inhibition of 11-beta-hydroxylase, an enzyme responsible for production of cortisol. For most healthy children this will not be a concern, but is not recommended for use in patients with septic shock or immuno-suppresion. Myoclonus and pain at injection site are other side effects of etomidate.

Propofol is an intravenous short-acting pure sedative with quick onset and recovery once administration is stopped. It requires continuous infusion carefully titrated to effect, which is best administered with an infusion pump. There is no reversal agent. It is manufactured with a lipid base and contains egg and soy products, therefore, allergies to either of these food products is an absolute contraindication for its use. Propofol is administered as a bolus dose of 0.5–1 mg/kg, fol-lowed by an infusion starting at 25–50 mcg/kg/min and titrated to effect. It is essential for practi-tioners administering propofol to have advanced airway and resuscitation skills, as airway obstruc-tion, shallow respirations, and hypotension are common. Propofol infusion syndrome, usually associated with infusions >48 hours, is the constel-lation of metabolic acidosis, acute renal failure, rhabdomyolysis, hyperlipidemia, and cardiac dys-function. The incidence of this syndrome is unknown. Propofol also causes pain at injection site; this can be limited by locking 1 cc of 1% lido-caine without epinephrine into the IV 10 minutes before propofol administration, or administering through a central line if available.

Analgesics

Fentanyl is the most commonly utilized opioid for procedural sedation. It is a powerful analgesic that is approximately 50–100 times more potent than morphine. When given intravenously, it has a rela-tive quick onset of action and short half-life which makes it an attractive choice. It is a potent analge-sic, usually dosed at 0.5–1 mcg/kg and repeated as necessary. The onset of analgesia is almost imme-diate and the effects last for 30–60 minutes. It is important not to administer fentanyl too rapidly; rapid infusions in smaller children predispose them to chest wall rigidity. In this case, positive pressure ventilation should be immediately per-formed, and an opioid antagonist should be pro-vided. In severe cases, muscle relaxation and intubation may be required.

Alfentanil, sufentanil and remifentanil are all congeners of fentanyl which are primarily utilized by anesthesiologists. Alfentanil is one-third the potency of fentanyl with a quicker onset and shorter duration of action. Sufentanil is 10 times the potency of fentanyl, and remifentanil about 2 times the potency. These are all very short-acting medications that demonstrate cardiovascular sta-bility, yet experience in pediatric procedural seda-tion outside the operating room is minimal.

Naloxone is the reversal agent of choice for all opioid overdoses. For children less than 20 kg, usual dosage is 0.1 mg/kg, and may be repeated every 2–3 minutes. For children greater than 5 years or 20 kg, 2 mg may be used. As its duration of effect is only 20–30 minutes, shorter than that of some opioids, one can anticipate needing repeat doses.

Other

Ketamine is considered a general anesthetic or a dissociative amnestic, and is a potent analgesic that renders the patient unconscious. Given intra-venously, the usual induction dose is 1–2 mg/kg with onset time of 1–3 minutes, and duration of 10–20 minutes. Hypertension, tachycardia, laryn-gospasm, hypersalivation, emergence reactions and nystagmus are some of the side-effects reported with its use. As ketamine causes increased intracranial and intraocular pressure, it is con-traindicated for patients with concern for these issues. It also lowers seizure threshold, and should not be utilized in patients with a seizure disorder. Ketamine is considered to have minimal respira-tory or cardiovascular depression. It is not con-traindicated for patients with asthma as it causes bronchodilation. For endoscopy, an anticholiner-gic can be administered concomitantly to decrease hypersalivation, such as atropine or glycopyrro-late. Emergence reaction or delirium may occur when the patient is recovering and manifest as confusion, fear and agitation. Although not fully supported by the literature, many advocate for pretreatment with a benzodiazepine or for the use of calming techniques during induction to decrease the possibility of emergence reaction.

Dexmedetomidine is an alpha-2 adrenergic agonist with sedative properties, and its use has been increasing in pediatrics. It is administered as a continuous infusion and should be delivered with an infusion pump, dosed at 0.2– 0.6 mg/kg/hour. Common side-effects during procedural sedation are hypo- or hypertension, bradycardia, and dry mouth. As the experience with dexmedetomidine grows in pediatrics, it may be seen more frequently as a valid choice for sedation.

Conclusions

Procedural sedation in children carries a significant number of considerations which depend on the developmental and chronological age of the patient, history of previous experiences, and individualized response to medication. In order to avoid complications, the setting for the procedure must be well equipped, and the staff performing procedural sedation must be adequately trained in pediatric pharmacology and resuscitation. Good communication between all practitioners during the procedure contributes to a safe and efficient environment, and the likelihood of procedural success.

Appendix 4.1 ASA physical status classification

Class I	A normal healthy patient
Class II	A patient with mild systemic disease (e.g. controlled reactive airway disease)
Class III	A patient with severe systemic disease (e.g. a child who is actively wheezing)
Class IV	A patient with severe systemic disease that is a constant threat to life
Class V	A moribund patient who is not expected to survive without the operation

FURTHER READING

Agus MS, Alexander JL, Mantell PA. (2006) Continuous non-invasive end-tidal CO2 monitoring in pediatric inpatients with diabetic ketoacidosis. *Pediatric Diabetes*, **7(4),** 196–200.

American Academy of Pediatrics, American Academy of Pediatric Dentistry, Coté CJ, Wilson S, and the Work Group on Sedation. (2006) Guidelines for Monitoring and Management of Pediatric Patients During and After Sedation for Diagnostic and Therapeutic Procedures: An Update. *Pediatrics*, **118,** 2587–2602.

Barbi E, Petaros P, Badina L, *et al.* (2006) Deep sedation with propofol for upper gastrointestinal endoscopy in children, administered by specially trained pediatricians: a prospective case series with emphasis on side effects. *Endoscopy* **38(4),** 368–375.

Coté CJ, Karl HW, Notterman DA, *et al.* (2000) Adverse Sedation Events in Pediatrics: Analysis of Medications Used for Sedation. *Pediatrics* **106,** 633–644.

Cravero JP, Blike GT, Beach M, *et al.* (2006) Incidence and nature of adverse events during pediatric sedation/anesthesia for procedures outside the operating room: report from the Pediatric Sedation Research Consortium. *Pediatrics*, **118(3),** 1087–1096.

Deitch DO, Miner J, Chudnofsky JR, *et al.* (2010) Does End Tidal CO_2 Monitoring During Emergency Department Procedural Sedation and Analgesia with Propofol Decrease the Incidence of Hypoxic Events? A Randomized, Controlled Trial. *Annals of Emergency Medicine*, **55(3),** 258–264.

Dial S, Silver P, Bock K, *et al.* (2001) Pediatric sedation for procedures titrated to a desired degree of immobility results in unpredictable depth of sedation. *Pediatric Emergency Care*, **17,** 414–420.

Doyle L, Colletti J. (2006) Pediatric Procedural Sedation and Analgesia. *Pediatric Clinics of North America*, **53,** 279–292.

American Heart Association 2005 American Heart Association Guidelines for Cardiopulmonary Resuscitation and Emergency Cardiovascular Care of Pediatric and Neonatal Patients: Pediatric Basic Life Support. (2006) *Pediatrics*, **117,** e989–e1004.

Friesen RH, Alswang M. (1996) End-tidal PCO2 monitoring via nasal cannulae in pediatric patients: accuracy and sources of error. *Journal of Clinical Monitoring and Computing*, **12(2)**, 155–159.

Gozal D, Gozal Y. (2008) Pediatric sedation/anesthesia outside the operating room. *Current Opinion in Anesthesiology*, **21(4)**, 494–498.

Hiller A, Olkkola KT, Isohanni P, *et al.* (1990) Unconsciousness associated with midazolam and erythromycin. *British Journal of Anaesthesia*, **65**, 826–828.

Howe TA, Jaalam K, Ahmad R, *et al.* (2009) The use of end-tidal capnography to monitor non-intubated patients presenting with acute exacerbation of asthma in the emergency department. *Journal of Emergency Medicine*, Mar 7 Epub ahead of print.

Krauss B, Green SM. (2006) Procedural sedation and analgesia in children. *Lancet*, **367**, 766–780.

Levine DA, Platt SL. (2005) Novel monitoring techniques for use with procedural sedation. *Current Opinions in Pediatrics*, **17(3)**, 351–354.

Malviya S, Voepel-Lewis T, Tait AR, *et al.* (2002) Depth of sedation in children undergoing computed tomography: validity and reliability of the University of Michigan Sedation Scale (UMSS). *British Journal of Anaesthesia*, **88**, 241–245.

Mattila MJ, Idanpaan-Heikkila JJ, Tornwall M, *et al.* (1993) Oral single doses of erythromycin and roxithromycin may increase the effects of midazolam on human performance. *Pharmacology and Toxicology* **73**, 180–185.

Maxwell LG, Yaster M. (1996) The myth of conscious sedation. *Archives of Pediatric and Adolescent Medicine*, **150**, 665–667.

Motas D, McDermott NB, VanSickle T, *et al.* (2004) Depth of consciousness and deep sedation attained in children as administered by nonanaesthesiologists in a children's hospital. *Paediatric Anaesthesia*, **14**, 256–260.

Olkkola KT, Aranko K, Luurila H, *et al.* (1993) A potentially hazardous interaction between erythromycin and midazolam. *Clinical Pharmacology & Therapeutics*, **53**, 298–305.

Patel KN, Simon HK, Stockwell CA, *et al.* (2009) Pediatric procedural sedation by a dedicated nonanesthesiology pediatric sedation service using propofol. *Pediatric Emergency Care*, **25(3)**, 133–138.

Thakkar K, El-Serag HB, Mattek N, *et al.* (2007) Complications of pediatric EGD: a 4-year experience in PEDS-CORI. *Gastrointestinal Endoscopy*, **5(2)**, 213–221.

von Rosensteil NA, Adam D. (1995) Macrolide antibacterials: drug interactions of clinical significance. *Drug Safety*, **13**, 105–122.

Wengrower D, Gozal D, Gozal Y, *et al.* (2004) Complicated endoscopic pediatric procedures using deep sedation and general anesthesia are safe in the endoscopy suite. *Scandinavian Journal of Gastroenterology*, **39(3)**, 283–286.

Wheeler DS, Vaux KK, Ponaman ML, *et al.* (2003) The safe and effective use of propofol sedation in children undergoing diagnostic and therapeutic procedures: experience in a pediatric ICU and a review of the literature. *Pediatric Emergency Care*, **19(6)**, 385–392.

Part Two

Basic Pediatric Endoscopy Techniques

5

Diagnostic upper gastrointestinal endoscopy

George Gershman

 KEY POINTS

- The correct preparation and position of the child before and during EGD are important safety issues.
- The proper assembling of the equipment is necessary to avoid malfunction of instruments during the procedure.
- Precise handling of the endoscope and a good knowledge of the anatomical landmarks are key for the best technique of esophageal

  intubation and endoscopic examination of the upper GI tract.
- Most complications of EGD are preventable with adequate preparation, appropriate patient selection, and proper technique.
- A basic knowledge of endoscopic anatomy and endoscopic signs of common, and some rare pathology, are the cornerstones of correct interpretation of endoscopic images.

Preparation for esophageal intubation

Once adequately sedated, the patient is placed in the left lateral decubitus position, with his or her head resting on a small pillow in a neutral position and the back supported by a folded pillow inserted between the patient and sidebars of the gurney.

The height of the gurney is adjusted to a level comfortable for the endoscopist and assisting nurse (optimal height corresponds to the endoscopist elbows). At the beginning of the procedure, the nurse should be standing behind the patient, with her left arm supporting the patient's head in the occipital area, and her right palm beneath the chin. This technique will help to secure the patient's head during insertion of the endoscope.

The endoscopist should stand at least one-foot away from the gurney or the distance corresponding to the length of the slightly flexed left arm pointed toward the patient's mouth. Such positioning is optimal for aligning the endoscope with the pharyngeal and esophageal axis and manipulations with the endoscope. Placement of a bite-guard is mandatory for all children, except infants without teeth.

The bite guard serves three important functions:

1. Protection of the endoscope;
2. Facilitation of proper positioning of the endoscope between the palate and the tongue;
3. Anchoring of the suction catheter.

A modern bite-guard consists of a plastic cylinder with a front hollow bumper and side-clips with

---

Practical Pediatric Gastrointestinal Endoscopy, Second Edition. George Gershman, Mike Thomson, Marvin Ament.
© 2012 Blackwell Publishing Ltd. Published 2012 by Blackwell Publishing Ltd.

an attached strip of ribbon, preventing it from sliding to the side.

Despite clever design, close attention should be paid to the position of the bite-guard to avoid mechanical damage of the endoscope when the child becomes more awake or agitated.

In younger children, insertion of a bite-guard is facilitated by adequate sedation. To avoid accidental trauma, both lips should be gently pulled in corresponding directions (up or down) protecting them from accidental entrapment between the teeth and the bite-guard.

Assembling the equipment and pre-procedure check-up

The following steps are necessary for proper assembly of the endoscopic equipment:

1. Insert the connection plug into a light source tightly. A faulty connection may result in a distorted image, loss of image or malfunction of the air-water delivery system.
2. Connect the video endoscope with the video processer by the special cable.
3. Use a special adapter, if one is available, to connect the old model fiberscope with the video processer to use a monitor.
4. Choose the appropriate mode (OES for fiberscopes and 100–200 for video endoscopes) for "Olympus Co" light sources (if applicable) and an additional cable for the 100 series video endoscopes. False connection or selection of the wrong mode will result in improper white balance, excessive brightness or loss of the endoscopic image (a "blind" screen).
5. Push the ignition button to activate the light source.
6. Check the white balance.
7. Fill the water container up to ¾ of its capacity with sterile water.
8. Fill the water channel by pressing and holding down the air-water valve and confirming vigorous water spurting from the nostril. If water is not running out at a decent pressure, check the status of the air pump: turn the on/off knob to the "on" position, adjust the pressure level, reassure a tight connection of the endoscope with the light source and the water container to the endoscope. Check the integrity of the "O" ring for older style water containers. If the problem persists, tighten the cap of the water container and determine if the air-water valve is properly mounted. Consider sequential replacement of an air-water valve, water container and the endoscope, if all other options have been exhausted.
9. Adjust the air pump to medium intensity while avoiding excessive distention of the stomach. Excessive insufflation could result in a patient's irritability and retching, secondary to increased intra-abdominal pressure, elevation of the left hemi-diaphragm and decreased tidal volume, especially in infants and toddlers. Excessive use of air increases the risk of vomiting and aspiration. In our opinion, the high air pressure setting should not be used for routine EGD in children.
10. Check and adjust the intensity of the suction. If it is inadequate, check the suction system in a stepwise fashion. First, make sure that the suction switch is in the "On" position; the suction cable is tightly connected to the endoscope and the suction canister. If suction is still inadequate, reassemble the suction canister properly. Then, check the suction valve: pull it out for visual inspection, dip it in water and reinsert it back by pressing down into a suction nostril of a control panel until a soft click occurs. Replace the endoscope if all previous steps have failed.
11. Wipe the lens of the endoscope with alcohol swab if the image is blurry.

Endoscope handling

The endoscopist holds the control panel of the endoscope in the left slightly extended palm by the 4th and 5th fingers with the connecting tube hanging behind the thumb (Figure 5.1). The index and the middle finger are positioned comfortably above the suction and air-water valves respectively (Figure 5.2). This allows the endoscopist to use the thumb for rotation of the large up/down [U/D] knob in a clockwise or counterclockwise

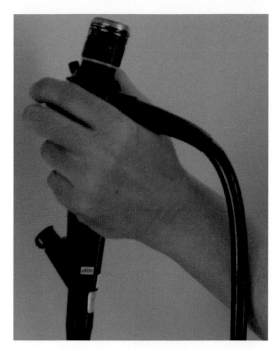

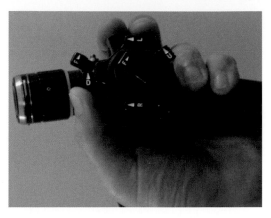

Figure 5.3 Manipulations with the R/L and U/D knobs. The thumb is the main tool for rotation of the U/D and R/L knobs.

Figure 5.1 Control panel handling. The control panel is in the left palm between the 4th and 5th fingers. Slight extension of the arm and the connecting tube hanging behind the thumb balances the weight of the control panel and further secures the correct grip.

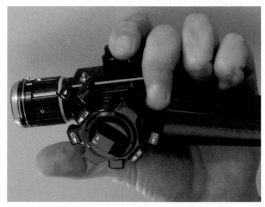

Figure 5.4 Technique of the extensive rotation of the control knobs. The middle finger can serve the function of the locker during extensive rotation of the knobs: ratchet-wheel technique.

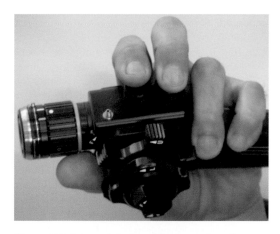

Figure 5.2 Approach to the air/water and suction buttons. The index and the ring fingers are free to work with the air/water and suction buttons.

direction (Figure 5.3). The middle finger can assist with additional rotation by locking the knob from above and leaving the thumb free for continuous movement from below (e.g. a ratchet-wheel) (Figure 5.4).

The experienced endoscopist can also use the thumb for simultaneous adjustment of the small right/left |R/L| knob. Lateral deflection of the bending portion of the endoscope can also be produced by twisting the left hand and/or forearm in clockwise or counterclockwise direction. The generated force is then transmitted from the control panel to the shaft of the endoscope.

The effectiveness of the torque technique is directly related to the degree of straightening of the working part of the endoscope between the control panel and the bite-guard. Moving the right or left shoulder forward reinforces counterclockwise and clockwise rotations, respectfully. Thus,

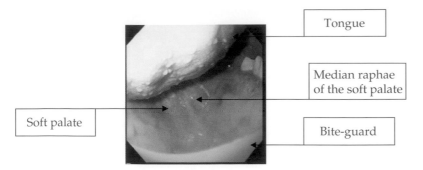

Tongue

Median raphae
of the soft palate

Soft palate

Bite-guard

Figure 5.5 The initial phase of the esophageal intubation. The endoscopist should concentrate on the proper positioning of the scope in the oral cavity: the view of the tongue and the soft palate through the bite guard.

appropriate handling of the U/D knob, in addition to the positioning of the endoscope using the left arm, is sufficient for precise orientation without frequent manipulations with the R/L knob.

The R/L knob, however, is useful for target biopsies, the U-turn maneuver, and intubation of the second portion of the duodenum.

The left index and middle fingers control the suction and air-water valves respectively. The endoscopist uses the right hand to advance, withdraw, and rotate the shaft of the endoscope. In addition, the right hand is used to manipulate the biopsy forceps or other accessories.

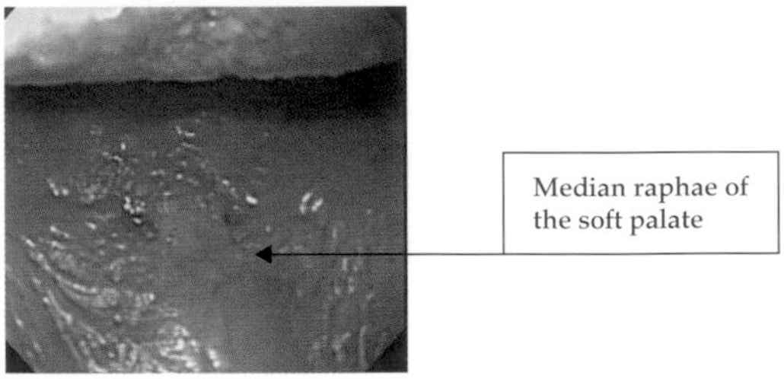

Median raphae of
the soft palate

Figure 5.6 The correct approach to the pharynx. The midline of the tongue and the palate shows the correct direction of the insertion.

Techniques of esophageal intubation

Three different techniques exist for esophageal intubations: direct observation, blind, and finger-assisted. The direct observation technique is the preferred method of pediatric upper GI endoscopy with the forward view endoscopes due to its superiority and safety. After all of the preparations have been made, and the endoscope has been found to be properly functioning, it is lubricated to the 15 cm mark and handled by the endoscopist as described above. The endoscopist holds the control panel in the left hand and the shaft in the right hand between the thumb, index, and middle finger at the 20 cm mark. The bending section of the endoscope should be straightened to achieve vertical movement when the U/D knob is used. Just before insertion of the scope into the mouth, the tip of the endoscope should be bent slightly downward. It will mark the plane of the endoscope, which should be aligned with the longitu-

dinal axis of the pharynx by clockwise or counterclockwise rotation.

Initially, the endoscopist should devote his full attention to the proper placement of the endoscope into the patient's mouth in order to facilitate a smooth insertion of the endoscope into the pharynx and prevent accidental trauma (Figure 5.5). This is especially important in infants and toddlers due to the relatively small space in the oral cavity and easy displacement of the tongue toward the pharynx by the bite-guard.

The rule of thumb is to concentrate on the child (not on the monitor) until the endoscope is placed properly along the midline of the tongue and the tip of the scope is no longer visible (Figure 5.6). If the tongue is flipped up or sticking out through the bite-guard, attempts to insert the endoscope may push the tongue toward the pharynx increasing the risk of apnea and accidental trauma of the buckle or pharyngeal mucosa, due to lateral displacement of the instrument. In this specific instance, it is useful to remove the bite-guard, fit it over the shaft, slide it back and transfer the endoscope to the assistant, who must keep it parallel to the longitudinal pharyngeal axis.

Meanwhile, the endoscopist inserts the left index finger into the child's mouth and using it as a tongue blade, pushes the tongue inferiorly and anteriorly, while placing the endoscope over the tongue with the right hand. Then, the bite-guard is fitted back into the mouth. Finally, the endoscopist takes over the control panel and adjusts the position of the endoscope as described above. At this point, all further manipulations with the scope should be carried out under direct observation of the picture on the monitor. Remember, that the endoscopic image is reversed due to bending of the instrument. In other words, the relatively pale tongue with its rough texture occupies the upper portion of the screen, while the bright-pink and smooth palate appears at the bottom of the monitor (Figure 5.7). Move the endoscope slowly forward along the midline and gently angle it down by rotating the U/D knob counterclockwise. This will facilitate sliding into the pharynx over the root of the tongue, which may be seen transiently

as a papillary structure (Figure 5.8). The lumen of the oropharynx could be lost momentarily just before the pharynx is revealed. While adequately angled, the endoscope is slowly inserted forward. The first structure to emerge will be the epiglottis, however, the appearance of the posterior pharyngeal wall should be also anticipated. The epiglottis will occupy the upper part of the screen as a crescent-shaped structure (Figure 5.9). Failure to find the epiglottis indicates that the endoscope was advanced too far anteriorly (above the epiglottis), or too close to the cricoarytenoid cartilages, or was angled laterally. Always use the rule of thumb: pull the endoscope back until orientation is fully restored. Pull the endoscope back to the first recognizable structure, for example, the uvula pointed up from the bottom of the screen, the laterally located tonsils or the "median raphae" of the tongue at the top of the monitor. Reposition the shaft of the endoscope along the midline, push it forward slowly and rotate the U/D knob

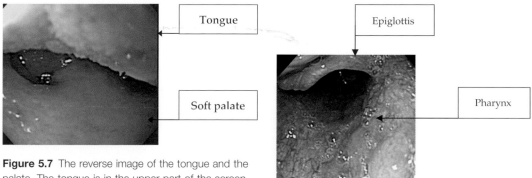

Figure 5.7 The reverse image of the tongue and the palate. The tongue is in the upper part of the screen while the soft palate occupies the low part of the monitor. Beginners should use to the reversed images created by the endoscopes.

Figure 5.9 The initial view of the epiglottis. The epiglottis should be found and seen clearly before esophageal intubation is attempted.

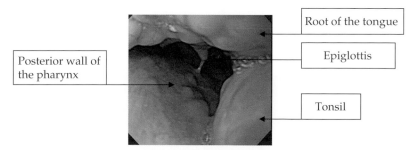

Figure 5.8 The root of the tongue. The root of the tongue appears as the rough texture, papilla structure. It may be seen briefly or not at all during routine procedure. However, careful examination of this area and tonsils should be attempted in children with suspected post-transplantation lymphoproliferative disorder.

counterclockwise simultaneously. Stay on the same track until the larynx is clearly viewed. Stop advancing if resistance is felt or if the picture becomes diffusely pink and blurry.

The larynx has a triangular shape with the epiglottis above, two small spherical structures of arytenoid cartilage at the bottom, and aryepiglottic fold on a side (Figure 5.10). The true vocal cords can be occasionally seen as a white/silver upside down letter "V" (Figure 5.11). A close view of the vocal cords is a warning sign of excessive deviation of the endoscope anteriorly. Remember that the esophageal orifice is hiding behind the cricoarytenoid cartilages, i.e. at the very bottom of the

screen. In order to reach this point, the tip of the endoscope should be angled downward toward the posterior wall of the pharynx by rotation of the U/D knob in clockwise direction. The opened cricopharyngeal portion of the esophagus can be seen briefly during swallowing as a dark ring slightly lateral of the larynx.

Direct midline intubation of the esophagus is practically impossible due to significant pressure generated by the larynx toward the posterior pharyngeal wall. This resistance will push the endoscope either to the right or left of the larynx (Figure 5.12). If it is pushed to the right, rotate the shaft clockwise to about ¼ turn. If it is pushed to the

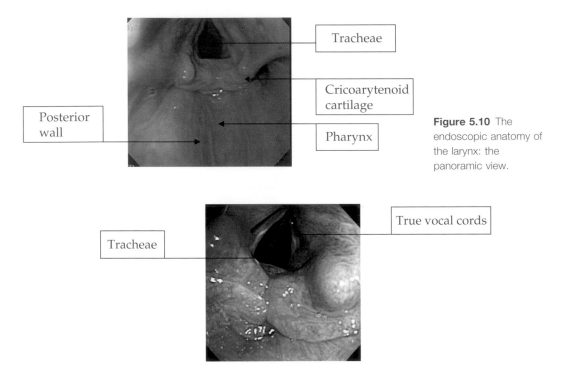

Figure 5.10 The endoscopic anatomy of the larynx: the panoramic view.

Figure 5.11 The endoscopic appearance of the vocal cords. A close capture of the vocal cords indicates that the tip of the scope is advanced too far anteriorly. The shaft must be pulled back a few centimeters immediately and the tip should be deviated down toward the posterior wall.

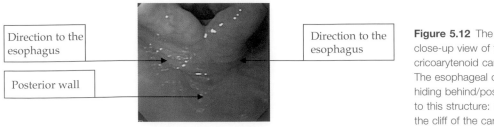

Figure 5.12 The close-up view of the cricoarytenoid cartilages. The esophageal orifice is hiding behind/posteriorly to this structure: below the cliff of the cartilage.

left, adjust the shaft to the same degree counterclockwise (Figure 5.13). In either case, advance the shaft forward slightly until the mucosal fold appears crossing the upper part of the screen in a diagonal fashion (Figure 5.14). If the direction of insertion is unchanged at this point, the endoscope will enter the "periform recess". Rotate the shaft in the opposite direction and angle the tip of the endoscope up by rotating the U/D knob counterclockwise (Figure 5.15). If the resistance diminishes, continue advancing the endoscope along the mucosa. Spontaneous opening of the esophagus helps to adjust the position of the endoscope and simplifies the intubation process. In case of persistent resistance or loss of orientation, pull the endoscope back to the level of the arytenoids cartilage and repeat the intubation from the opposite side of the larynx.

In neonates and small infants, once it has been already inserted into the cervical esophagus, additional rotation of the endoscope is necessary to overcome resistance and reduce the force pushing it further into the esophagus.

During the swallowing process, the larynx moves superiorly to protect the airway. It is useful to pull the endoscope back with the swallow and advance it quickly forward through the briefly opened pharyngeal portion of the esophagus. When the tip of the endoscope is submerged

between the cricoid cartilage and posterior wall of the pharynx longer than 10–15 seconds, it may induce irritability and agitation even in well-sedated patients. Apnea and/or bradycardia, especially in infants and toddlers, may also occur due to constant pressure on the larynx and irritation of the nearby superior laryngeal nerve. If intubation of the esophagus lasts more than 20 seconds, it is wise to pull the endoscope out until the child regains normal breathing.

In addition, resistance to the passage of the endoscope, the presence of light in the lateral neck, or loss of a clear picture warrants the withdrawal of the endoscope.

To facilitate subsequent esophageal intubations, an endoscopist should wait for spontaneous opening of the esophageal orifice or use air insufflations and or brief (one or two seconds) water irrigations. To avoid aspiration, this technique should be used only, when the tip of the endoscope has been inserted behind the larynx and deviated from the midline.

Exploration of the esophagus, stomach and duodenum

After a successful intubation of the upper esophageal sphincter, the endoscope should be advanced

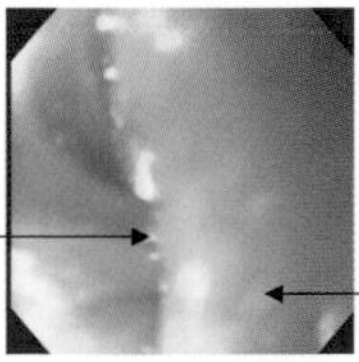

Esophageal orifice — Larynx

Figure 5.13 Side-view of the grove between the lateral wall of the larynx and pharynx. The shaft was rotated counterclockwise wise to approach the esophageal orifice. Direct intubation of the esophagus along the midline is impossible due to extensive pressure between the posterior wall of the larynx and anterior wall of the pharynx.

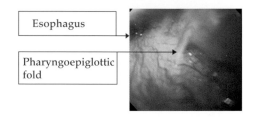

Esophagus —

Pharyngoepiglottic fold

Figure 5.14 The pharyngoepiglottic fold. It signals to switch rotation and deviate the tip of the scope upward.

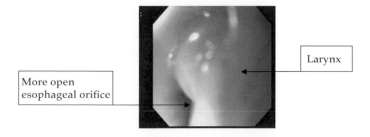

More open esophageal orifice — Larynx

Figure 5.15 Close-up view of the esophageal orifice. Rotation in the opposite direction allows positioning the tip of the scope toward the esophagus and away from the "piriform recess".

strictly along the lumen. The cervical esophagus is collapsed by tonic contractions of the longitudinal and circular fibers of striated muscles. Because of this, it is only partially seen during antegrade insertion of the endoscope. Therefore, air insufflation is necessary to keep the tip of the endoscope a safe distance from the esophageal wall. A more detailed examination of the cervical esophageal is feasible under general anesthesia with muscle relaxants, e.g. during foreign body removal. Advancement of the endoscope toward the thoracic inlet is facilitated by slight clockwise rotation.

The thoracic portion of the esophagus is normally patent, except during brief peristaltic activity. It makes a detailed examination of the entire tubular esophagus quite easy without air insufflation. The distention of the esophagus with air is indicated only in few occasions such as extra luminal compression, foreign bodies, esophageal varices and severe esophagitis. Intermittent clockwise or counter clockwise rotations of the endoscope are necessary to keep the shaft in the middle of the esophageal lumen. A central position of the endoscope is optimal for a panoramic view of the esophagus.

The lumen of the thoracic esophagus is narrowed down at the area of the so-called second physiological narrowing created by the left main bronchus. It is always unilateral (Figure 5.16). Bilateral narrowing of the thoracic esophagus is pathological and further work-up should be considered to rule out a double aortic arch or aberrant subclavian artery.

The useful landmark of the distal esophagus is a pulsation of the left atrium. The distal esophagus acquires a funnel shape right above the diaphragm (Figure 5.17). It narrows down and deviates to the left, passing through the diaphragmatic notch (the third physiological narrowing). The border between the relatively pale esophageal and bright gastric mucosa, the so-called "Z-line", is slightly irregular (Figure 5.18). The location of the "Z-line" in relation to the hiatal notch has normal variations. In general, elevation of the Z-line" by 2 cm or more above the diaphragm is abnormal. The only reliable endoscopic sign of the diaphragm is sequential constriction of the lumen during inspiration and relaxation/opening of the same segment during expiration. Respiratory excursion of the diaphragm is blunted in a deeply sedated child with shallow breathing, especially during antegrade approach. The location of the diaphragm in relation to the "Z-line" becomes more obvious during retrograde observation (U-turn maneuver).

To follow the natural course of the abdominal portion of the esophagus, the endoscope has to be

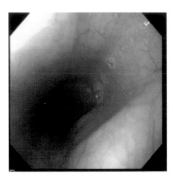

Figure 5.16 The second physiological narrowing of the esophagus. It does not have sharp borders and is always unilateral.

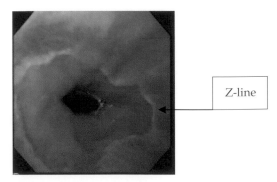

Z-line

Figure 5.18 "Z"-line. The junction between the pale esophageal and richer colored gastric mucosa is slightly irregular. It is located at the level or within 2 cm above the hiatal notch.

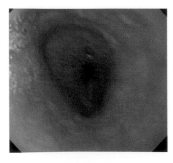

Figure 5.17 The distal esophagus. It tapers down toward the hiatal notch.

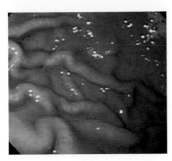

Figure 5.19 Prominent fold of the greater curvature of the stomach. Appearance of these folds is the sign of a successful intubation of the stomach.

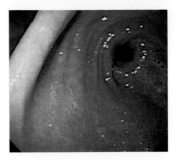

Figure 5.21 Gastric angularis. The detail image of the angularis can be easily obtained during withdrawal phase of the procedure: 1. Position the tip of the scope at the level of the distal body. 2. Rotate the scope counterclockwise and advance forward.

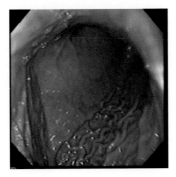

Figure 5.20 Panoramic view of the gastric body. It can be achieved by clockwise rotation of the shaft and elevation of the tip of the scope.

slowly advanced and rotated counter-clockwise with simultaneous elevation of the tip of the instrument. The straightforward approach to the stomach will result in a loss of orientation due to the close proximity of the posterior wall of the cardia or upper body. The stomach is recognized by the folds of the greater curvature between 5 and 7 o'clock as well as a pool of mucus (Figure 5.19). At this point, the endoscope should be rotated clockwise and bent downward until appearance of a panoramic view of the gastric body is achieved (Figure 5.20). Four slightly outlined folds between 1 and 3 o'clock highlight the lesser curvature. These folds disappear quickly during insufflation.

It is important to minimize the amount of air pumped into the stomach. It is especially important in neonates and infants, who are quite sensitive to gastric distention and may become irritable, start retching and develop respiratory distress or bradycardia.

Additional clockwise rotation and upward deflection of the tip of the endoscope will facilitate the advancement of the instrument toward the incisura angularis. The junction between the gastric body and antrum is marked by a prominent incisura angularis from above and a loss of folds of the greater curvature from below (Figure 5.21). At this point, it is useful to elevate the tip and advance the endoscope further toward the antrum.

Resistance or loss of orientation warrants pulling back. In cases of a so-called "cascade" stomach, it is difficult to reach the pylorus just by pushing the endoscope forward. Instead, move the tip of the endoscope upwards, advance it forward, rotate the shaft clockwise and pull it back. Repeat this maneuver and push the endoscope slightly deeper each time until the pylorus appears on the screen.

A normal pylorus looks like a ring, which disappears during peristalsis. The length of the normal pylorus channel during relaxation is approximately 3 to 5mm.

For successful intubation of the pylorus, the endoscope should be advanced along the prepyloric folds. The tip has to be bent slightly downward to avoid flipping into a retroflexed (U-turn) position (Figure 5.22).

If the pylorus is lost during peristalsis, it is useful to either wait until it opens up spontaneously or to pull the endoscope 3 to 4cm backward to regain a panoramic view of the prepyloric antrum.

Gentle advancement is enough to pass the endoscope through the pylorus. In rare cases, attempts to bypass the pylorus will move the endoscope away from the target.

In such instances, it is useful to pull the endoscope back into the gastric body, decompress the

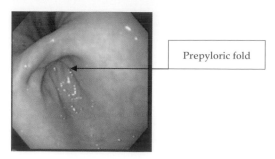

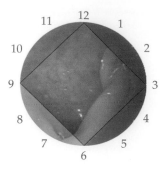

Figure 5.22 Panoramic view of the antrum. At this stage of the procedure the tip of the scope should deviated down to prevent flipping of the shaft into U-turn position. The prepyloric folds are pointed toward the pylorus.

Figure 5.24 Endoscopic mapping of the duodenal bulb during insertion phase of the procedure. Anterior wall is located between 6 and 9 o'clock; Posterior wall is located between 12 and 3 o'clock; Lesser curvature or medial wall is located between 9 and 12 o'clock; Greater curvature or lateral wall is located between 3 and 6 o'clock.

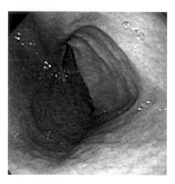

There is a "blind" zone in the proximal part of the duodenal bulb between the 3 and 6 o'clock position. Rotating the patient into the prone position facilitates exploration of this area.

The walls of the duodenal bulb are labeled traditionally as the anterior, posterior, lesser and greater curvatures (Figure 5.24).

Certain corrections in orientation within the duodenal bulb should be made in respect to the stage of the procedure: the antegrade phase is always associated with coiling of the endoscope within the stomach and distortion of normal anatomy. Alternatively, the endoscope is more or less straightened during the retrograde stage of the procedure where the configuration of the duodenal bulb approaches to a normal pattern (Figure 5.25).

An accurate location of lesions in the duodenal bulb is important for patients with bleeding duodenal ulcers. Bleeding ulcers on the posterior wall of the distal portion of the duodenal bulb or the superior duodenal angle are associated with a high risk of recurrence due to intense blood supply to the area and close proximity of the pancreas.

Figure 5.23 Panoramic view of the duodenal bulb. It is useful for correct engagement of the endoscope beyond the superior duodenal angle.

stomach and approach the pylorus from as close as possible. The goal of the following maneuver is to align the tip of the endoscope with the center of the pylorus. It can be achieved by constant pressure on the pylorus and rotation of the R/L knob toward the visible portion of the pylorus until the endoscope begins moving toward the center of the pyloric ring. Sometimes, it is useful to pull the endoscope back slightly when it is almost embraced by the pylorus.

Passage of the pylorus is manifest by disappearance of resistance. The endoscopist must be careful to avoid blind trauma of the duodenal bulb due to rapid advancement of the endoscope.

The duodenal bulb should be examined carefully before exploration of the second portion of the duodenum. The endoscope has to be pulled back toward the pylorus slowly and deviated to the right to achieve a panoramic view of the duodenal bulb (Figure 5.23).

"Pull and twist technique"

Intubation of the second portion of the duodenum requires:

- Straightening of the endoscope and
- Clockwise rotation

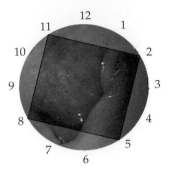

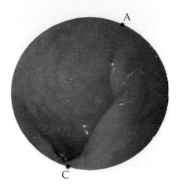

Figure 5.25 Mapping of the walls of the duodenal bulb after reduction of the gastric loop. Anterior wall is now located between 5 and 8 o'clock; Posterior wall is now located between 2 and 11 o'clock; Lesser curvature or medial wall is now located between 8 and 11 o'clock; Greater curvature or lateral wall is now located between 2 and 5 o'clock.

Figure 5.26 Appearance of the transitional zone between the duodenal bulb and the superior duodenal angle. AC line reflects the usual configuration of this transitional zone.

The goal of the first maneuver is restoration of the normal anatomy of the stomach, which is always disturbed by the coiled endoscope within the stomach on its way to the duodenum. The second element of the technique is clockwise rotation of the shaft.

It is necessary to achieve an axial alignment between the stomach and the duodenum and straightening of a twisted superior duodenal angle.

Upon entering the duodenal bulb, the lumen of the transitional zone between the distal duodenal bulb and the superior duodenal angle appears as a slot, which lies quite often in a plane of the "AC" line (Figure 5.26).

In this scenario, exploration of the second portion of the duodenum begins by advancing the endoscope forward and positioning the endoscope just below the AC line. The next step involves bending the tip of the endoscope up and to the right in the 5 o'clock direction.

This will anchor the endoscope to the superior duodenal angle. Finally, rotate the shaft clockwise roughly 90 degrees and pull it back simultaneously until the duodenal lumen is clearly visible.

If the duodenal folds are sharply demarcated, but the duodenal lumen is still obscure, rotate the endoscope counter-clockwise about a quarter turn and orient the tip in the 10–11 o'clock direction.

Intubation of the second portion of the duodenum can be challenging if the transitional zone

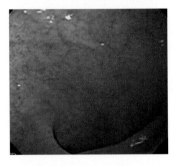

Figure 5.27 Horizontal configuration of the transitional zone between the duodenal bulb and the superior duodenal angle. Decompression of the stomach and reduction of the gastric loop should precede an exploration of the second portion of the duodenum. Counterclockwise rotation may facilitate intubation of the duodenum beyond the duodenal bulb.

between the distal duodenal bulb and superior duodenal angle is almost horizontal (Figure 5.27).

In this case, try a standard "pull and twist" technique first. If unsuccessful, pull the endoscope back to the upper portion of the gastric body, decompress the stomach and repeat duodenal intubation. The keys to success are minimal insufflation and avoidance of pushing the endoscope straightforward against increasing resistance. If the technique is not working, position the tip of the endoscope in the middle of the duodenal bulb and rotate the endoscope counter-clockwise. It might straighten the axis of the proximal duodenum and "unlock" the superior duodenal angle. While the duodenal lumen becomes wider, continue counter-clockwise rotation and pull the endoscope back simultaneously until the second portion of the duodenum is reached.

Intubation of the second portion of the duodenum in neonates and infants is quite simple with a thin 6 mm endoscope. The 8 and 9 mm pediatric endoscopes are more rigid and difficult to straighten during duodenoscopy in neonates or infants. An attempt to perform the "pull and twist" maneuver usually results in displacement of the endoscope back into the stomach. Instead, advance the endoscope gently toward the superior duodenal angle and move the tip to the right. If resistance is minimal, continue advancement. Rotate the endoscope counter-clockwise slightly (about 15 to 20 degrees) as soon as the "crescent" of the duodenal lumen appears on the screen, and adjust the position using the up/down knobs to achieve a panoramic view of the second portion of the duodenum. Advance the endoscope forward until the duodenal lumen begins moving away due to increased resistance and looping of the endoscope in the stomach.

The hallmark of the second portion of the duodenum is the papilla of Vater (Figure 5.28). During the antegrade stage of the procedure, the major papilla is usually found between 8 and 10 o'clock on the medial wall of the second portion of the duodenum. During withdrawal of the endoscope from the distal duodenum, the location of major papilla is shifted toward the 12 o'clock position.

It is not always easy to find the major papilla or to obtain the detailed images with the forward view endoscopes.

To overcome this limitation, the tip of the endoscope should be positioned almost above and perpendicular to the major papilla (Figure 5.29).

It is more practical to perform this maneuver during the retrograde phase of the duodenoscopy. After an examination of the distal duodenum is completed, pull the endoscope back and angle it up slowly in the 12 o'clock direction until the longitudinal fold is revealed (Figure 5.30). At this point, the major papilla can be reached either by withdrawal for an additional 3 to 4 cm and gentle counter-clockwise rotation, or by careful advancement and orientation of the endoscope upward and to the right using both control knobs with simultaneous counter clockwise torque.

More detailed images of the papilla of Vater can be obtained with a side view duodenoscope (Figure 5.31).

The hallmark of the third portion of the duodenum is the superior mesenteric artery responsible for a prominent pulsation of the right part of the duodenal wall.

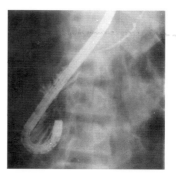

Figure 5.29 Retro-flexion of the scope in the duodenum. This technique allows a detailed examination of the major duodenal papilla.

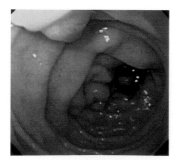

Figure 5.28 Major duodenal papilla. It is the hallmark of the second portion of the duodenum. It is seen more clearly during withdrawal phase at 11–12 o'clock location.

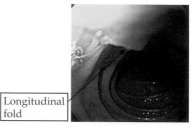

Longitudinal fold

Figure 5.30 The longitudinal fold. It is the best guide to the major duodenal papilla.

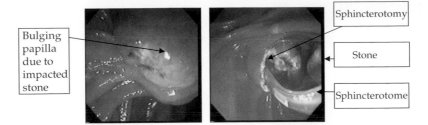

Bulging papilla due to impacted stone

Sphincterotomy

Stone

Sphincterotome

Figure 5.31 The major duodenal papilla. The side-view duodenoscope allows obtaining the detail image of the major duodenal papilla and performing endoscopic retrograde cholangiopan-creatography (ERCP) and sphincterotomy.

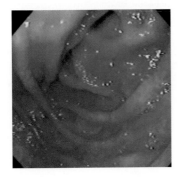

Figure 5.32 The endoscopic appearance of the duodenum at the level of the ligament of Treitz.

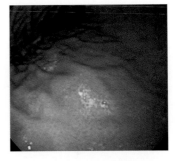

Figure 5.33 The view of the gastric body during initial phase of retroflexion maneuver.

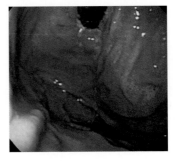

Figure 5.34 Appearance of the cardia after partial withdrawal of the shaft during retroflexion maneuver.

The lumen of the fourth portion of the duodenum is narrowed at the level of ligament of Treitz (Figure 5.32).

The small duodenal papilla is located 3 to 4 cm proximal to the major one. It can be found in the right upper corner of the lumen between the 1 and 2 o'clock position. It is a smooth, 4 to 5 mm structure, which resembles a sessile polyp.

The withdrawal phase of upper GI endoscopy is the best for detailed observation of the entire duodenum, stomach, and the esophagus.

Retrograde inspection of the proximal stomach or the so-called U-turn maneuver is the best technique for careful exploration of the gastric cardia and fundus. It is reasonable to perform it at the end of examination except for children with portal hypertension or acute bleeding from the stomach.

The U-turn technique consists of a few steps: first, position the tip of the endoscope in the middle of the gastric body and orient it toward the anterior wall in the 10 o'clock direction. Second, bend the tip of the endoscope further up and advance the shaft forward until the incisura angularis appears, separating the gastric body on the left, from the antrum on the right part of the screen (Figure 5.33). Third: pull the endoscope back and rotate it clockwise to achieve a close up view of the fundus (Figs. 5.34, 5.35).

For a detailed image of the cardia, target biopsy or precise hemostasis, find the grooves between the shallow folds of the lesser curvature during counter-clockwise rotation and pull the endoscope back slowly. Recognition of the "Z-line" indicates the end of withdrawal (Figure 5.36). This

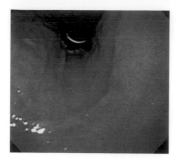

Figure 5.35 Detailed view of the cardia after additional withdrawal of the scope.

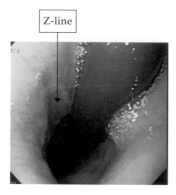

Figure 5.36 Appearance of the Z-line signals the end of withdrawal part of the retroflexion technique.

part of U-turn maneuver should be performed with caution to avoid an accidental impaction of the sharply bended tip of the endoscope in the distal esophagus.

To get away from the cardia safely push the endoscope forward, rotate it clockwise and return the control knobs in neutral position. Check and unlock the controlled knobs if they lock accidentally to avoid a blind trauma of the gastric mucosa. Decompress the stomach as much as possible before withdrawal. Careful examination of the esophagus should be carried out at the end of the procedure.

Biopsy technique

Histological and histochemical analysis is crucial for definitive diagnosis of many diseases involving the GI tract, for example, reflux or eosinophilic esophagitis, chronic gastritis, celiac disease and chronic inflammatory bowel disease. A correct interpretation of regular microscopy slides is problematic without adequate tissue samples and, virtually impossible, without proper mounting of the specimens in children with villous atrophy or dysplasia.

It is always feasible to obtain an adequate tissue samples, even with small pediatric size biopsy forceps, if an endoscopist is familiar with the appropriate technique. There are three rules of endoscopic biopsy:

1. It is not a blind procedure.
2. The more that biopsy forceps are advanced away from the tip of the endoscope the harder they are to control.
3. Forceful pushing of the forceps up against the wall is a dangerous and ineffective way to obtain an adequate tissue sample.

The technique of esophageal biopsy is more complicated than either gastric or duodenal mucosal sampling. It is related to a tangential position of the forceps along the esophageal wall and the relatively narrow space within the tubular esophagus.

The most common indication for esophageal biopsy in children is diagnosis of esophagitis. For correct interpretation, each biopsy should be labeled using the Z-line as the reference point. To avoid confusing results in children with suspected reflux related esophagitis, the biopsies should be taken at least 2 cm above the gastro-esophageal junction. Two good samples are usually sufficient.

The proper technique of the esophageal biopsy consists of few steps. First, the endoscope is positioned 1–2 cm above the target. Then, the bending segment of the endoscope is configured into an L-shape position by rotation of the control knobs upwards and to the right. The goal of this maneuver is orientation of the forceps, perpendicular to the mucosa. The biopsy forceps is advanced just enough to be fully open. Finally, suction is applied, forcing mucosa into the biopsy cap before it closes. The protocol of esophageal biopsy sampling for specific diseases will be discussed in the following section of the chapter.

The larger volume of the stomach and duodenum makes biopsy process less complicated, unless the target lesion is located in the gastric cardia or posterior wall of the proximal portion of the duodenal bulb, and the distal segment of the superior duodenal angle.

To obtain an adequate sample from the target lesion, the biopsy forceps should be positioned as much perpendicular to the surface of mucosa as possible. An application of excessive force to the forceps compromises safety, sample volume and quality of the biopsy, and should be avoided. In general, target biopsy for different areas within the stomach requires different approaches. Thus, biopsy of the lesions within the gastric cardia and subcardia areas are more accurate during U-turn maneuver. Biopsies from the antrum of the stomach are more efficient if taken when the endoscope is partially withdrawn into the distal portion of the gastric body with the tip deflected upwards.

The biopsy from the anterior wall of the duodenal bulb should be taken when the endoscope is position just beyond the pylorus. Biopsy from the distal portion of the duodenal bulb required slightly dipper insertion.

Biopsy from the second and the third portion of the duodenum provides better samples if taken from the edge of duodenal folds with minimal imbedding into the mucosa.

The number and the sites of the gastric and duodenal biopsies are determined by suspected GI pathology. For example, biopsies from four different sites are recommended to confirm *Helicobacter Pylori* infection: the prepyloric antrum, the lesser curvature of the antrum, the body, and the cardia.

Biopsies of gastric ulcers or erosions are usually taken from the edges, although specimens from the base are essential for diagnosis of some opportunistic viral infection. Special attention should be paid to the first biopsy: the lesion may become covered with blood and subsequent target biopsies could be difficult to obtain.

The best site for a duodenal biopsy is the edge of the valvulae conniventes. A perpendicular orientation of the forceps to the mucosal folds, eliminates the needs for deep and forceful imbedding of the biopsy cap into the tissue, prevents mucosal trauma and sampling artifacts and guarantees the best tissue samples.

Although it is debatable, at least 4 tissue samples from the second or the third portion of the duodenum are recommended for diagnosis of celiac sprue.

Recently, the water-immersion technique has been described. This technique consists of rapid instillation of 20 ml of water into the duodenal bulb and the second portion of the duodenum after air aspiration from the duodenum. Water magnifies the mucosal surface especially the villi. Based on the appearance, duodenal villi can be classified in three distinguished patterns: normal pattern, when villi are numerous, regular, finger-like structures; partial villous atrophy, when villi are shortened and diminished; and marked villous atrophy, when villi are rare, very short or undetectable.

Preliminary results showed that the water-immersion technique improves an accuracy of endoscopic assessment of the mucosal pattern and may reduce the need for multiple mucosal sampling for diagnosis of celiac sprue.

It was already mentioned, that proper orientation and mounting of tissue specimens is crucial for correct histological diagnosis of celiac sprue, inflammatory bowel disease, and dysplasia in patients with long-standing ulcerative colitis, Barrett's esophagus and polyps. The proper tissue mounting technique on a fine synthetic mesh adds not more than 5–7 minutes to the endoscopic procedure. The orientation of tissue samples is more precise with a magnifying glass lamp. Several steps are involved in proper mounting technique:

- Wearing of tight-fitting gloves free of talcum.
- Gentle transferring of a specimen from the open forceps to the index finger with or without the help of dissecting needle.
- Uncurling of a specimen with a light touch of the side of the dissecting needle until the cleavage surface is exposed.
- Recognition of the surface area: mucosal site of the specimen is more reddish and shiny.
- Complete uncurling of the specimen facing submucosal site up.
- Transferring the specimen from the index finger to the mesh, resting on the thumb of the same hand:
  - Touching the supporting mesh with the half of the specimen
  - Sweeping the visible part of the specimen to the mesh by placing a side of the dissecting needle between the biopsy specimen and the index finger
  - Moistening of the needle with water
  - Pushing of the remaining part of the specimen away from the index finger by the side of the needle
  - Placing the mesh with mounted specimen upside down into the fixative solution to prevent it from floating off the supporting mesh.

The labeled bottle with fixative solution should contain no more than 2–3 biopsy specimens from each site of GI tract.

Plastic mesh is a suitable supporting material for different fixative techniques except formalin-fixed biopsy specimens due to floating off effect. The choice of supporting material for formalin fixation is the prerogative of the particular pathology laboratory.

Complications

Complications related to sedation for pediatric endoscopy is discussed in Chapter 4.

Complications associated with handling of the endoscope during EGD can be divided into mild, requiring no therapeutic intervention and severe, mandating hospitalization. The true incidence of mild complications such as transient sore throat, bloating and abdominal discomfort is unknown.

Serious complications include perforation, bleeding and infections. The reported incidence of such complications is low across pediatric and adult literature. According to American Society for Gastrointestinal Endoscopy (ASGE) and British Society of Gastroenterology (BSG) guidelines, perforations associated with EGD in adults is 0.03% to 0.13%. Large cohort retrospective or prospective studies in pediatric patients who suffered from iatrogenic esophageal perforation during EGD are not available. However, a review of pediatric literature supports the overall consensus, that the incidence of perforation related to EGD in children is also low.

Moderate to severe bleeding during diagnostic EGD is extremely rare and usually occurs after biopsy in children with unrecognized coagulopathy.

Transient bacteremia is uncommon following diagnostic upper GI endoscopy and is rarely of clinical significance. According to revised guidelines of the American Heart Association and American Society for Gastrointestinal Endoscopy, antibiotic prophylaxis of infective endocarditis (ID) is not recommended for endoscopic procedures, except for patients with established GI-tract infections in which enterococci may be part of the infecting bacterial flora, and one of the following conditions: a prosthetic cardiac valve, history of previous ID, cardiac transplant recipients, unrepaired cyanotic congenital heart diseases (CHD), completely repaired CHD with prosthetic material and repaired CHD with residual defects at the site of a prostatic patch or device.

Indications for upper endoscopy and associated pathology

There are three general categories of indications for GI endoscopy:

1. Urgent (diagnostic and therapeutic).
2. Elective / diagnostic.
3. Elective/Therapeutic.

Specific indications for pediatric EGD are listed in Table 5.1.

Table 5.1 Indications for pediatric upper GI endoscopy

Urgent	Elective/diagnostic	Elective/therapeutic
GI bleeding	Recurrent upper abdominal pain	Portal hypertension (non-bleeding)
Caustic ingestion	Dysphagia/Odynophagia	Placement of gastrostomy tube
Foreign body ingestion	Vomiting	Polyps
	Weight loss	Esophageal stricture
	Anemia/occult blood loss	Achalasia
	Chronic diarrhea	
	Radiographic evidence of mucosal lesions	
	Evidence of mass lesion by upper GI series or CT scan	
	Polyposis syndromes	

Table 5.2 Age-related indications for upper GI endoscopy

Neonates and non-crawling infants	Crawling infants	School-age and teenagers
Hematemesis	Recurrent vomiting	Recurrent abdominal pain
Melena	Hemocult-positive stool	Failure to thrive
Obstructive apnea	Foreign bodies	Typical symptoms of GERD
Recurrent vomiting	Caustic ingestion	Dysphagia and food impaction
Chronic diarrhea	Chronic diarrhea Hematemesis Recurrent abdominal pain	Iron deficiency anemia Chronic diarrhea Hematemesis Caustic ingestion Foreign bodies

The spectrum of indications for EGD varies between the different age groups (Table 5.2).

The age-related difference in indications to EGD simply reflects the age related variations of GI pathology.

Indications for urgent endoscopy

Bleeding

Upper gastrointestinal bleeding in children is probably the most serious condition requiring urgent endoscopy.

The goal of upper GI endoscopy in children with melena or hematemesis is finding the source of bleeding and endoscopic hemostasis. Before endoscopy, however, several questions should be answered: Is the patient stable? Does the child have upper GI bleeding or epistaxis? What is the optimal time for endoscopy?

A good history, quick assessment of skin, tissue perfusion, pulse, blood pressure, presence of old or fresh blood at the nostrils or oropharynx and level of consciousness, provide enough information to answer the first two questions.

Good venous access must be established for adequate fluid resuscitation. Blood should be typed and screened. Transfusion of pocket red blood cells or donor's blood is usually reserved for children with moderate to severe acute bleeding. Repeated measurements of pulse and blood pressure are indirect but useful criteria of adequate fluid resuscitation.

The patient with recurrent hematemesis is at risk for aspiration, and protection of the airways is an important component of the therapy. This may be achieved by reverse Trendelenburg position, repeated aspiration of oropharyngeal contents, and/or endotracheal intubation of unconscious patients and children with tachypnea due to hypoxia and metabolic acidosis.

Gastric lavage is a routine procedure targeting initial/temporary hemostasis and assessment of bleeding activity. It is important to remember, that absence of blood in the stomach does not rule out an active bleeding from the duodenum or the proximal jejunum. Gastric lavage should be performed with room-temperature saline, through a large diameter oral-gastric tube, until the returned fluid is clear or contains significantly less blood. It usually takes about 10 minutes to assess the effectiveness of the gastric lavage. Most of the time, the bleeding will stop or decrease significantly. The diagnostic yield of EGD is best if performed as soon as the patient becomes stable or within 24 hours of the onset of bleeding.

If the gastric lavage is ineffective but the patient is stable after initial resuscitation, EGD is indicated to localize the source of bleeding and create at least a temporary hemostasis.

The upper GI endoscopy is also useful for developing a treatment plan based on the detected

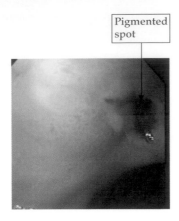

Figure 5.37 Pigmented spot. This is the sign of the recent bleeding with low probability of recurrent bleeding.

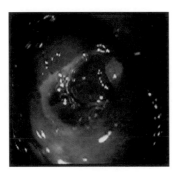

Figure 5.38 An adherent clot. The discovery of these stigmata of recent bleeding warrants the higher risk of recurrent bleeding and required endoscopic hemostasis and close observation.

source of variceal or non-variceal bleeding, for example, peptic, drug-, or stress-induced ulcers, versus hemorrhagic gastritis, versus portal hypertension.

Upper endoscopy provides important information regarding the risk of recurrent bleeding from ulcer and an indication for hospitalization. Presence of pigmented spots (Figure 5.37) and well-organized clot (Figure 5.38) is associated with a low probability of recurrent bleeding and justifies outpatient treatment. A visible vessel, spurting of blood from the ulcer, or a large, poorly organized blood clot with or without active bleeding are the warning signs of significant bleeding and a high risk of recurrence. In addition, the location of

the ulcer on the posterior wall of the duodenum is another negative prognostic factor.

The causes of bleeding vary in the different age groups (Table 5.3).

The most common endoscopic finding in neonates with upper GI bleeding is stress or sepsis related gastric or duodenal ulcers. The rare cause of hematemesis in neonates is hemorrhagic gastritis.

In infants and toddlers, the spectrum of diseases causing hematemesis or melena is broader: acute drug-induced gastritis or duodenitis; secondary gastric and duodenal ulcers due to stress, sepsis, or increased intracranial pressure; reflex esophagitis; prolapse gastropathy or Mallory-Weiss tear; esophageal varices, or opportunistic infections in immuno-compromised patients.

The frequency of aspirin-induced gastric and duodenal lesions in children is substantially less now than in the past. However, they still do occur because many over-the-counter "cold medications" contain salicylates. Additionally, non-steroidal anti-inflammatory (NSAIDs) drugs may also cause gastritis and ulcers in children.

Two types of aspirin- or NSAID-induced lesions can be found. Type 1: acute gastritis with multiple separate or confluent spots of erythema, petechiae and erosions with rims of erythema and Type 2: "punch-out" ulcers in the stomach and duodenum. The other type of drug-induced lesion is hemorrhagic gastritis. The hallmark of hemorrhagic gastritis is subepithelial hemorrhage, with or without mucosal edema. It may be either localized or widespread. In severe cases, a large area of gastric surface may be bleeding actively.

Although peptic ulcer disease is relatively uncommon in pediatric patients, it comprises at least one-half of the cases of bleeding from the upper gastrointestinal tract in school age children. The majority of bleeding ulcers are located within the duodenal bulb (Figure 5.39). In general, most episodes of bleeding (at least 80%) cease spontaneously, but, if the bleeding is arterial, the incidence of re-bleeding increases significantly and may potentially become life-threatening.

If blood spurting or a visible vessel has been found, the risk of recurrent bleeding is high, even after initially successful endoscopic hemostasis. These patients require careful observation and treatment with a high-dose of Proton Pump Inhibitors given as a continuous infusion for 48–72 hours. The specific therapy is indicated if *Helicobacter pylori* is found. The recurrence

Table 5.3 Common causes of GI bleeding in children

Age	Upper GI Bleeding	Low GI bleeding
Neonates (0 to 30 days)	Swallowed maternal blood Hemorrhagic disease of the newborn Stress ulcers/sepsis Hemorrhagic gastritis	Necrotizing enterocolitis Midgut vollulus Anal fissure Hirschsprung's disease Vascular malformation
Infants (30 days to 6 months)	Cow milk or soy protein allergy Esophagitis Mallory-Weiss tear Portal hypertension	Anal fissure Allergic proctitis or enterocolitis Nodular lymphoid hyperplasia Intussusception
Infants and children (6 months to 6 years)	Epistaxis Esophagitis Portal hypertension Drug induced ulcers Gastritis	Anal fissures Intussusception Meckel's diverticulum Intestinal lymphoid hyperplasia Polyps Infectious colitis Hemolytic uremic syndrome Henoch-Schonlein purpura
Children and teenagers (7 years to 18 years)	Drug-induced gastropathy and ulcers Peptic ulcer Esophagitis Gastritis Portal hypertension	Infectious colitis Ulcerative colitis Crohn's disease Polyps Polyposis Hemorrhoids

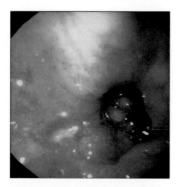

Figure 5.39 Active bleeding from the duodenal ulcer.

usually occurs during the first three days after the initial episode of bleeding. The second look endoscopy is not recommended for stable children. Clinical signs of re-bleeding warrant repeat EGD. Therapeutic endoscopy is not indicated for chil-dren with a non-bleeding ulcer with a pigmented spot or a flat, well-organized thrombus.

Indications for elective/diagnostic endoscopy

Chronic recurrent abdominal pain

Recurrent abdominal pain (RAP) is the most common indication for EGD simply because it occurs in 10–17% of children between 5–14 years. More than 90% of children with RAP have "functional" abdominal pain. If the clinical scenario is indicative for organic causes of pain, EGD with biopsy is the best tool for diagnosis of peptic ulcer, gastritis, celiac sprue or other underlying disorders.

Esophagitis associated with gastroesophageal reflux disease

Persistent symptoms, associated with primary and secondary esophagitis associated with gastro-esophageal reflux disease (GERD), are the most common indication for EGD in infants and, perhaps, toddlers. Endoscopic classification of reflux esophagitis in children consists of five types of findings or grades ranging from 0 to 4. Grade 0 is associated with the normal appearance of the esophageal mucosa (Figure 5.40). Grade 1 confines focal or circumferential lesions such as erythema, edema, exudate and loss of vascular pattern. Mild circumferential erythema of the distal esophageal mucosa right above the "Z" line is normal for neonates and should not be associated with grade 1 lesions. Endoscopic descriptions of esophageal mucosa in children with grade 0 and 1 lesions are quite subjective and require a morphological verification. Two mucosal biopsies are recommended at least 2 cm above the "Z" line. Grade 2 mucosal changes are associated with non-circumferential lineal erosions (Figure 5.41). More advanced circumferential lesions constitute Grade 3 esophagitis (Figure 5.42). Grade 4, or the most severe form of reflux esophagitis presents with ulcers (Figure 5.43) or stricture (Figure 5.44). Multiple circumferential step-wise biopsies are indicated for children with grade 2–4 lesions to rule out Barrett's esophagus (BE). This classification reflects the fact that EGD alone has low sensitivity and specificity for diagnosis of non-erosive forms of reflux esophagitis in children.

The main advantage of EGD is a combination of visual inspection of the esophagus, target biopsy and assessment of entire upper GI tract, which often leads to the discovery of synchronous lesions in the stomach and duodenum.

Strictures due to reflux esophagitis are usually short and located in the distal esophagus. Uncom-

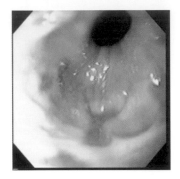

Figure 5.41 Grade 2 endoscopic findings consistent with esophagitis. The hallmark of grade 2 lesions is non-circumferential lineal erosions.

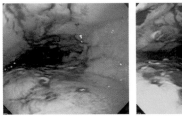

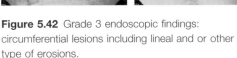

Figure 5.42 Grade 3 endoscopic findings: circumferential lesions including lineal and or other type of erosions.

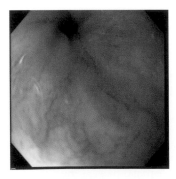

Figure 5.40 Normal endoscopic appearance of the esophageal mucosa. A biopsy is necessary to confirm a normal morphology.

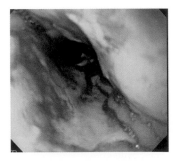

Figure 5.43 Esophageal ulcer as one of the element of endoscopic classification consistent with Grade 4 esophagitis.

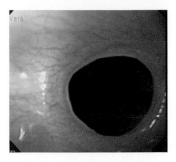

Figure 5.44 Esophageal stricture. Esophageal stricture due to reflux esophagitis usually appears as a short, white or silver colored, crescent-like or ring-type scar in the distal esophagus surrounding by pale or inflamed mucosa.

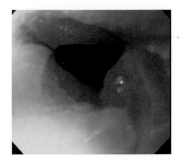

Figure 5.45 Stricture of the middle esophagus in the child with repaired tracheo-esophageal fistula and severe gastroesophageal reflux and failed fundoplication. The irregular shape of the stricture is secondary to esophagitis and healed ulcer.

plicated esophageal stricture appears as white, crescent-like scars surrounded by pale mucosa or inflamed edematous mucosa. Esophageal stricture becomes asymmetrical if complicated by a co-existing ulcer (Figure 5.45).

Classification, based on the diameter of the strictures in adults, includes three grades. Grade one (low-grade stricture from 11 to 13 mm wide) implicates a "narrow esophagus" and passage of a standard upper endoscope with resistance. Grade two (intermediate-grade stricture from 7 to 10 mm) is associated with passage of 6 mm endoscope only. Grade three (high-grade stricture less than 7 mm) makes it impossible to advance a 6 mm scope beyond the stricture. The classification can be adopted into pediatric practice with some correction to the size of pediatric upper endoscopes.

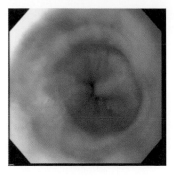

Figure 5.46 Schatzki's ring. Type B or mucosal rings are more common entity, which is associated with dysphagia. These short lesions within the 2 cm of the distal esophagus can be missed on endoscopy. Care should be taken to minimize insufflation and secondary over distension of the distal esophagus to avoid false negative results. The esophagram may be very useful in children with dysphagia and negative endoscopy.

Schatski's ring should be considered if a narrowing is short, located just above the Z-line and is surrounded by normal appearing esophageal mucosa (Figure 5.46). It could be missed during endoscopy. An esophagram with barium is indicated in children with dysphagia of solid food and negative upper GI endoscopy.

On rare occasions, a severe stenosis of the middle esophagus may be caused by tracheobronchial remnants. This type of stenosis is usually symmetrical but more elongated compared with stricture secondary to esophagitis. Translucent cartilages and absence of inflammation support the diagnosis.

Barrett's esophagus

Barrett's esophagus (BE) is a well-known complication of chronic gastroesophageal reflux disease associated with increased risk of malignancy. Although BE is rare in children more than ten cases of esophageal cancer related to BE in children have been described. There are two conflicting definitions of BE. The American College of Gastroenterology defines BE as

> "a change in the esophageal epithelium of any length that can be recognized at endoscopy and is confirmed to have intestinal metaplasia by biopsy of the tubular esophagus and excludes intestinal metaplasia of the cardia"

At the same time, The British Society of Gastroenterology defines BE as:

> "a segment of columnar metaplasia (whether intestinalized or not) of any length, visible endoscopically above the gastroesophageal junction and confirmed histologically."

This definition highlights that "intestinal metaplasia can always be identified providing a sufficient number of biopsies are taken over an adequate time-scale." This statement is supported by the fact that the appearance of goblet cells within the intestinal metaplasia is an age-related process, showing an exponential increase in incidence from 50% in pediatric BE to 84% in adult BE.

Three types of epithelium can be found in the tubular esophagus in patients with BE: gastric cardia type, gastric fundic type, and intestinal metaplastic type with goblet cells. Although all 3 types of mucosa may coexist in patients with chronic GERD, it has been demonstrated that only intestinal metaplastic mucosa may progress to dysplasia. Intestinal metaplasia is characterized by a change in the mucosa, to the extent that it morphologically, and histochemically, resembles the normal mucosa of either the small or large bowel.

Several conditions are associated with BE including neurological impairment, chronic lung disease (in particular, cystic fibrosis) and repaired esophageal atresia. It has recently been suggested that adult obesity and obesity at a young age increases risk of BE and esophageal adenocarcinoma.

During endoscopy, suspicious tongue-like lesions in the distal esophagus (Figs. 5.47 and 5.48)

are the target for multiple, multilevel biopsies from "Z"-line up. At least 2 samples should be taken from each level. Staining of sulfo- and sialo-mucins with Alcian blue at pH 2.5 is the standard technique for identification of the goblet cells. However, recent studies indicate that acidic mucins may occur normally in the glandular epithelium of the cardia and distal esophagus independent of the presence of intestinal metaplasia.

New data suggests that the homeobox gene Cdx2 could be a better marker of developing intestinal differentiation, even when histologic evidence of intestinal metaplasia is lacking. Some data indicates that Cdx2 expression increases in stepwise fashion from squamous to cardia and oxyntocardia mucosa to BE with intestinal metaplasia. Endoscopic surveillance at 3–4 year intervals have been proposed for children over 10 years of age with BE without dysplasia.

Endoscopic sign of hiatal hernia is cephalad displacement of the Z-line by 2 cm or more above the diaphragmatic notch. The diagnosis requires precise recognition of the diaphragmatic notch by respiratory movements: closure during inspiration and opening with expiration. These movements are often blunted in the deeply sedated child and difficult to recognize during the antegrade phase of the procedure. Observation of the cardia with retroflexion technique helps to locate the diaphragmatic notch and clarify the relationship with the "Z"-line.

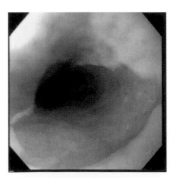

Figure 5.48 Barrett's esophagus. Circumferential lesions can imitate displacement of the "Z"-line and create a false impression of hiatal hernia. The random biopsies with 4 biopsy specimens taken at least every 1–2 cm of esophageal mucosa with additional biopsy specimens taken of any mucosal abnormality is recommended.

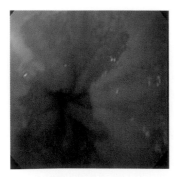

Figure 5.47 Barrett's esophagus: tongue-like lesions spreading from the "Z"-line upwards.

Esophagitis unrelated to GERD

by Alberto Ravelli

Eosinophilic esophagitis

Introduction

Eosinophilic esophagitis is a clinicopathological entity characterized by a prominent eosinophilic infiltrate of the esophageal mucosa, which results in symptoms very similar to that of gastroesophageal reflux disease (GERD), more notably vomiting and failure-to-thrive in infants, dysphagia and food impaction in older children and adults. According to a recent consensus produced by an expert panel of pediatric and adult gastroenterologists, the diagnosis of eosinophilic esophagitis can be established when an eosinophilic count of >15 eosinophils/HPF is found which is not responsive to a course of high-dose proton pump inhibitors and/or intraesophageal pH monitoring is normal.

Eosinophilic esophagitis is a relatively novel disease. The first formal description was published in 1995 in a group of infants who suffered from what appeared to be a severe GERD refractory to medical and surgical therapy, but who eventually responded to dietary treatment with an elemental formula. Numerous subsequent publications confirmed these features, but also showed that eosinophilic esophagitis can present at any age, and the presence of previous or concurrent manifestations of allergy in the patient and a positive family history of atropy are common.

The disease affects males much more commonly than females, and seems to be present almost worldwide, since reports have come from all continents except Africa. The prevalence seems to be increasing – 2 to 27 per 100 000 individuals in Switzerland – and the incidence in the pediatric population was 1:10 000 children per year in the Midwest USA.

Etiology and pathogenesis of eosinophilic esophagitis are still unclear. Translational and basic science research suggests that this disease is sparked by food or aeroallergens. Several reports showed a familial clustering of the disease, and a genetic predisposition is suggested by one recent study which showed that the gene encoding for the eosinophil-specific chemoattractant eotaxin-3 was the most highly induced gene in patients with eosinophilic esophagitis compared to healthy controls and individuals with GERD.

Treatment is based, either on dietary measures such as an elemental formula in small infants and an exclusion diet in children, or pharmacological intervention such as topical or (less commonly) systemic steroids. Each therapy can achieve a good clinical and histological response but symptoms – and the related eosinophilic infiltrate of the esophageal mucosa – tend to recur following treatment withdrawal, so long-term treatment is a major problem.

Endoscopy

Upper GI endoscopy with biopsy is a must in the work-up of suspected eosinophilic esophagitis, as the demonstration of the prominent eosinophilic infiltrate is essential for the diagnosis. Endoscopy is especially indicated in the presence of signs and symptoms reported in Table 5.4.

Eosinophilic esophagitis can be characterized by a number of macroscopic abnormalities of the esophagus, including longitudinal furrowing and/or shearing of the mucosa (Figure 5.49), "crêpe paper" appearance of the mucosa, raised white specks and/or whitish exudates on the mucosal surface, or transient or fixed rings (so-called "trachealization" of the esophagus, Figure 5.50), Schatzki's ring, stricture, felinization, friability and edema of the mucosa.

With the possible exception of longitudinal furrowing/shearing and the "crêpe paper" mucosa, none of the reported features is pathognomonic of eosinophilic esophagitis since they have been reported in other esophageal diseases. On the one hand, findings such as longitudinal furrowing and shearing, trachealization and raised white specks or exudates have been consistently and universally reported in eosinophilic esophagitis. Therefore, a very high index of suspicion for eosinophilic esophagitis should be maintained in any patient with GERD-like symptoms in whom such abnormalities are seen at endoscopy, and in the appropriate clinical context the presence of more than one of these findings, is strongly suggestive of eosinophilic esophagitis. On the other hand, some studies have reported a normal appearing esophageal mucosa in patients with histological evidence of eosinophilic esophagitis. It is likely that the ability to detect subtle but typical abnormalities such as furrowing and "crêpe paper" appearance of the esophageal mucosa is related to such variables as the refinement of endoscopic equipment and the experience and knowledge of the operator. In any case, careful inflation of the esophagus usually helps emphasize the less prominent features.

Table 5.4 Clinical manifestations suggestive of eosinophilic esophagitis in pediatric patients

Infants*	Small children*	Older children and adolescents*
Vomiting, regurgitation	Regurgitation	Recurrent food impaction
Food aversion/refusal	Upper abdominal pain	Dysphagia
Failure to thrive	Heartburn	Refractory GERD**
Refractory GERD**	Dysphagia	GERD symptoms with normal pH study
GERD symptoms with normal pH study	Refractory GER**	
	GERD symptoms with normal pH study	

*The suspicion is stronger if the patient is male and has a personal and/or family history of atropy.
**Empiric diagnosis (i.e., no endoscopy or pH study done).

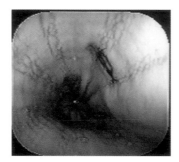

Figure 5.49 The lineal furrows sign. This endoscopic finding is suspicious for eosinophilic esophagitis. The definitive diagnosis is made on the basis of 15 or more eosinophils per squire field on light microscopy.

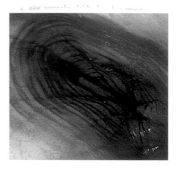

Figure 5.50 Circular folds in the tubular esophagus are a common finding in children with eosinophilic esophagitis.

Biopsy

Regarding biopsy procurement, a number of issues should be remembered about eosinophilic esophagitis. First, the typical histological abnormalities can also be found in endoscopically normal esophageal mucosa (up to 30% in a study on nearly 400 children), although, once again, as endoscopists become increasingly aware of subtle abnormalities, the number of endoscopically normal cases will probably be reduced. Second, mucosal specimens should be fixed in preservatives other than Bouin's (e.g. formalin) as this may result in reduced identification of eosinophils. Third, multiple biopsies should be taken from both the distal and proximal esophagus, and espe-

cially from areas of macroscopic abnormalities, since the sensitivity of biopsies is directly related to their number. Finally, it is also always advisable to take biopsies from the stomach and duodenum irrespective of their endoscopic appearance, in order to rule out – in the appropriate clinical context – eosinophilic gastroenteritis or other causes of GI eosinophilia such as drugs, parasites and Crohn's disease.

Histology

As mentioned above, a number of >15 eosinophils per high power field (40×) in at least one biopsy is required to confirm the diagnosis of eosinophilic esophagitis. More often, the number of eosinophils exceeds 20/HPF, and up to a few hundred eosinophils/HPF have been reported. Eosinophils are more often spread within the esophageal epithelium, but sometimes they are clustered on the epithelial surface, resulting in eosinophilic abscesses, and this is more often found where raised white specks or whitish exudates are seen at endoscopy.

Infectious esophagitis

Infectious esophagitis is a frequent cause of dysphagia and odynophagia in immunocompromised children. The most common types of infectious esophagitis are candida, cytomegalovirus (CMV) or herpes simplex virus (HSV). Endoscopy with brush cytology, biopsy and tissue culture is the most reliable diagnostic methods.

Candida esophagitis may present with erythematous mucosa covered by scattered or confluent white, cream-colored, thick plaques with greatest density in the distal esophagus (Figure 5.51).

Shallow, well-circumscribed ulcerations surrounded by normal mucosa are the hallmark of CMV esophagitis. Deep ulcers can be found in the middle or distal esophagus. Histological signs of CMV are basophilic, intracellular inclusions, a clear halo surrounding the nucleus and the presence of multiple smaller periodic acid-Schiff positive intracytoplasmic inclusions.

Herpes simplex virus is the most common cause of herpetic esophagitis. The disease may be started with herpetic lesion(s) on the lips or buccal mucosa followed by odynophagia or dysphagia.

The endosopic hallmark of herpetic esophagitis is aphthoid-like ulcers with a raised erythematous margin and gray or yellowish base. These ulcers are typically seen in the middle or upper esophagus. In advanced disease, large, confluent ulcers with yellowish exudate at the base may occur (Figure 5.52).

To obtain adequate tissue samples with the replicating HSV, the biopsy should be taken from the edge of the ulcerations as the HSV viral cytopathic effect is reliably found in the squamous cells. Histological analysis reveals typical Cowdry type-A intranuclear inclusion bodies, multinucleate giant cells, ballooning of the cells, and chromatin margination.

Caustic ingestion

Despite precautions, corrosive injuries still occur, usually as tragic accidents. These incidents take place mostly in young children under 5-years old or during suicide attempts by teenagers. Lye ingestion induces severe injuries primarily in the esophagus; although strong acid may create more diffuse lesions, including the stomach or duodenum. Sodium hydroxide in different preparations induces rapid liquefaction necrosis with deep [even full thickness] injuries. Respiratory distress, esophageal perforation or periesophageal inflammation with subsequent mediastinitis and peritonitis are the most serious short-term complications of caustic ingestion.

Immediate and long-term outcomes are directly related to the degree of the burn. The absence of visible lesions on the lips, oral or pharyngeal mucosa does not correlate with the absence of

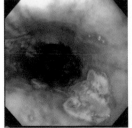
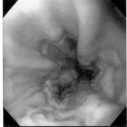

Figure 5.52 Herpetic esophagitis. The triad such as erythema, aphthoid-like ulcers and exudates are suggestive of viral esophagitis. The presence of the multinucleated giant cells with prominent eosinophilic intranuclear inclusions and chromatine margination are diagnostic.

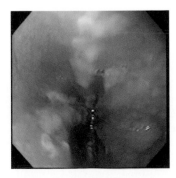

Figure 5.51 Candida esophagitis: characteristic white, thick plaques in the distal esophagus.

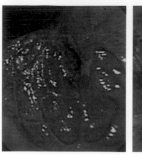
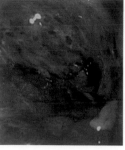

The lumen is very narrowed due to severe spasm

Figure 5.53 Severe fibrosis and narrowing of the antrum in teenager 2 months after ingestion of a strong acid solution.

Figure 5.54 Severe spasm of the duodenal bulb induced by an active ulcer.

esophageal or gastric injuries. As soon as the patient is stabilized, an EGD should be performed under general anesthesia. Superficial mucosal chemical injury manifests with erythema, edema with minimal mucosal peeling.

For a more severe injury, the sloughing of mucosa will be more extensive and associated with hemorrhagic exudates, islands of mucosal debris, or ulcerations. The hallmark of severe esophageal burns is the presence of an eschar or deep ulcers. It is common to find that the lumen of the esophagus in severe cases is completely obliterated due to severe spasms and marked transmural edema of the esophageal wall. In general, endoscopy is not indicated or should be aborted in suspected severe caustic esophagitis.

Children with an acid-based caustic ingestion are prone to more severe injuries of the stomach or duodenum and increased risk of perforation and fibrosing gastropathy (Figs. 5.53a and b).

Patients with no visible mucosal injuries or grade 1 lesions can be discharged home. Patients with grade 2 or higher lesions caused by caustic ingestions must be hospitalized for at least 24–48 hours.

Withholding oral feeding, parenteral nutritional support, broad-spectrum antibiotics and steroids are the conventional therapies for patients with the moderate to severe burns. Naso-gastric tube placement is indicated for preservation of esophageal lumen in case of stricture development and necessity of esophageal dilatation.

Peptic ulcers

Peptic ulcer disease occurs predominantly in middle and high school-age children (especially boys). In the vast majority of children, peptic ulcers are located in the duodenal bulb. An active peptic ulcer induces significant spasms and rigidity of the duodenal bulb (Figure 5.54). It could be aggravated by scarring from previous relapses or by manipulations with the endoscope per se. Under these circumstances, maximal attention should to be paid to indirect endoscopic signs such as convergence of mucosal folds, severe erythema or edema of the duodenal mucosa. Glucagon may be used to reduce a spasm of the duodenum. It is not unusual to find multiple or "kissing" duodenal ulcers in children with peptic disease. That is why a thorough examination of the opposite wall has to be carried out if an ulcer or a scar has been detected.

Gastritis

During endoscopic examination of the stomach, several mucosal patterns may be found: pink and smooth gastric mucosa with visible vessels more prominent in proximal areas; gastric mucosa with focal or diffuse erythema, edema, petechiae, and erosions; nodular appearing mucosa and ulcers. The diagnostic value of these findings is determined by the clinical scenario and histological analysis of the tissue samples. For example, if the clinical history is positive for salicylates or NSAIDs ingestion, the presence of erosions in the stomach is diagnostically important. However, gastric erosions have also been found in asymptomatic volunteers. As another example, endoscopic characteristics of the gastric mucosa, such as erythema, edema, or petechiae do not necessarily indicate inflammation. Tissue sampling would be required for a confirmed diagnosis of acute or chronic gastritis. This is especially important for detection of *helicobacter pylori* (HP), as it may substantially change the approach to the therapy.

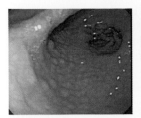
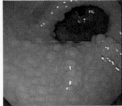

Figure 5.55 *Helicobacter Pylori* Gastritis. The most common endoscopic sign of HP gastritis is antral or diffuse nodularity.

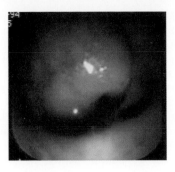

Figure 5.57 CMV gastritis. The intense inflammation in the prepyloric antrum may simulate a submucosal mass effect.

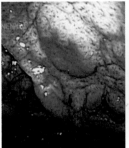
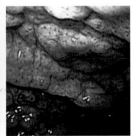

Figure 5.56 Multiple irregular nodules in a 14-year-old boy with recurrent abdominal pain and anemia. Biopsy revealed presence of a thickened subepithelial collagen layer.

Although numerous uniformed nodules in the gastric antrum are present in about 50% of HP-colonized children, this endoscopic sign (Figure 5.55) is no substitute for histological identification of S-shaped bacteria on the surface of gastric mucosa [stained by Warthin Starry or Giemsa technique].

Diffuse nodularity of the gastric body, especially along the greater curvature with extension of the lesions toward the antrum in children with RAP and anemia, could be a sign of collagenous gastritis. The mucosal pattern of this rare disease consists of multiple irregular grooves and numerous, flat nodules different in size (Figs. 5.56a, 5.56b). The presence of a thickened subepithelial collagen layer, which is more than 10 μm and inflammatory cell infiltrate in the lamina propria is diagnostic.

Multiple biopsies are necessary to avoid false-negative results due to patchy distribution of collagen deposition.

A finding of gastric erosions or ulcers in immunocompromised children is always suspicious for opportunistic infection. CMV induced inflammation is usually patchy and deep. It may appear as an irregular, edematous, nodular area most often in the distal body or antrum. Multiple shallow ulcers can be found. If inflammation occupies the antrum or prepyloric area of the stomach, it may cause gastric outlet obstruction and can occasionally mimic a submucosal mass (Figure 5.57). The presence of cytomegalic cells in tissue biopsies stained by H&E is considered the gold standard for establishing a diagnosis of CMV GI disease. When the diagnosis is uncertain, additional immunohistochemical methods may be useful in confirming the presence of CMV. However, the number of tissue samples appears to be especially important. When histology involved multiple sections of 8–10 biopsies, the frequency of diagnosing CMV by histology could be greater than by culture.

Herpetic gastritis may be found in children with HIV infection or post bone marrow or liver transplantation. EGD shows small shallow ulcers with whitish or yellowish exudates at the base. Ulcers may coalesce and be surrounded by erythematous mucosa. Biopsies from the base of the ulcer and surrounding mucosa are necessary to confirm herpetic infection.

Hypertrophic gastropathy or Menetrier's disease

Mentrier's disease is a rare cause of protein-losing enteropathy in children, but over the last decade the number of published cases has doubled. The exact etiology of the disease is unknown. CMV infection has been documented in one third of pediatric cases.

In children with Menetrier's disease, EGD shows an enormous amount of gelatinous mucus in the stomach, giant gastric rugae in the fundus or gastric body that remain unchanged despite vigorous insufflation, and edematous mucosa often with shallow ulceration. Histological signs of Menetrier's disease are: mucus filled dilated gastric glands; basilar cystic changes, and mixed infiltration of lamina propria with neutrophils, lymphocytes, eosinophils and plasma cells occasionally. A unique feature of Menetrier's disease in children is complete resolution of the symptoms and pathological changes of the gastric mucosa with adequate therapy in the majority of patients.

Crohn's disease

Current data suggests that involvement of the upper GI tract in pediatric patients with Crohn's disease occurs more often than previously thought. The rate of positive findings of noncaseating granuloma in the stomach or duodenum in unselected patients with Crohn's disease is higher than in selected patients with presumptive symptoms of upper GI tract involvement: dysphagia, aphthoid lesions in the mouth, epigastric pain, weight loss, nausea, and vomiting or blood loss. In addition, 11.4–29% of patients with onset of Crohn's disease may have isolated inflammation of the stomach and duodenum. Thus, routine use of EGD in patients with suspected Crohn's disease is indicated.

Endoscopic findings of skipped lesions such as aphthous ulcers, nodularity, thickening of mucosal folds, rigidity or narrowing of the antral portion of the stomach or proximal duodenum are suggestive for Crohn's disease. Serpiginous or longitudinal ulcers are rarely seen in children but, if found, may be helpful to distinguish it from peptic disease.

The goal of a histological evaluation of the stomach and the duodenum in children with suspected Crohn's disease is confirmation of chronic inflammation and a finding of noncaseating granulomas, which occur in 30–40% of cases. There is no significant difference in the detection of granulomas in biopsies taken from endoscopically normal or abnormal areas of gastric or duodenal mucosa. Because of this multiple samples of endoscopically normal or altered mucosa have to be obtained to increase the diagnostic value of the procedure.

However, the absence of noncaseating granulomas does not rule out Crohn's disease. The presence of focal inflammation with "crypt abscesses", focal lymphoid aggregates and fibrosis may support the diagnosis of Crohn's disease in children with suggestive history. Discovery of inflammation in the upper GI tract of children with confirmed Crohn's disease in the small or large intestine may justify adjustment of or changes in existing therapy.

Hypertrophic pyloric stenosis (HPS)

In typical cases, HPS can be easily diagnosed by clinical symptoms, physical examination, and the presence of metabolic alkalosis. Palpation of a pyloric mass is conclusive and does not require further investigation.

If a pyloric mass is not detected or palpation is equivocal, an ultrasonic scan (US) is the procedure of choice. Despite the high accuracy of US, false negative results have been described (especially during early stages of the disease). In this situation, an upper gastrointestinal endoscopy may be a good alternative to an upper gastrointestinal series. The advantages of EGD consist of direct assessment of the pylorus and coexistent conditions such as esophagitis, hiatal hernia, or gastritis that may interfere with the postoperative recovery. The obvious disadvantages are invasiveness and a high cost compared with sonography or upper GI series. However, the very low rate of serious complications, elimination of radiation exposure, as well as an earlier diagnosis and shorter hospitalization, may compensate for any initial expenses and risk of the procedure.

The most reliable endoscopic sign of HPS is a bulging of the tight pylorus into the pre-pyloric antrum with the mucosal folds converted toward the depressed center of the pyloric channel (Figure 5.58). In the early stage of the disease, when a muscle hypertrophy is not as "stiff" and allows some relaxation, a diameter of pyloric ring less than 5 mm, an elongation and irregularity of the pyloric channel are diagnostically significant.

Inability to advance the endoscope beyond the pylorus should be interpreted in favor of HPS only in conjunction with the other endoscopic signs of pyloric stenosis. Concomitant findings of esophagitis or gastritis may help to predict and prevent such complications as recurrent vomiting or bleeding in the early postoperative period.

Gastric tumors and bezoar

Gastric tumors in children are rare and usually benign. Ectopic pancreases and hyperplastic polyps are the most common gastric tumors in children. Ectopic pancreas is often asymptomatic and, in most children, is an incidental finding during EGD or upper GI series. True prevalence of ectopic pancreas in children is unknown. In the stomach, ectopic pancreas is located on the greater curvature of the antrum and appears as a small, less than 1 cm, dome-shaped lesion with the central depression (Figure 5.59). It is usually covered by normal gastric mucosa. Sometimes, the lesions may be less protruded toward the gastric lumen and may appear as "bagel" or "doughnut" structure. A biopsy is not indicated as an ectopic tissue arises from the submucosal or subserosal layers.

A small hyperplastic gastric polyp is usually asymptomatic unless it is located near the pylorus, causing gastric outlet obstruction or anemia due to recurrent prolapse into the duodenal bulb. More often, a hyperplastic polyp in children is single, sessile, less than 1 cm in length and located in the antrum or the proximal aspect of the enlarged fold of the cardia (Figure 5.60). It is not considered as pre-malignant. Endoscopic polypectomy is indicated only if the patient is symptomatic or the polyp is bigger than 1 cm and ulcerated. Endoscopic surveillance after polypectomy is unnecessary if the diagnosis of hyperplastic polyp is confirmed histologically.

The presence of multiple gastric polyps is the sign of polyposis syndrome. In children with Gardner's syndrome, small sessile polyps are usually located in the gastric fundus. In generalized juvenile polyposis or Peutz-Jeghers syndrome, gastric polyps may be dispersed throughout the stomach (Figure 5.61). The polyps could be removed in one or several endoscopic sessions. Sometimes, the number of polyps precludes a complete eradication. In these cases, the largest polyps should be removed. In children with Peutz-Jeghers syndrome, gastric polyps coexist with multiple hamartomas in the duodenum or proximal jejunum (Figure 5.62). Some of these polyps could be quite large, reaching 4 or 5 cm. Such polyps are the common cause of chronic small bowel intussusceptions and the leading cause of

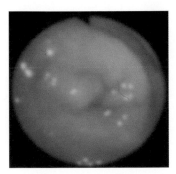

Figure 5.58 Hypertrophic pyloric stenosis. Bulging pylorus is reliable endoscopic sign of infantile hypertrophic pyloric stenosis.

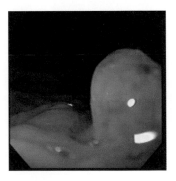

Figure 5.60 Inflammatory polyp of the enlarged fold of the cardia.

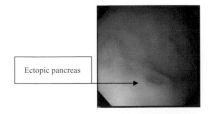

Ectopic pancreas

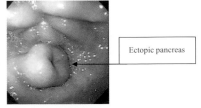

Ectopic pancreas

Figure 5.59 Ectopic pancreas in the stomach. The "doughnut" shaped small lesion is located on the greater curvature of the antrum. It is usually an incidental finding during EGD.

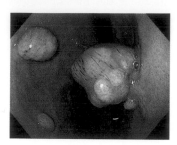

Figure 5.61 Multiple hamartomas of the stomach in a patient with Peutz-Jeghers syndrome. Biannual surveillance endoscopy with polypectomy of polyps 10mm or bigger is indicated.

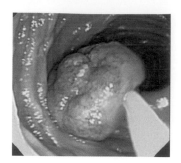

Figure 5.62 Hamartoma in the duodenum. These lesions are usually multiple and required repeat polypectomies. The risk of complication is proportional to the size of the polyp. Surgery should be considered in a patient with polyps of 4cm or bigger to avoid severe bleeding or perforation.

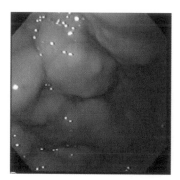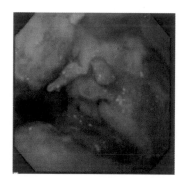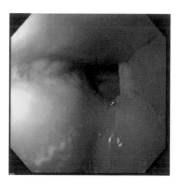

Figure 5.63 Non-Hodgkin's lymphoma. Induration of the gastric wall and multiple deep ulcerations are always suspicious for malignancy. Left image: malignant infiltration of the gastric folds; Middle image: ulcerated malignant mass; Right image: malignant infiltration of the pylorus.

intermittent abdominal pain. Polypectomy of these hamartomas is a technically challenging procedure, and carries a high risk of severe arterial bleeding and perforation.

Malignant tumors of the stomach account for only 5% or less of all malignant neoplasm in children. The most common malignant gastric tumors in children are non-Hodgkin or Burkitt's lymphoma or gastric involvement in lymphoproliferative disorder after solid organs or bone marrow transplantation (Figs. 5.63–5.65).

Gastric bezoar must be included in differential diagnosis because it may simulate clinical symptoms of malignancy, especially if a palpable mass or anemia is present. These symptoms are related to large trichobezoar, which may virtually occupy the entire stomach and proximal duodenum

(Rapunzel syndrome), causing irritation of the gastric mucosa, secondary gastric ulcers, and anemia. Surgical removed or extracorporeal shock way lithotripsy is indicated.

Effectiveness of Coca-Cola lavage for children with gastric Phytobezoar has been proven.

Celiac sprue

Partial and total villous atrophy may be the endpoint of different pathological processes, including celiac sprue, giardiasis, cow's milk allergy, post-infectious inflammation, and immunodeficiency. Clinical manifestations of these diseases are non-specific.

For more than three decades jejunal capsule biopsy was the cornerstone for diagnosis of celiac

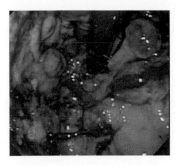 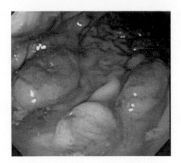 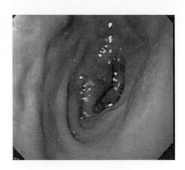

Figure 5.64 Burkitt's lymphoma of the stomach and the small intestine. Loose teeth were the presenting symptom. EGD was performed to evaluate progressive weight loss, abdominal pain and anemia. Multiple erythematous nodules with or without ulcerations and infiltration of the gastric wall were found. The diagnosis was confirmed morphologically of the gastric and bone marrow biopsies. Left picture: multiple ulcerated masses in the proximal stomach; Middle picture: ulcerated masses along the greater curvature of the stomach; Right picture: focal malignant infiltration of the duodenum.

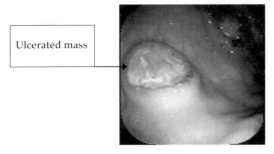 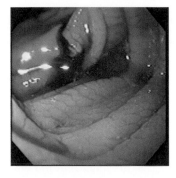

Figure 5.65 Multiple ulcerated gastric mass in patient with lymphoproliferative disorder following liver transplantation.

Figure 5.66 Mosaic pattern of the duodenal mucosa in the child with untreated celiac sprue.

sprue. But it is time-consuming, requires fluoroscopy, and is associated with failure of adequate tissue sampling. It has been replaced by endoscopic biopsies in adults and children. Endoscopic assessment of the duodenal mucosa in conjunction with chromoendoscopy and water-immerging technique targets the biopsy minimizing the false negative results in patients with patchy distribution of villous atrophy. In addition, accidental discovery of mucosal changes suggestive of celiac sprue during EGD in children is not uncommon. The main endoscopic sign of celiac sprue in children is a mosaic pattern of the duodenal and jejunal mucosa and "scalloping" of the valvulae conniventes (Figs. 5.66, 5.67).

In the active phase of celiac disease, the duodenal mucosa appears grayish, edematous and a

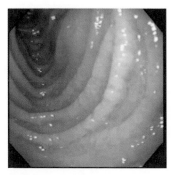

Figure 5.67 Scalloping of the duodenal and/or jejunal folds. This endoscopic sign is more prominent in the distal duodenum or jejunum. An application of the vital stains such as methylene blue augments this mucosal pattern.

mosaic with an increased vascular pattern in the proximal duodenum. Duodenal folds are coarse and have scalloped appearance. Mucosa between the duodenal folds has a mosaic or honeycomb pattern. These endoscopic signs are usually more prominent in the distal duodenum or proximal jejunum. Although duodenal or jejunal mucosa are not friable, biopsy is associated with slightly more intensive bleeding.

The final diagnosis of celiac sprue is histological. At least four biopsies from the distal portion of duodenum are required. All specimens have to be properly oriented for correct assessment of the villous and cryptal pattern.

Complete regeneration of atrophic mucosa is expected within 6 months in children on a strict gluten-free diet. In noncompliant children, especially adolescents, mucosal atrophy may be clinically silent.

Intestinal lymphangiectasia

by Alberto Ravelli

Intestinal lymphangiectasia is a diffuse or segmental dilatation of the enteric lymphatic vessels which may cause protein-losing enteropathy. It can be either primary (idiopathic) or secondary. Primary intestinal lymphangiectasia (also known as Waldmann's disease) is a rare condition characterized by dilated intestinal lymphatic vessels causing leakage of lymph into the bowel lumen and protein-losing enteropathy, which, in turn, results in hypoalbuminemia, hypogammaglobulinemia and lymphopenia. The etiology is also unknown. Primary intestinal lymphangiectasia is usually diagnosed in infants and small chil-

dren but, occasionally, it can be detected for the first time in older children and even adults. Very rare familial forms have also been described and several syndromes have been linked with intestinal lymphangectasia including Von Recklinghausen's, Turner's, Noonan's, Klippel-Trenaunay-Weber's, Hennekam's and the yellow nail syndrome.

Secondary intestinal lymphangiectasia is more often seen in adults and is related to an elevated lymphatic pressure as may occur in lymphoma, constrictive pericarditis, cardiac surgery, inflammatory bowel disease, systemic lupus erythematosus, and malignancies.

Endoscopy with biopsy is the cornerstone of the diagnosis in primary intestinal lymphangiectasia. The endoscopic features of lymphangiectasia consist of numerous white-yellowish spots incorporated into the edematous small bowel mucosa and enlarged folds (Figs. 5.68a and b). However, this finding is not entirely specific of primary lymphangiectasia, as scattered white spots along the duodenal mucosa (Figure 5.69) have also been reported in other small bowel disorders, such as infestation by the parasite *Giardia Lamblia* and chronic non-specific duodenitis. Therefore, duodenal biopsies should always be taken when such abnormalities are seen.

In the majority of cases, upper GI endoscopy with biopsy is sufficient to make the diagnosis. However, intestinal lesions may be segmental and sometimes located distal to the duodenum and the duodeno-jejunal flexure. In primary lym-

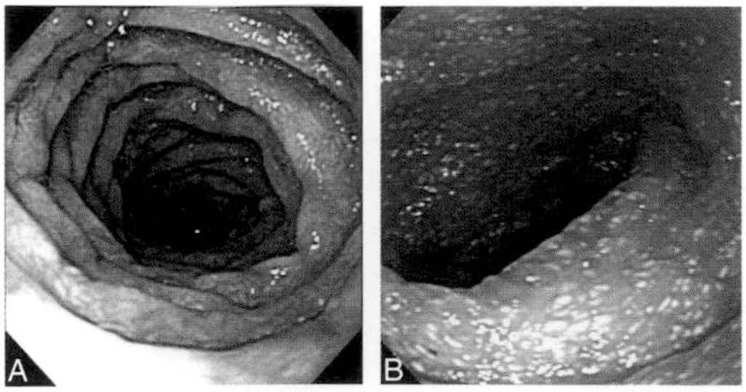

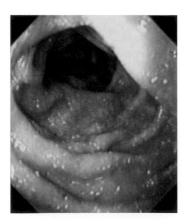

Figure 5.68 (A) Severe edema and multiple dilated lacteals in the proximal jejunum in infant with LAE (B) Multiple dilated lacteals in the small bowel suggestive but not diagnostic of LAE.

Figure 5.69 Scattered whitish spots in the second and the third portion of the duodenum is not specific for LAE. Clinical correlation and histological verification is a key for correct interpretation.

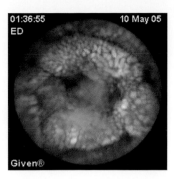

Figure 5.70 In primary intestinal lymphangiectasia, whitish and edematous villi in the jejunum are clearly shown by capsule endoscopy.

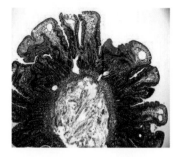

Figure 5.72 A duodenal biopsy from a child with primary intestinal lymphangiectasia shows mild to moderate dilatation of mucosal and submucosal lymphatic vessels – some of which look like small intra-villus cysts (H&E, 10x).

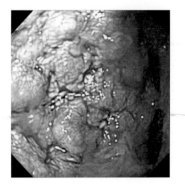

Figure 5.71 Dilated lacteals and edema of the terminal ileum in a child with LAE.

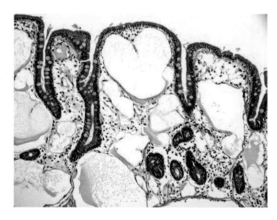

Figure 5.73 A duodenal biopsy from another child with intestinal lymphangiectasia shows severely dilated lymphatic vessels with abundant lymphatic fluid within and below the villi, which cause shortening and broadening of villi, thus giving the impression of partial villus atrophy (H&E, 20 x).

phangiectasia the magnitude and density of endoscopic findings also varies, and can be maximal in the jejunum, where villi often appear creamy or yellow (Figure 5.70). Furthermore, it may be relevant for prognostic and therapeutic purposes to define the extension of the disease within the gut. Therefore, if upper endoscopy and biopsies are negative or inconclusive but the clinical suspicion is strong, video capsule endoscopy or enteroscopy should be used to establish the diagnosis of lymphangiectasia and to define its location and extension. Wireless capsule endoscopy – which is easier to use, less invasive and more widely available than enteroscopy – can be effectively used to assess the extent of lymphangiectasia in children. In one of our patients who was 19 months old and weighed 19 kg, the procedure was carried out successfully after placing the capsule in the duodenum with an endoscope (personal observation).

The retrograde ileoscopy can also reveal the involvement of the terminal ileum (Figure 5.71).

The histological examination of biopsies taken from the small bowel shows moderately to severely dilated mucosal and submucosal lymphatic vessels – often with a cystic appearance – and the presence of lymphatic fluid as major features (Figure 5.72). The lymphatic vessels located along the villus axis may also be grossly dilated, and although primary intestinal lymphangiectasia does not usually cause mucosal atrophy, these changes may cause shortening and broadening of villi, thereby, giving the impression of a partial villous atrophy (Figure 5.73).

Push enteroscopy

> **KEY POINTS**
>
> • Endoscopy of the proximal jejunum is feasible with standard endoscopic equipment.
> • The average depth of intubation is 50 cm beyond the ligament of Treitz.
> • Jejunoscopy does not required special sedation and add only few minutes to the procedural time of routine EGD.
> • It is effective endoscopic procedure for a well-defined cohort of children.

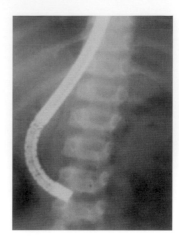

Figure 5.74 The scope is positioned along the lesser curvature of the stomach while the tip is in the second portion of duodenum. The modified pull and twist technique prevents formation of a big gastric loop and optimal conditions for intubation of the duodenum and proximal jejunum.

Push enteroscopy/ jejunoscopy

Over the last decade, significant progress has been made in the field of small bowel endoscopy. It was associated primarily with capsule endoscopy and double balloon enteroscopy. At the same time, push enteroscopy has lost its leading role in diagnosis of obscure or occult GI bleeding and non-surgical treatment of small bowel polyps. However, it may be useful in some circumstances.

Indications include:

• Jejunal biopsy.
• Polypectomy of the polyps in the proximal jejunum.
• Placement of gastro-jejunal feeding tube.
• Endoscopic jejunostomy.

Three types of standard endoscopes are suitable for pediatric push enteroscopy. A pediatric panendoscope is ideal for infants, toddlers, and children 7 years and younger. An adult size (less than 10 mm) panendoscope and a pediatric colonoscope are more appropriate for children under 12 years of age and teenagers respectfully. Long specially designed enteroscopes can be used if available, but do not provide significantly deeper intubation of the small bowel.

Technique

The procedure is started after the patient is adequately sedated (*see* Chapter 4). The initial phase

of push enteroscopy is similar to standard EGD (*see* Chapter 5).

Once an endoscope is in the stomach, it is advanced along the greater curvature. Increasing resistance of the gastric wall leads to coiling of the endoscope and gastric distention. When the endoscope is finally in the second portion of the duodenum, the resistance reaches the level, which precludes further intubation: pushing the shaft forward inducing paradoxical movement of the duodenal lumen away from the tip. To overcome this problem, the endoscope should be positioned along the lesser curvature of the stomach before or right after exploration of the duodenum.

The goal of the maneuver is to straighten the scope as much as possible between the esophagus and duodenum (Figure 5.74).

Once the tip is beyond the incisura angularis, it is elevated sharply; the shaft is rotated clockwise by 30–45 degree and pulled back. As the result, the endoscope moves toward the lesser curvature and the pylorus. Appearance of the prepyloric folds at 12 o'clock position is a sign to pull back more, until the pylorus is fully open and allows the endoscope to slip into the duodenum (Figure 5.75). Immediate clockwise rotation facilitates advancement of the scope into the second portion of the duodenum. Additional clockwise rotation and gentle pulling back propel the tip close to the ligament of Treitz (Figure 5.76). If the duodenum is not successfully

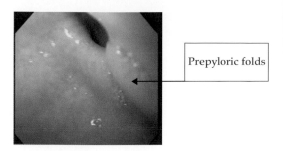

Prepyloric folds

Figure 5.75 The pylorus is in the upper pole of the screen. The tip is adjusted according the direction of prepyloric folds.

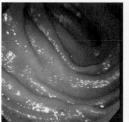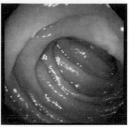

Figure 5.77 The proximal jejunum. The prominent villous pattern and multiple mucosal folds with less space between the folds compared with the duodenum pattern are seen.

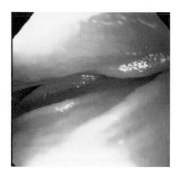

Figure 5.76 The distal duodenum at the level of the ligament of Treitz. The lumen of this area may look like a slot or disappear during transition into the proximal jejunum.

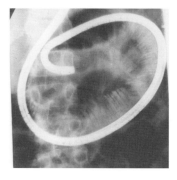

Figure 5.78 The tip is in proximal jejunum 20–30 cm below the level of a ligament of Treitz.

explored with, "pull and twist" technique can be used (*see* Chapter 5). Minimal insufflation is an important element of the technique. The corkscrew maneuver is the key for effective sliding beyond the duodeno-jejunal junction: the tip of the endoscope is deflected toward the underlying mucosa pushing the intestinal wall down while the shaft is rotated clockwise. Additional to and fro movements help to create an optimal angle for the endoscope to slip into the jejunum. Temporary disappearance of the lumen is expected at this stage of procedure and further progress is assessed by sliding mucosa. To regain the lumen, the shaft is rotated clockwise and pulled back repetitively. The folds of the proximal jejunum are less prominent but more frequent than in the duodenum. The villous pattern of mucosa is more prominent in the jejunum than in the duodenum (Figure 5.77). Increased resistance and coiling usually occurs when the tip has advanced approximately 20 to 30 cm beyond the ligament of Treitz. At this point, the jejunum starts deviating from left hypochondrium to the right (Figure 5.78). A supine

position is more useful for deeper jejunal exploration. After the patient is turned supine, a quick search for an excessive coiling is performed by palpation. If a loop is found, it should be reduced by clock- or counterclockwise rotation, pulling the shaft back and trance abdominal pressure. Before further jejunal intubation, a gentle pressure should be applied by the assistant to the epigastric area to prevent coiling of the endoscope in the stomach. Repeated torque, push and pull back movements drive the shaft into the deeper jejunum up to 80 to 100 cm beyond the ligament of Treitz (Figure 5.79).

More accurate estimation of the length of jejunal intubation is possible during the withdrawal phase of the procedure by counting the number of intestinal segments (the length of the segment between two adjacent narrowing of the intestinal lumen is about 7 to 10 cm).

The push enteroscopy adds 10 to 15 minutes to the duration of routine EGD.

The procedure may be associated with mild pain or abdominal discomfort during the early

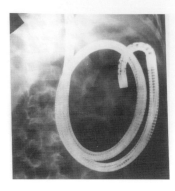

Figure 5.79 The endoscope is in proximal jejunum at 80 cm to 100 cm.

recovery phase. Serious complications such as perforation or bleeding have not been reported. Few petechiae in the jejunum and or stomach can be seen.

 FURTHER READING

Barkin J, Lewis B, Reiner D *et al.* (1996) Diagnostic and therapeutic jejunoscopy with a new, longer enteroscope. *Gastrointestinal Endoscopy*, **38,** 55–58.

Darbari A, Kalloo AN, Caffari C. (2006) Diagnostic yield, safety, and efficacy of push enteroscopy in pediatrics. *Gastrointestinal Endoscopy*, **64,** 224–228.

Gershman G, Boxer VO, Belmer SV *et al.* (1992) Jejunoscopy: endoscopic markers of celiac disease and truc response to a gluten free diet in children. *Gastrointestinal Endoscopy*, **38,** 233.

Gershman G, Thomson M. (2006) Enteroscopy: push and intraoperative. In: Winter HS, Murphy S, Mougenot JF, *et al.* (eds) *Atlas of Pediatric Gastrointestinal Endoscopy*. pp. 73–80. BC Decker: Hamilton, Ontario.

Lewis B. Enteroscopy. (2000) *Gastrointestinal Endoscopy Clinics in North America*, **10**(1), 101–116.

Technique of diagnostic gastrointestinal endoscopy

Cotton PB, Williams CB, Hawes RH, *et al.* (2008) Upper endoscopy: diagnostique techniques. In: *Practical Gastrointestinal Endoscopy: The Fundamentals*, (6th edn). pp. 37–60. Wiley-Blackwell, Oxford, UK.

de Boissieu D, Dupont C, Barbet JP, *et al.* (1994) Distinct features of upper gastrointestinal endoscopy in the newborn. *Journal of Pediatric Gastroenterology & Nutrition*, **18,** 334–338.

Dupont C, Kalach N, de Boissieu D, *et al.* (2005) Digestive endoscopy in neonates. *Journal of Pediatric Gastroenterology & Nutrition*, **40,** 406–420.

Fox VL. (2008) Patient preparation and general consideration. Gastrointestinal endoscopy. In: Walker WA, Goulet O, Kleinman RE, *et al.* (eds) *Pediatric Gastrointestinal Disease*, (5th edn). pp. 1259–1264. BC Decker, Hamilton, Ontario.

Gershman G, Ament ME. (1999) Pediatric upper gastrointestinal endoscopy: state of the art. *Acta Paediatric Taiwan*, **40,** 369–392.

Gershman G, Ament ME. (2002) Pediatric upper gastrointestinal endoscopy, endoscopic retrograde cholangiopancreatography, and colonoscopy. In: Lifschitz H (ed). *Pediatric Gastroenterology and Nutrition in ClinicalPpractice.* pp. 799–846, New York: Dekker.

Gershman G. (2007) Diagnostic upper endoscopy technique. In: Gershman G, Ament ME (eds) *Practical Pediatric Gastrointestinal Endoscopy.* pp. 60–77. Blackwell, Malden, Massachusetts.

Murphy MS. (2006) Diagnostic upper gastrointestinal endoscopy. In: Winter HS, Murphy MS, JF Mougenot JF, *et al*, (eds). *Pediatric Gastrointestinal Endoscopy Textbook and Atlas*. pp. 65–72 BC Decker, Hamilton, Ontario.

Schaeppi MG, Mougenot JF, Dominique CB. (2008) Upper gastrointestinal endoscopy. Gastrointestinal endoscopy. In: Walker WA, Goulet O, Kleinman RE, *et al.* (eds) *Pediatric GastrointestinalDdisease*, (5th edn). pp. 1265–1284, BC Decker, Hamilton, Ontario.

Biopsy

Brindley N, Sloan JM, McCallion WA. (2004) Esophagitis: optimizing diagnostic yield by biopsy orientation. *Journal of Pediatric Gastroenterology & Nutrition*, **39,** 262–264.

Cohen J. (2004) The impact of tissue sampling on endoscopy efficiency. *Gastrointestinal Endoscopy Clinics of North America*, **14**(4), 725–734.

Genta RM, Graham DY. (1994) Comparison of biopsy sites for the histological diagnosis of helicobacter pylori: a topographic study of H. pylori density and distribution. *Gastrointestinal Endoscopy*, **40**(3)**,** 342–345.

Gillett P, Hassal E. (2000) Pediatric gastrointestinal mucosal biopsy. Special considerations in children. *Gastrointestinal Endoscopy Clinics of North America*, **10**(4)**,** 669–712.

Lewin KJ, Riddell RH, Weinstein WM. (1992) Part 1: Technique: Biopsy specimen, handling and processing. In: *Gastrointestinal Pathology and its Clinical Implications*. (Vol 1) pp. 8–13, Igaku-Shoin, New York.

Oberhuber G, Granditsch G, Vogelsang H. (1999) The histopathology of celiac disease: the time for a standardized report scheme for pathologist. *European Journal of Gastroenterology & Hepatology*, **11,** 1185–1194.

Weinstein WM. (2000) Mucosal biopsy techniques and interaction with the pathologist. *Gastrointestinal Endoscopy Clinics of North America*, **10**(4)**,** 555–572.

Complications

ASGE guideline. (2008) Antibiotic prophylaxis for GI endoscopy. *Gastrointestinal Endoscopy* **67,** 791–798.

Riley S, Alderson D. (November 2006) Complications of upper gastrointestinal endoscopy. *British Society of Gastroenterology.* www.bsg.org.uk. [accessed on Oct 18, 2010.]

Rothbaum RJ. (1996) Complications of pediatric endoscopy. *Gastrointestinal Endoscopy Clinics of North America*, **6**(2)**,** 445–459.

Indications

Franciosi J, Fiorino K, Ruchelli E, *et al.* (2010) Changing indications for upper endoscopy in children during a 20-year period. *Journal of Pediatric Gastroenterology & Nutrition*, **51,** 443–447.

Guariso G, Meneghel A, Visona Dolla Pozza L, *et al.* (2010) Indications for upper gastrointestinal endoscopy in children with dyspepsia. *Journal of Pediatric Gastroenterology & Nutrition*, **50,** 493–499.

Lee KK, Anderson MA, Baron TH, *et al.* (2008) Modifications in endoscopic practice for pediatric patients. ASGE Standards of Practice Committee. *Gastrointestinal Endoscopy*, **67,** 1–9.

Thakkar K, Gilger MA, Shulman RJ. (2007) EGD in children with abdominal pain. *American Journal of Gastroenterology*, **102,** 654–661.

Thakkar K, Chen L, Tatevian N, *et al.* (2009) Diagnostic yield of oesophagogastroduodenoscopy in children with abdominal pain. *Aliment Pharmacology & Therapeutics*, **30,** 662–669.

NSAIDs, stress and peptic ulcers

ASGE guideline. (2010) The role of endoscopy in the management of patients with peptic disease. *Gastrointestinal Endoscopy*, **71,** 663–68.

Autret-Leca E, Bensouda-Grimaldi L, Maurage C, *et al.* (2007) Upper gastrointestinal complications associated with NSAIDs in children. *Therapie*, **62,** 173–176 (French).

Dohil R, Hassall E. (2000) Peptic ulcer disease in children. In: Tytgart GN, (Ed) *Baillieres Best Practice & Research in Clinical Gastroenterology*, **14,** 53–73.

Dowd JE, Cimaz R, Fink CW. (1995) Nonsteroidal anti-inflammatory drug-induced gastrointestinal injury in children. *Arthritis & Rheumatism*, **38,** 1225–1231.

Edwards MJ, Kollenberg SJ, Brandt ML, *et al.* (2005) Surgery for peptic ulcer disease in children in the post-histamine2-blocker era. *Journal of Pediatric Surgery*, **40,** 850–854.

Gisbert JP, Calvet X. (2009) Review article: helicobacter pylori-negative duodenal ulcer disease. *Aliment Pharmacology & Therapeutics*, **30,** 791–815.

Goyal A, Treem WR, Hyams JS. (1994) Severe upper gastrointestinal bleeding in healthy full-term neonates. *American Journal of Gastroentrology*, **89,** 613–616.

Kalach N, Bontems P, Koletzko S, *et al.* (2010) Frequency and risk factors of gastric and duodenal ulcers or erosions in children: a prospective 1-month European multicenter study. *European Journal of Gastroenterology & Hepatology*, **22,** 1175–1181.

Koletzko S, Richy F, Bontems P, *et al.* (2006) Prospective multicenter study on antibiotic resistance of Helicobacter pylori strains obtained from children living in Europe. *Gut*, **55,** 1711–1716.

Li Voti G, Acierno C, Tulone V, *et al.* (1997) Relationship between upper gastrointestinal bleeding and non-steroidal anti-inflammatory drugs in children. *Pediatric Surgery International*, **12,** 264–265.

O'Laughlin JC, Hoftiezer JW, Ivery KJ. (1981) Effect of aspirin in the human stomach in normals: endoscopic comparison of damage produced in one hour, 24 hours, and 2 weeks after administration. *Scandinavian Journal of Gastroenterology*, **67**(16)**,** 211–214.

Peura DA. (2000) The problem of Helicobacter pylori-negative idiopathic ulcer disease. In: Tytgart GN, (Ed). *Baillieres Best Pracice Research and Clinical Gastroenterology*, **14,** 109–117.

Reveiz L, Guerrero-Lozano R, Camacho A, *et al.* (2010) Stress ulcer, gastritis, and gastrointestinal bleeding prophylaxis in critically ill pediatric patients: A systematic review. *Pediatric Critical Care Medicine*, **11,** 125–132.

Esophagitis

Boyce HW. (1992) Hiatus hernia and peptic diseases of the esophagus. In: Sivak MV, (ed) *Gastroenterologic Endoscopy*. (2nd edn, Vol. 1), pp. 582–587. WB Saunders Company, Philadelphia.

El-Segar HB, Bailey NR, Gilger M, *et al.* (2002) Endoscopic manifestations of gastroesophageal reflux disease in patients between 18 months and 25 years without neurological deficits. *American Journal of Gastroenterology*, **97,** 1635–1639.

Rudolph CD, Mazur LJ, Liptak GS, *et al.* (2001) Guidelines for evaluation and treatment of gastroesophageal reflux in infants and children. Recommendations of the North American Society for Pediatric Gastroenterology and Nutrition. *Journal of Pediatric Gastroenterology & Nutrition*, **32(Suppl 2),** S1–31.

Salvatore S, Hauser B, Vandemaele K, *et al.* (2005) Gastroesophageal reflux disease in infants: how much is predictable with questionnaires, ph-metry, endoscopy and histology? *Journal of Pediatric Gastroenterology & Nutrition*, **40,** 210–215.

Vandenplas Y. (2000) Diagnosis and treatment of gastroesophageal reflux disease in infants and children. *Canadian Journal of Gastroenterology*, **14(D),** 26D–34D.

Barrett's esophagus

Cohen MC, Ashok D, Gell M, *et al.* (2009) Pediatric columnar lined esophagus vs Barrett's esophagus: Is it the time for consensus definition? *Pediatrics & Developmental Pathology*, **12,** 116–126.

Hassall E, Dimmick JE, Magee JF. (1993) Adenocarcinoma in childhood Barrett's esophagus. Case documentation and need for surveillance in children. *American Journal of Gastroenterology*, **88,** 282–288.

Hassal E. (1997) Columnar lined esophagus in children. *Gastroenterology Clinics of North America*, **26,** 533–548.

Hassall E. (2008) Cardia-type mucosa as an esophageal metaplastic condition in children: Barrett esophagus, gastric mucosa-positive? *Journal of Pediatric Gastroenterology & Nutrition*, **47,** 102–106.

Eosinophilic esophagitis

Aceves SS, Newbury RO, Dohil R, *et al.* (2007) Distinguishing eosinophilic esophagitis in pediatric patients: clinical, endoscopic, and histologic features of an emerging disorder. *Journal of Clinical Gastroenterology*, **41,** 252–256.

Blanchard C, Wang N, Rothenberg ME. (2006) Eosinophilic esophagitis: pathogenesis, genetics, and therapy. *Journal of Allergy and Clinical Immunology*, **118,** 1054–1059.

Collins MH. (2008) Histopathologic features of eosinophilic esophagitis. *Gastrointestinal Endoscopy Clinics of North America*, **18,** 59–71.

Furuta GT, Liacouras CA, Collins MH, *et al.* (2007) Eosinophilic esophagitis in children and adults: a systematic review and consensus recommendations for diagnosis and treatment. *Gastroenterology*, **133,** 1342–1363.

Kelly KJ, Lazenby AJ, Rowe PC *et al.* (1995) Eosinophilic esophagitis attributed to gastroesophageal reflux: improvement with an amino acid-based formula. *Gastroenterology*, **109,** 1503–1512.

King J, Khan S. (2010) Eosinophilic esophagitis: perspectives of adult and pediatric gastroenterologists. *Digestive Diseases & Sciences*, **55,** 973–982.

Liacouras CA, Spergel JM, Ruchelli E, *et al.* (2005) Eosinophilic esophagitis: a 10-year experience in 381 children. *Clinical Gastroenterology & Hepatology*, **3,** 1198–1206.

Mishra A, Hogan SP, Brand EB, *et al.* (2001) An etiological role for aeroallergens and eosinophils in experimental esophagitis. *Journal of Clinical Investigation*, **107,** 83–90.

Schaefer ET, Fitzgerald JF, Molleston JP, *et al.* (2008) Comparison of oral prednisone and topical fluticasone in the treatment of eosinophilic esophagitis: a randomised trial in children. *Clinical Gastroenterology & Hepatology*, **6,** 165–173.

Spergel JM, Brown-Whitehorn TF, Beausoleil JL, *et al.* (2008) Fourteen years of eosinophilic esophagitis: clinical features and prognosis. *Journal of Pediatric Gastroenterology & Nutrition,* **48,** 30–36.

Viral esophagitis

Baroco AL, Oldfield EC. (2008) Gastrointestinal cytomegalovirus disease in the immunocompromised patients. *Current Gastroenterology Reports,* **10,** 409–416.

Feiden V, Borchard F, Bürrig KF, *et al.* (1984) Herpes oesophagitis. I. Light microscopical and immunohistochemical investigations. *Virchows Archives of Pathology Anatomy & Histopathology,* **404,** 167–176.

Ramanathan J, Rammouni M, Baran J Jr, *et al.* (2000) Herpes simplex virus esophagitis in the immunocompetent host: an overview. *American Journal of Gastroenterology,* **95,** 2171–2176.

Rodrigous F, Brandäo N, Dugue V, *et al.* (2004) Herpes simplex virus esophagitis in immunocompetent children. *Journal of Pediatric Gastroenterology & Nutrition,* **39,** 560–563.

Thomson M. Esophagitis. (2008) In: Walker WA, Goulet O, Kleinman RE, *et al.* (eds). *Pediatric Gastrointestinal Disease,* (5th edn) pp. 87–104, BC Decker, Hamilton, Ontario.

Caustic ingestion

Kay M, Wyllie R. (2009) Caustic ingestions in children. *Current Opinion in Pediatrics,* **21,** 651–654.

Mas E, Olives JP. (2008) Toxic and traumatic injuries of esophagus. In: Walker WA, Goulet O, Kleinman RE, *et al.* (eds). *Pediatric Gastrointestinal Disease,* (5th edn). 105–116, BC Decker, Hamilton, Ontario.

Riffat F, Cheng A. (2009) Pediatric caustic ingestion: 50 consecutive cases and a review of the literature. *Diseases of the Esophagus,* **22,** 89–94.

Wilsey MJ Jnr, Scheimann AO, Gilger MA. (2001) The role of upper gastrointestinal endoscopy in the diagnosis and treatment of caustic ingestion, esophageal strictures, and achalasia in children. *Gastrointestinal Endoscopy Clinics of North America,* **11**(4)**,** 767–787.

Gastropathy, HP gastritis and viral gastritis

Ashorn M, Rägö T, Kokkonen J, *et al.* (2004) Symptomatic response to helicobacter pylori eradication in children with recurrent abdominal pain: double blind randomized placebo-controlled trial. *Journal of Clinical Gastroenterology,* **38,** 646–650.

Black DD, Haggitt RC, Whitington PF. (1988) Gastroduodenal endoscopic-histologic correlation in pediatric patients. *Journal of Pediatric Gastroenterology & Nutrition,* **7,** 353–358.

Borelli O, Hassall E, Cucchiara S, *et al.* (2003) Inflammation of the gastric cardia ["carditis"] in children with acid peptic disease. *Journal of Pediatrics,* **143,** 520–4.

Bujanover Y, Konikoff F, Baratz M. (1993) Nodular gastritis and helicobacter pylori. *Journal of Pediatric Gastroenterology & Nutrition,* **16,** 120–124.

Dixon M, Genta R, Yardley J, *et al.* (1996) Classification and grading of gastritis. The updated Sydney system. *American Journal of Surgical Pathology,* **20,** 1161–1181.

Dohil R, Hassal E, Jevon G, *et al.* (1999) Gastritis and gastropathy of childhood. *Journal of Pediatric Gastroenterology & Nutrition,* **29,** 378–394.

El-Zimaaity H, Graham D. (1999) Evaluation of gastric mucosal biopsy site and number for identification of Helicobacter pylori on intestinal metaplasia: role of the Sydney system. *Human Pathology,* **30,** 72–77.

Guarner J, Herrera-Goepfert R, Mohar A, *et al.* (2003) Diagnostic yield of gastric biopsy specimens when screening for preneoplastic lesions. *Human Pathology,* **34,** 28–31.

Guarner J, Kalach N, Elitsur Y, *et al.* (2010) Helicobacter pylori diagnostic tests in children: review of the literature from 1999 to 2009. *European Journal of Pediatrics,* **169,** 15–25.

Hassall E, Dimmick J. (1991) Unique features of helicobacter pylori disease in children. *Digestive Diseases & Sciences,* **36,** 417–423.

Hassall E. (2002) Getting to grips with gastric pathology. *Journal of Pediatric Gastroenterology & Nutrition,* **34,** S46–S50.

Ooi CY, Lamberg DA, Day AS. (2008) Other causes of gastritis. Gastritis. In: Walker WA, Goulet O, Kleinman RE, *et al.* (eds) *Pediatric Gastrointestinal Disease,* (5th edn). pp. 165–174, BC Decker, Hamilton, Ontario.

Pashankar DS, Bishop WP, Mitros FA. (2002) Chemical gastropathy: a distinct histopathological entity in children. *Journal of Pediatric Gastroenterology & Nutrition,* **53,** 653–657.

Prieto G, Polanco I, Larrauri J, *et al.* (1992) Helicobacter pylori infection in children: clinical, endoscopic and histological correlations.

Journal of Pediatric Gastroenterology & Nutrition, **14,** 420–425.

Collagenous gastritis

Kamimura K, Kobayashi M, Narisava R, *et al.* (2007) Collagenous gastritis: endoscopic and pathologic evaluation of the nodularity of gastric mucosa. *Digestive Diseases & Sciences*, **52,** 995–1000.

Leung ST, Chandan VS, Murray JA, *et al.* (2009) Collagenous gastritis. Histopathologic features and associations with other gastrointestinal diseases. *American Journal of Surgical Pathology*, **33,** 788–798.

Ravicumara M, Ramani P, Spray CH. (2007) (Collagenous gastritis: a case report and review. *European Journal of Pediatrics*, **166,** 769–773.

Menetrier disease

Blackstone MM, Mittal M. (2008) The edematous toddler. *Pediatric Emergency Care*, **24,** 682–684.

Eisenstat DDR, Griffiths AM, Cutz E, *et al.* (1995) Acute cytomegalovirus infection in child with Menetrier disease. *Gastroenterology*, **109,** 592–595.

Kovacs AA, Churchill MA, Wood D, *et al.* (1993) Molecular and epidemiologic evaluations of cluster of cases of Menetrier's disease associated with cytomegalovirus. *Pediatric Infectious Diseases Journal*, **12,** 1011–1014.

Megged O, Schlesinger Y. (2008) Cytomegalovirus-associated protein-losing gastropathy in childhood. *European Journal of Pediatrics*, **167,** 1217–1220.

Sferra TJ, Pawel BR, Qualman SJ, *et al.* (1996) Menetrier disease of childhood: role of cytomegalovirus and transforming growth factor alfa. *Journal of Pediatrics*, **128,** 213–219.

Crohn's disease

Lenaerts C, Roy CC, Vaillancourt M, *et al.* (1989) High incidence of upper gastrointestinal tract involvement in children with Crohn's disease. *Pediatrics*, **83,** 777–781.

Mashako MNL, Cezard JP, Navarro J, *et al.* (1989) Crohn's disease lesions in the upper gastrointestinal tract: correlation between clinical, radiological, endoscopic and histological features in adolescents and children. *Journal of Pediatric Gastroenterology & Nutrition*, **8,** 442–446.

Ruuska T, Vaajalathi P, Arajarvi P, *et al.* (1994) Prospective evaluation of upper gastrointestinal mucosal lesions in children with ulcerative colitis and Crohn's disease. *Journal of Pediatric Gastroenterology*, **19,** 181–186.

Turner D, Griffiths AM. (2007) Esophageal, gastric, and duodenal manifestations of IBD and the role of upper endoscopy in IBD diagnosis. *Current Gastroenterology Reports*, **9,** 475–478.

Ectopic pancreas

Christodoulidis G, Zacharoulis D, Barbanis S, *et al.* (2007) Heterotopic pancreas in the stomach: A case report and literature review. *World Journal of Gastroenterology*, **13,** 6098–6100.

Ormarsson OT, Gudmundsdottir I, Marvik R. (2006) Diagnosis and treatment of gastric heterotopic pancreas. *World Journal of Surgery*, **30** 1682–1689.

Gastric tumors and bezoar

Attard TM, Yardley JH, Cuffari C. (2002), Gastric polyps in pediatrics: an 18yr hospital based analysis. *American Journal of Gastroenterology*, **97,** 298–301.

Attard TM, Cuffari C, Tajouri T, *et al.* (2004) Multicenter experience with upper gastrointestinal polyps in pediatric patients with familial adenomatous polyposis. *American Journal of Gastroenterology*, **99,** 681–686.

Benes J, Chumel J, Jodl J, *et al.* (1991) Treatment of a gastric bezoar by extracorporeal shock wave lithotripsy. *Endoscopy*, **23,** 346–348.

Gorter RR, Kneepkens CM, Mattens EC, *et al.* (2010) Management of trichobezoar: case report and literature review. *Pediatric Surgery International*, **26,** 457–463.

Goyal A, Langer JC, Zutter N, *et al.* (1999) Primary gastric plasmocytoma: a rare cause of hypertrophic gastritis in adolescent. *Journal of Pediatric Gastroenterology & Nutrition*, **29,** 424–430.

Harris GJ, Laszewski MJ. (1992) Pediatric primary gastric lymphoma. *Southern Medical Journal*, **85,** 432–434.

Jones GC, Coutinho K, Anjaria D, *et al.* (2010) Treatment of recurrent Rapunzel syndrome and trichotillomania: case report and literature review. *Psychosomatics*, **51,** 443–446.

McGill TW, Downey J, Westbrook D, *et al.* (1993) Gastric carcinoma in children. *Journal of Pediatric Surgery*, **28,** 1620–1621.

Sanna CM, Loriga P, Dessi E, *et al.* (1991) Hyperplastic polyp of the stomach simulating hypertrophic pyloric stenosis. *Journal of Pediatric Gastroenterology & Nutrition,* **13,** 204–208.

Ziring DA, Gershman G, Hui W. (2004) Successful dissolution of gastric phytobezoar using coca-cola lavage: a pediatric experience. *Journal of Pediatric Gastroenterology & Nutrition,* **39**(1), s343.

Celiac sprue

Bonamico M, Mariani P, Thanasi E, *et al.* (2004) Patchy villous atrophy of the duodenum in childhood celiac disease. *Journal of Pediatric Gastroenterology & Nutrition,* **38,** 204–207.

Cammarota G, Cazzato A, Genovese O, *et al.* (2009) Water-immersion Technique during Standard Upper Endoscopy. *Journal of Pediatric Gastroenterology & Nutrition,* **49,** 411–416.

Corazza GR, Caletti GC, Lazzari R *et al.* (1993) Scalloped duodenal folds in childhood celiac disease. *Gastrointestinal Endoscopy,* **39,** 543–545.

Hill ID, Dirks MH, Liptak GS, *et al.* (2005) Guidelines for the diagnosis and treatment of celiac disease in children: recommendations of the North American Society for Pediatric Gastroenterology, Hepatology and Nutrition. *Journal of Pediatric Gastroenterology & Nutrition,* **40,** 1–19.

Oderda G, Forni M, Morra I, *et al.* (1993) Endoscopic and histological findings in the upper gastrointestinal tract of children with coeliac disease. *Journal of Pediatric Gastroenterology & Nutrition,* **16,** 172–177.

Rashid M, MacDonald A. (2009) Importance of duodenal bulb biopsies in children for diagnosis of celiac disease in clinical practice. *BMC Gastroenterology,* **9,** 78.

Ravelli AM, Tobanelli P, Minelli L, *et al.* (2001) Endoscopic features of celiac disease in children. *Gastrointestinal Endoscopy,* **54,** 736–742.

Ravelli I, Villanacci V, Monfredini C, *et al.* (2010) How Patchy Is Patchy Villous Atrophy? Distribution Pattern of Histological Lesions in the Duodenum of Children with Celiac Disease. *American Journal of Gastroenterology,* **105,** 1203–1210.

Sanfilippo G, Patane R, Fusto A, *et al.* (1986) Endoscopic approach to childhood celiac disease. *Acta Gastroenterology Belgium,* **49,** 401–408.

Venkatesh K, Abou-Taleb A, Cohen M, *et al.* (2010) Role of Confocal Endomicroscopy in the Diagnosis of Celiac Disease. *Journal of Pediatric Gastroenterology & Nutrition,* **51,** 274–279.

Intestinal lymphangiectasia

Biyikoglu I, Babali A, Çakal B, *et al.* (2009) Do scattered white spots in the duodenum mark a specific gastrointestinal pathology? *Journal of Digestive Diseases,* **10,** 300–304.

Chamouard P, Nehme-Schuster H, Simler JM, *et al.* (2006) Videocapsule endoscopy is useful for the diagnosis of intestinal lymphangiectasia. *Digestive Liver Disease,* **38,** 699–703.

Fang YH, Zhang BL, Wu JG, *et al.* (2007) A primary intestinal lymphangicctasia patient diagnosed by capsule endoscopy and confirmed at surgery: a case report. *World Journal of Gastroenterology,* **13,** 2263–2265.

Rivet C, Lapalus MG, Dumortier J, *et al.* (2006) Use of capsule endoscopy in children with primary intestinal lymphangiectasia. *Gastrointest inal Endoscopy,* **64,** 649–650.

Suresh N, Ganesh R, Sankar J, *et al.* (2008) Primary intestinal lymphangiectasia. *Indian Pediatrics,* **46,** 903–906.

Thomson M, Fritscher-Ravens A, Mylonaki M, *et al.* (2007) Wireless capsule endoscopy in children: a study to assess diagnostic yield in small bowel disease in pediatric patients. *Journal of Pediatric Gastroenterology & Nutrition,* **44,** 192–197.

Vignes S, Bellanger J. (2008) Primary intestinal lymphangiectasia (Waldmann's disease). *Orphanet Journal of Rare Diseases,* **3,** 5.

Waldmann TA, Steinfeld JL, Dutcher TF, *et al.* (1961) The role of the gastrointestinal system in "idiopathic hypoproteinemia". *Gastroenterology,* **41,** 197–207.

6

Therapeutic upper GI endoscopy

George Gershman

 KEY POINTS

- Therapeutic endoscopic procedures are safe and effective in the hands of a well-trained endoscopist.

- Each procedure required a comprehensive knowledge of indications, technique and complications.

Pneumatic dilatation of benign esophageal strictures

Three chronic conditions are responsible for benign esophageal strictures in the majority of pediatric patients: severe reflux esophagitis, corrosive esophagitis and esophageal atresia.

Indications for balloon dilatations of benign esophageal strictures are:

- Short strictures of the distal esophagus in children with severe GERD.
- Short strictures of cervical and tubular esophagus related to caustic ingestion.
- Short stricture after repaired esophageal atresia.

Long stricture of the esophagus is an indication for endoscopic stent therapy. The technique of this procedure will be discussed in Chapter 11.

The endoscopic balloon dilation of short strictures does not require fluoroscopy. The length of narrowed esophagus in children with a simple (symmetrical) or complex (asymmetrical and tight) strictures is estimated by esophagram prior to endoscopic dilatation. Some corrections should be made for X-ray magnification and edema and spasm of adjacent esophagus.

The most popular "through-the-scope" type of device is CRE™ Wire guided Balloon Dilator (Boston Scientific Co, USA). It is available in three different lengths: 3 cm, 5 cm, and 8 cm. The short one is more vulnerable to slip away from the stricture during dilation. A 5 cm dilator is the more "stable" during dilatation in pediatric patients.

The diameter of the balloon is regulated by the attached water filled mechanical pump. It can be adjusted by changes of the recommended pressure settings.

Dilators are available in 4 different sizes: 6–7–8 mm, 8–9–10 mm, 12–13.5–15 mm, and 18–19–20 mm.

The procedure is started with proper sedation and intubation of the esophagus in the standard fashion. The diameter of the stricture is estimated visually. The initial size of the balloon should not exceed the diameter of the stricture by more than 2 mm. The maximal diameter of CRE™ dilator chosen for sequential technique should not be greater than three times the diameter of the stricture. Three dilatations per session are safe.

The dilator is lubricated with silicone spray. An additional 1 or 2 ml of silicone oil can be injected into the biopsy channel. The dilator with the attached guidewire is inserted into the biopsy channel, advanced into the esophagus and positioned above the stricture.

The position of the endoscope is adjusted to align it with the axis of the stricture. The guidewire is gently pushed for approximately 10 cm beyond the stricture.

A dilator is advanced over the guidewire with minimal resistance until the entire balloon is passed beyond the stricture (only the black delivery system and edge of transparent balloon are visible). Then, the dilator is pulled back to position the middle portion of the balloon across the stricture. A small portion of the black delivery system should be kept outside the tip of the endoscope to prevent expansion of the balloon within the biopsy channel (Figure 6.1). The optimal duration of dilatation is not established. In our practice, we keep the balloon inflated for 30 seconds. If three sequential dilatations per session are chosen, the total dilatation time is not exceeded 1 minute. Repeat treatments are necessary with two to three weeks intervals to dilate the stricture, ideally up to 15 mm. Dysphagia for solids and food impaction is usually resolved when the esophageal diameter is more than 12 mm.

Perforation is uncommon after balloon dilation of benign esophageal stricture. The reported frequency is less than 3%. This complication can occur when an inappropriate size of dilator or prolonged dilation time has been used, especially in children with complex strictures. Medical treatment of the perforation is very effective. It requires withholding all oral feeding for 7–14 days, parenteral nutrition, treatment with protein pump inhibitors and broad-spectrum antibiotics to prevent mediastinitis.

Pneumatic dilation in achalasia

Pneumatic dilation (PD) in achalasia is an effective and safe procedure if performed by an experienced gastroenterologist. However, even in the good hands, esophageal perforation can occur.

It is quite unlikely that a practicing pediatric gastroenterologist will come across more than a few children with achalasia because the disease is rare (the reported incidence across the western world ranges from 0.4 to 1.1 per 100 000 people) and usually becomes clearly apparent in teenagers.

It may be reasonable to refer children with achalasia for pneumatic dilation to a tertiary center.

However, a pediatric gastroenterologist should be familiar with the effects of pneumatic stretching of lower esophageal sphincter (LES), principles of technique, outcome and post-procedure care.

First of all, pneumatic dilation works by rupturing some fibers of the circular muscle incorporated in LES. The magnitude of muscle rupture is related to pressure, diameter of the dilator and time of dilatation. Due to the complexity of a special configuration, variable thickness of LES and lack of experimental data from animal models, it is virtually impossible to calculate exact time and pressure to produce a desirable affect in particular patient. It was proposed, that a mucosal layer become responsible for integrity of esophageal wall after mechanical stretching and rupture of circular muscle fibers. Similar effect was reproduced after balloon dilation of the small and large bowel.

In general, high pressure associated with use of large size balloons and prolonged duration of the dilation increases the risk of perforation due to excessive damage of the esophagus. Progressive ischemic necrosis of the esophageal mucosa could explain so-called delayed perforation and false negative results of an immediate post procedure chest and abdominal films and an esophagram with water-soluble contrast.

Two techniques of PD have been described: traditional or so-called fluoroscopic-guided technique and recently reported endoscope-guided PD without fluoroscopy, which is not validated in children.

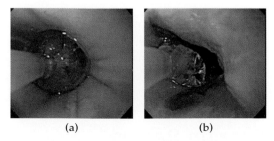

(a)   (b)

Figure 6.1 Dilatation of the benign esophageal stricture. The dilator is placed across the stricture, filled with water (a) and then deflated (b).

The child should be well prepared before dilation to decrease risk of aspiration with residual food in the dilated and poorly emptying esophagus. Liquid diet for 24 hours and overnight fasting are recommended.

Pneumatic dilatation is quite a painful procedure. That is why PD requires deep sedation or general anesthesia without muscle relaxant.

The initial steps are similar for fluoroscopic- and endoscope-guided PD:

1. Complete aspiration of residual liquid and solid food from the dilated esophagus;
2. Advancement of the endoscope into the middle of the gastric body;
3. Insertion of a guidewire (Microvasive, Boston Scientific Corp, Boston, MA) into the antrum through the biopsy channel;
4. An "exchanged" procedure: a guidewire is pushed slowly forward while the endoscope is pulled back synchronously until completely removed from the mouth.

A few additional steps are involved in the fluoroscopic-guided technique. The Rigiflex 30 mm diameter dilator (Microvasive, Boston Scientific Corp, Boston, MA) is prepared by injecting a small amount of diluted water-soluble dye into the balloon, spreading it manually and aspirating it completely. Then a well-lubricated dilator is inserted into the mouth and slowly advanced into the esophagus over the guidewire under fluoroscopy until two radio-opaque markers in the middle of the balloon traverse the diaphragm. Then, the dilator is pulled back slowly until the markers appeared 1 cm above the diaphragm. The position of the balloon is secured by holding the dilator firmly up against the bite block, preventing a displacement of the balloon into the stomach.

During inflation, a high pressure zone of low esophageal sphincter creates an hourglass-shaped fluoroscopic image of the balloon dilator. This so-called "waist" disappears once the pressure within the balloon reaches 7 to 12 psi.

There is no consensus on the duration of inflation. However, the long sessions increase the risk of mucosal ischemia and subsequent perforation.

Based on our experience, a 45 second's single 30 mm balloon technique is optimal for children younger than 12 years old. For teenagers and adolescents, we prefer a double-balloon technique with initial 30 seconds inflation of 30 mm dilator followed by the 15 seconds inflation with 35 mm balloon unless a significant amount of blood (more than few streaks or small clots) is observed after the first part of procedure.

The endoscope-guided technique eliminates exposure to the radiation. The technique requires a few additional steps:

1. Marking the mid-section of the Regiflex balloon dilator with the thick colored marker;
2. Passing the balloon over the guidewire into the stomach;
3. Reinsertion of the endoscope to control the position of the balloon in the esophagus;
4. Pulling the balloon back into the esophagus until the color mark reaches the gastroesophageal junction;
5. Inflation of the balloon up to 12 psi and maintaining the balloon inflated until the appearance of the ischemic ring at the low esophageal sphincter.

Once again, this technique was not validated in children.

A careful observation for at least 4 hours and post-procedure chest X-ray is mandatory. Persistent chest pain for more than one hour and fever should be considered as the red flags of complication and indication for treatment even without a proven pneumomediastinum or radiographic signs of perforation.

The major complication of PD is esophageal perforation. In large pediatric and adult studies, the reported rate of this complication is under 5%. Conservative management of perforation with broad-spectrum antibiotics, proton pump inhibitors, withholding of oral feeds and parenteral nutrition is very effective and carries less risk of morbidity associated with early surgery.

Immediate symptomatic improvement after the first dilatation occurs in the majority of adults and children.

Two or three sessions are usually necessary to achieve sustained (5 or more years) remission. Large scale, long-term follow up studies proved that sustained remission is achievable in 40 to 78% of adults with achalasis. The results are less satisfactory in children. Heller's or laparoscopic myotomy should be considered after three failed PD attempts.

Foreign Bodies

Children with foreign bodies in the upper GI tract require either urgent care or cautious observation.

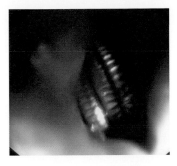

Figure 6.2 Three coins (quarters) in the cervical esophagus. This two-year-old girl was symptom free at the time of endoscopic coins removal.

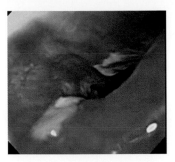

Figure 6.4 Pressure necrosis of the cervical esophagus. It consists of symmetrical lineal lesions on the lateral walls of the cervical esophagus.

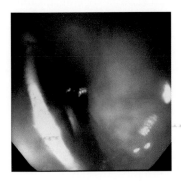

Figure 6.3 The locker key is in the cervical esophagus. The toddler swallowed the foreign body 4 hours before he was brought to the emergency room. The child was symptom free.

Indications for urgent care are:

- Esophageal foreign body.
- Sharp foreign body in the esophagus, stomach and duodenum.

Coins

Crawling infants and toddlers are the most common patients registered in the emergency room with coin and other small objects in the cervical esophagus (Figures 6.2 and 6.3).

They could be symptomatic; gagging, drooling, coughing, wheezing and breathing with strider or symptom-free. All symptomatic patients require urgent endoscopic intervention.

A few strategies are recommended for asymptomatic children with coins in the cervical esophagus:

- 12 hours observation.
- Foley catheter removal technique.

- Pushing the coin into the thoracic esophagus.
- Delayed endoscopic procedure.

In our opinion, these approaches are problematic.

First of all, an accurate estimation of the time of ingestion is not always possible.

Second, spontaneous migration of a coin into the stomach is quite unlikely over time, especially in infants.

Third, significant pressure necrosis of the cervical esophageal (Figure 6.4) can occur as early as 4 to 6 hours after coin ingestion (personal observation). This complication requires hospitalization and treatment with naso-gastric feeding and antibiotics for 5 days.

Last, the Foley catheter technique carries a small, but life-threatening risk of a coin dislodgment into the larynx and asphyxia.

We manage all asymptomatic children with a coin in the cervical esophagus according to the algorithm shown in Figure 6.5.

Endoscopic removal of a coin from the cervical esophagus can be done under deep sedation. However, general anesthesia with muscle relaxants not only protects the airways but provides the optimal conditions for safe endoscopic removal of a foreign body.

Technique of coin removal

The esophagus is intubated in standard fashion (*see* Chapter 5). A coin is identified almost immediately if it is still in the cervical esophagus (occasional dislodgement can occur during endotracheal intubation).

The main challenge during coin removal is the high pressure produced by striated muscle of the cervical esophagus.

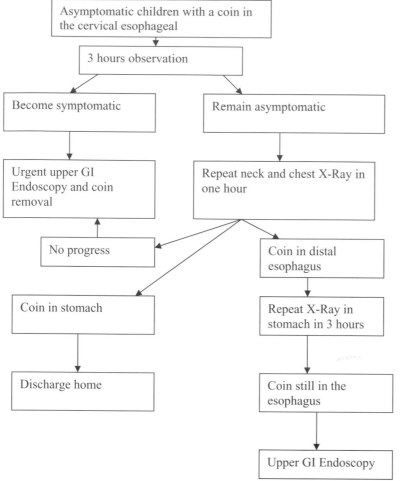

Figure 6.5
Asymptomatic children with a coin in the cervical esophagus: treatment algorithm.

Many devices have been used to extract coins from the cervical esophagus: regular biopsy forceps, "alligators", a snare with a net etc.

According to our experience, the foreign body retriever (Olympus Ltd.) is the only device that can grasp a coin between "teeth" and hold it tightly enough to overcome any resistance of the upper esophageal sphincter during removal. The key to success is the proper positioning of the retriever, right behind the edge of the middle part of the coin (Figure 6.6).

Delicate manipulations with the shaft and control knobs help to align the retriever with the coin. Slight opening of the retriever indicates the correct position of the branches in respect to the coin. The retriever should be repositioned until the coin is trapped between the branches. The tip of a scope is kept in about 1 cm from the coin creating enough space for safe manipulation.

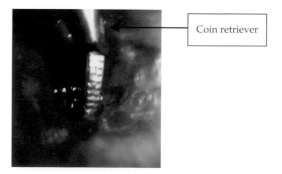

Coin retriever

Figure 6.6 Removal of the coin using a coin retriever device. The key to success is proper placement of the retriever in the middle of the coin edge.

During capture, the low branch of the device slides along the posterior wall of the cervical esophagus behind the coin. However, it does not create a blind trauma because a sharp tooth at the end of the branch is facing the coin. To eliminate any risk of accidental mucosal laceration, precise positioning of the retriever is mandatory before any attempt to close it.

If opened branches are not strictly perpendicular to a coin and are off-center, the coin is most likely to escape from the device. Once a coin grasped and secured, the retriever is kept tight and pulled back to bring the coin to the tip of the scope.

Coiling the external portion of the retriever around the left thumb allows the retriever to anchor and secure the position of the coin at the tip during withdrawal of the endoscope. Both control knobs should be released free. Some clock or counterclockwise torques facilitates escape of the coin from the esophagus and the pharynx. If the coin is lost in the mouth, remove a bite-guard and inspect the mouth using the right index finger. If the coin is not found, reinsert the endoscope into the esophagus and repeat the procedure.

Disc battery

A retained disk battery in the esophagus is a true medical emergency. Serious life-threatening complications including tracheo-esophageal and aorta-esophageal fistula and neck abscess can occur (Figure 6.7). A disk battery creates a deep tissue necrosis in a few hours (Figures 6.8 and 6.9). A tremendous spasm of the cricopharyngeal muscle makes the situation even worse. A disc battery has a smooth edge. It further complicates removal due to a lack of appropriate grasping devices. Careful washing and aspiration of necrotic debris helps to find the battery and assess the damage.

Attempts to push a battery into the thoracic esophagus are never successful. Multiple trials usually fail before successful grasping and removal of a disc battery with the retriever.

Rigid esophagoscopy is an option if a well-trained specialist is available.

V-shape and other sharp objects

Any V-shape object in the esophagus, such as an open safety pin with the sharp edge pointed cephalad (Figure 6.10) has to be gently brought into the stomach, reversed and removed in a retrograde fashion.

Any ingested sharp objects should be urgently removed from the stomach or duodenum (Figure 6.11).

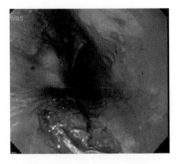

Figure 6.8 A disc battery in the cervical esophagus.

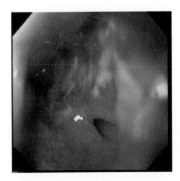

Figure 6.7 Tracheo-esophageal fistula. This complication has occurred in a 2-year-old toddler, who swallowed a 20 mm disc battery approximately 12 hours before it was removed.

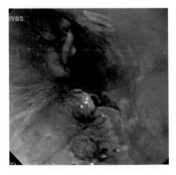

Figure 6.9 View of the cervical esophagus after the battery was removed 5 hours after ingestion. Severe tissue necrosis has already occurred.

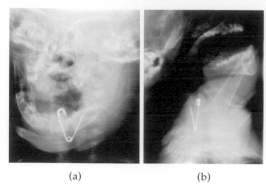

(a)   (b)

Figure 6.10 (a) Open safety pin in the cervical esophagus. (b) It was transferred into the stomach, reversed and then safely removed using a rat tooth grasper and protective rubber hood device.

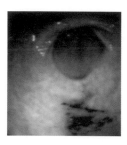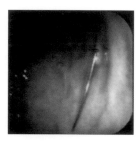

Figure 6.11 A pin in the duodenum. A 15-year-old girl swallowed a pin accidentally. She was followed-up in the outside emergency room for two days. A battery of flat film showed a retained pin in the duodenum. Superficial mucosal trauma was found in the antrum. A pin was discovered and removed from the duodenum uneventfully.

Improvised protective devices, e.g. a cylinder from the variceal bending set or plastic tube, can be attached to the tip. A grasped sharp object is pulled into the protective shield and removed with the endoscope.

Endoscopic hemostasis

by Jorge H. Vargas

Acute, moderate to severe bleeding from the upper GI tract in infants and children may arise from one of the following causes:

- Portal hypertension
- Medication, sepsis or stress-induced gastric and duodenal ulcers
- Peptic ulcer disease

- Mallory-Weiss tear
- Vascular Malformations.

Urgent upper GI endoscopy is the procedure of choice for children with active or recent upper GI bleeding. The primary goal of the procedure is finding the source of bleeding to establish an endoscopic hemostasis.

Methods of endoscopic hemostasis can be classified into three categories:

- Non-Thermal Hemostasis
- Constrictive, Mechanical devices
- Thermal Coagulation.

"Non-thermal" hemostasis

"Non-thermal" endoscopic hemostasis can be achieved by injection of sclerosing substances, or polymeric glue (e.g. histoacryl or cyanoacrylate) or vasoconstricting agents either directly into the bleeding vessel or into surrounding tissue.

Sclerotherapy

Not long ago, sclerotherapy was the most effective and only alternative to the surgical shunting procedure for children with portal hypertension. Recently, for the most part, it has been replaced by variceal banding. However, sclerotherapy is still the procedure of choice for infants and children under 5 years of age.

Indications for sclerotherapy

- Active bleeding from esophageal varices
- History of recent upper gastrointestinal bleeding
- A failed shunting procedure
- Prophylactic sclerotherapy.

The goal of sclerotherapy varies from temporary hemostasis in children waiting for liver transplantation to complete obliteration of varices in children with an extrahepatic block of a portal flow.

The data regarding primary prophylactic sclerotherapy in children is limited and inconclusive. It is fair to say than the subject remains controversial.

Sclerotherapy can be performed during acute variceal bleeding, but it is associated with high risk of complications.

The patient has to be stabilized hemodynamically before the procedure. Octreotide drip is routinely used to lower the pressure in the portal system. If the intensity of hematemesis excludes urgent endoscopy, the Sengstaken-Blakemore tube is indicated.

General anesthesia with endotracheal intubation is the method of choice for initial endoscopy and sclerotherapy in children with variceal bleeding. Deep sedation is optional for follow-up sessions. Antibiotics are used routinely before the procedure to reduce the risk of bacteremia.

The procedure consists of two parts: the diagnostic panendoscopy to confirm the sources of bleeding within the upper GI tract and therapeutic injection of the sclerosing agent. Many different agents have been used for sclerotherapy. The most favored agents in pediatrics are Ethanolamine and Polidocanol. We use them at half the strength to reduce the incidence of ulceration and strictures (from 6 to 14%).

Injection technique

The sclerosing agent can be injected directly into the vessel (intravariceal) or adjacent tissue (paravariceal) or both through a 21 or smaller 23–25-gauge needle. The first injection targets the varices just above the Z-line (Figure 6.12). Three to six subsequent injections are performed in a spiral fashion within 5 cm of the distal esophagus. If there is no sign of active bleeding, tortuous varices with cherry red spots or "red wale" marks are the first targets, as they carry a higher risk of rupture (Figure 6.13). In infants, the volume of Ethanolamine is limited to 0.5 ml per spot. In older children, a larger volume can be used safely (up to 1.5 ml per site but not more than 8 ml per session). A dose of Polidocanol should not exceed 0.4 mL/kg. The signs of sufficient injection are discoloration and swelling of the varix or adjacent tissue. However, under no circumstances should the volume of

sclerosing agent exceed the safety limits. Injection of a sclerosant while retrieving a needle may prevent bleeding from a site of injection. Simple advancement of the endoscope into the stomach creates sufficient pressure for hemostasis if oozing has occurred. Decompression of the stomach after each injection is necessary to prevent aspiration. Three to six injections per session are typically performed based on the patient's size, as well as the degree or severity of the varices.

Initial endoscopic hemostasis is successful in more than 80% of cases.

Repeat sessions of sclerotherapy are necessary for complete obliteration of varices. Usually, it is performed twice in the first month, followed by a monthly injection until complete obliteration is achieved. The schedule is modified if a deep esophageal ulcer occurs. The incidence of recurrent variceal bleeding after sclerotherapy fluctuates between 8 and 31%. The bleeding may be severe but is usually controlled endoscopically. The majority of uncontrolled bleeding is related to gastric varices, or severe hypertensive gastropathy. The risk of re-bleeding is high in children with liver disease and very low in those with portal vein thrombosis.

An average of 4–6 sessions of sclerotherapy is necessary to complete obliteration of esophageal varices.

Several complications of sclerotherapy have been described.

The most frequent side-effects are transient chest pain, dysphagia and low-grade fever. More serious but rare complications such as cerebral abscess, perforation with mediastinitis, respiratory

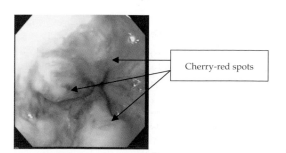

Figure 6.12 Cherry red spot. The varices with this mark carry a high risk of bleeding.

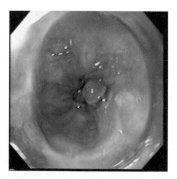

Figure 6.13 Portal hypertension. Appearance of the varices in the distal esophagus after the bending procedure was performed.

distress syndrome, anaphylaxis and spinal cord damage have been reported.

Small shallow esophageal ulcers can occur at the site of injection but are not usually associated with significant morbidity and heal spontaneously on treatment with sucralfate, H_2 blockers or proton pump inhibitors. Deep ulcers may be the source of bleeding or esophageal stricture and must be treated aggressively. An esophageal stricture due to sclerotherapy is managed by balloon dilatation. Transient changes of esophageal motility and gastroesophageal reflux have been described in adults but the real incidence of these complications in children is unknown.

Sclerotherapy with polymeric glues

Injection of polymeric glues is reserved for endoscopic sclerotherapy of bleeding gastric and large esophageal varices. For a detailed description of the technique please *see* Chapter 12.

Preparation for the procedure consists of thorough lubrication of the suction channel, mixing of the components, refrigerated eburilate and ethioldol in a 1:1 ratio, and loading it into a 19 or 23-gauge needle. A drop of glue is squeezed out prior to injection, to ensure liquidity of the polymeric mixture. One milliliter of cyanoacrylate is injected directly into the varix. Withdrawal of the needle during injection prevents needle embedment. Usually, only one needle per site is used.

Epinephrine injection therapy

Epinephrine in saline (1: 10 000) is the most commonly used vasoconstrictive agent for hemostasis in children with non-variceal bleeding. It is injected into the bleeding site through the 21–25-gauge needle (21G needle and 23–25G needles are suitable for endoscopes with 2.8 mm and 2 mm biopsy channels respectively). In our practice, we routinely use short 4 mm length needles. The needle should be primed (filled in with epinephrine) before insertion into the biopsy channel to prevent air embolism.

Injection of epinephrine can be used as a monotherapy: bleeding AVMs or bleeding after polypectomy, or in combination with thermal or constrictive types of endoscopic hemostasis, in case of active bleeding from an ulcer with a visible vessel.

According to The British Society of Gastroenterology Endoscopy Committee guidelines, injection of epinephrine as a mono-therapy will lead to a primary hemostasis in up to 95% of adult patients. However, bleeding will recur in 15 to 20% of them. Efficacy of epinephrine injection in pediatric patients has not been established.

Indications for epinephrine injections are:

• Bleeding ulcer
• Bleeding arteriovenous malformation
• Bleeding after polypectomy

The injection technique should be adjusted to the specific cause of bleeding, e.g. a bleeding ulcer with a visible vessel requires peripheral four quadrants injections, followed by direct injection into the bleeding vessel. In contrast, target injection into the bleeding spot is an initial step of endoscopic hemostasis caused by AVMs or bleeding from the stock or the base of the polyp after polypectomy. The amount of epinephrine solution should not exceed 16 ml (recommended adult dose). In our practice, we rarely inject more than 4 ml of epinephrine solution per session to avoid local ischemia or perforation.

Constrictive, mechanical devices

Endoscopic variceal ligation

Endoscopic variceal ligation procedure (EVL) has been proven superior to endoscopic sclerotherapy (EST) in three categories:

1. Simplicity of the procedure.
2. Faster eradication of the varices with fewer sessions involved.
3. Lower rate of complications.

However, EVL is associated with more frequent recurrence of varices and difficulties in ligating small residual varices. The major limiting factor is the size of a banding device: it adds up 3 mm to the diameter of the endoscope, restricting the use of this device to children over 4 years of age, because of risk of trauma during the esophageal intubation.

The banding device consists of two cylinders. The outer cylinder is mounted on the tip of an endoscope. The inner cylinder has "O" rings (up to 10 rings in the last models), which can be released by a trigger unit attached to the biopsy channel and connected to the inner cylinder through the trip wire.

A diagnostic upper GI endoscopy has to be performed immediately prior to the banding procedure for verification of the source of recent bleeding and to design the plan of action (banding schedule). The proper placement of the first band is important for several reasons:

1. To achieve a maximal reduction in blood flow.
2. To avoid significant narrowing of the esophageal lumen, especially in very young patients.
3. To eliminate the need to advance the endoscope beyond the treated varix and prevent dislodgement of the rubber ring.

The technique of EVL consists of two elements:

1. Proper sealing of the target lesion by the device and creating an adequate negative pressure for suctioning the varix into the inner cylinder.
2. Strangulating the varix by the rubber band ("O" ring) using the trip wire.

The first element of EVL begins with the positioning of the endoscope just above the most distal varix and the creation of a gentle but steady contact with the varix without accidental trauma.

The second stage of the procedure requires adequate suctioning of the varix into the inner cylinder and then release of the rubber band when the vessel blinds the view (Figure 6.14). The suction is stopped and the next varix above is targeted.

The key of this stage is an optimal use of suction to avoid slipping of the "O" ring from the varix and excessive suction of the varix into the cylinder with subsequent deep ulceration and stricture. Three to six bands are applied in an upward spiral fashion every 1–2 cm. It is reasonable to limit the number of bands to 3 or less per session in the smallest patients, to avoid partial esophageal obstruction and secondary dysphagia.

Repeat EVL is necessary within 3–4 weeks and then continuously on a monthly basis until complete eradication of the varices is achieved. The most common complication of EVL is an esophageal ulceration. Unlike ulcers after ES, EVL-induced ulcers are usually more superficial. Transient chest pain, odynophagia and dysphagia have been reported.

Long-term efficacy of EVL in children is unknown. Preliminary results of short-term follow up data are compatible with the outcome of ES. An absence of systemic complications along with further modifications of the banding device could make EVL suitable, even for the infants and toddlers.

Hemostatic clips

Over the last few years, significant progress has been made in metal clip technology, which sparked its application for adult and pediatric patients with acute GI bleeding (Figure 6.15).

Single-use preloaded rotatable clips and clipping devices, which can be reopened and repositioned up to 5 times, are commercially available.

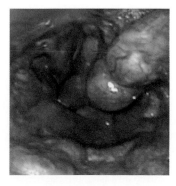

Figure 6.14 The target of the first sclerotherapy: esophageal varices just above the gastroesophageal junction.

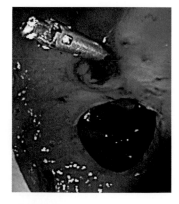

Figure 6.15 Hemoclip deployed at the base of bleeding ulcer.

The endoscope with 2.8 mm biopsy channels is necessary to accommodate a standard clipping device, which consists of a metal cable within a metal coil sheath covered by 2.2 mm Teflon catheter. However, we successfully used a 2-pronged clip (Resolution Clip, Boston Scientific) without Teflon catheter.

This approach allows suctioning and positioning of the clip while using the pediatric endoscopes with a 2 mm biopsy channel.

Indications for metal clip hemostasis are:

- A visibly bleeding vessel.
- Dieulafoy lesions.

The keys for successful application of a clipping device are:

- Good visibility of bleeding point.
- Precise positioning of the clip on a target lesion.
- Full opening of the clip before deployment.
- Minimal extension of the clipping device beyond the tip of the endoscope.
- Avoidance of excessive force while imbedding the clip into the tissue before deployment.
- Application of an additional clip if necessary.

The most challenging scenario for hemostatic clip therapy is bleeding from a large chronic ulcer on the posterior wall of the duodenal bulb, or the superior duodenal angle. In this case, it is wise to use a standard adult upper endoscope, which is more rigid compared with the pediatric one. It provides greater stability of the endoscope within the duodenum, better suction and visibility of target lesion positioning of the clip.

Primary hemostasis of a bleeding ulcer or Dieulafoy lesion can be achieved in the range of 84 to 100% respectively.

Complications associated with clipping hemostasis are quite rare.

Thermal coagulation

Thermal hemostasis embraces different methods, which target non-variceal causes of bleeding such as:

- ulcers with bleeding or non-bleeding visible vessels
- ulcers with an adherent clot
- Mallory–Weiss tear with active bleeding

- vascular malformations, e.g. Dieulafoy's lesions
- bleeding after polypectomy.

Three types of thermal devices are currently used in pediatric practice.

Bipolar or multipolar thermal devices

The heating unit of these devices consists of two (bipolar) or four to six (multipolar) active electrodes incorporated into a thermal probe. Advantages of the system are:

- Elimination of the needs for a grounding plate.
- Mechanical compression of the bleeding vessel.
- Large contact area.
- Low risk of tissue adherence to the probe and re-bleeding after pulling the probe back into the biopsy channel.
- Lesser deepness of thermal coagulation.
- Effective coagulation with tangential position of the probe, which is essential for hemostasis of bleeding duodenal ulcer.
- Capability of irrigation through the thermal probe.

Small (2.2 mm) and large (3.2 mm) bipolar or multipolar probes are commercially available. Large probes allow for the application of stronger pressure on a bleeding vessel and depth of coagulation.

The depth of coagulation is related to the power setting. Low-to-mid-range of setting (15–25 W) is preferable for deep coagulation. Escalating the power setting increases water evaporation and a diminished degree of coagulation.

Computer-controlled thermal probes (heater probes)

The device generates and controls heat up to 250 degrees Celsius by pulses of energy delivered to a silicon clip surrounded by a low heat-capacity metal envelope without any electric current in the tissue. The probe is supplemented by a three-water jets system.

The metal envelope warms up to the designed temperature in less than 0.2 seconds and cools off in less than 0.5 seconds. The computer controls the temperature and total energy delivered to the tissue. The endoscopist programs the computer to deliver a specific amount of energy from 5 to 30 j tailored to a specific bleeding source.

Advantages of the heater probe include:

- elimination of direct contact of the probe with the tissue
- no adherence to the tissue
- automatic control of energy delivered to the tissue
- adjustable depth of coagulation.

Bipolar/multipolar and heater probes have been used more often in pediatric patients than any other type of thermal hemostatic devices. Commercially available probes fit easily into the 2.8 biopsy channel of the pediatric endoscope. Both methods provide enough heat for coagulation of mesenteric arteries up to 2 mm in experimental models.

Argon plasma coagulation (APC)

Plasma coagulation is the result of ionization of a noble gas (argon is the cheapest one), which fills a small gap between the electrical electrode and the target tissue. Ionization of argon occurs when a high frequency current creates sufficient electric field strength.

Ionized argon conducts an electrical current and flows along the same pathway. The released energy induces desiccation and coagulation without carbonization and evaporation, which prevent deep tissue destruction. The depth of coagulation is proportional to the power setting and application time but almost never exceeds 3 mm. Holding a probe in one site for 5 seconds produces coagulation of 2–3 mm deep with the power setting of 30 to 60 W.

The advantages of APC coagulations are:

- larger area of coagulation compared with bipolar or multipolar probes
- decreased depth of tissue destruction.

The procedure carries a risk of perforation due to direct contact of the tissue with a probe, and stretching the bowel wall due to the accumulation of argon in the stomach, or the bowel. Thin (1.5 mm) probes are commercially available and suitable for small caliber pediatric endoscopes. This makes it possible to apply APC even in neonates and infants.

Two types of complications have been described in adults: perforation or submucosal emphysema due to direct contact of the probe with mucosa and flow of argon gas through the damaged mucosa.

Technique of thermal coagulation

Detailed description of endoscopic hemostasis with different thermal devices is beyond the scope of the chapter.

Before the procedure, a pediatric gastroenterologist should become familiar with the available equipment; proper setting of the coagulator and optimal treatment requirements for different types of bleeding lesions.

Bleeding from a nonvariceal lesion in the stomach or duodenum can be arterial from the visible vessel or venous/parenchymal. During endoscopy, the responsible vessel appears as a pyramid like "island" at the base of the ulcer. An observation of active forceful pulsating eruption of blood from the ulcer leaves no doubt about the arterial nature of bleeding. An immediate endoscopic intervention is required: creating pressure by forcing a bipolar or heater probe up against the bleeding vessel, followed by 4 pulses of 30 J using the heater probe or 8–10 seconds pulses with a power setting of 15–20 W on 50 W generator for bipolar or multipolar probe before repositioning the probe.

Coagulation is repeated until a visible vessel becomes flat and bleeding is stopped. The procedure is complicated by poor visibility, especially when the source of bleeding is located in the duodenum. Forceful irrigation and suction is more effective with therapeutic endoscope.

Finding a large blood clot at the site of bleeding is another challenging situation. The risk of worsening bleeding has to be weighed against the potential benefits before an attempt to remove an adherent clot to expose a bleeding vessel.

It requires careful washing out of blood and loose fibrin until the edge of the ulcer become visible. The next step is an injection of epinephrine under the clot in a circular fashion, decreasing the risk of bleeding during dislodgement of the clot from the ulcer, and to expose the underlying vessel for endoscopic hemostasis. Once again, this is a challenging procedure, which requires a highly skilful endoscopist and supportive team.

Presence of a non-bleeding vessel allows for better assessment of the lesion and more precise positioning of the hemostatic device. Thermal coagulation has minimal benefits for patients with a non-bleeding ulcer with a well-organized flat clot, red or black spots or gray fibrin in the ulcer base.

The power setting and force application should be adjusted in patients with angiodysplasia to avoid perforation. The APC technique is preferable in such circumstances.

Percutaneous endoscopic gastrostomy

by Robert Wyllie and Marsha Kay

Introduction

The first reported percutaneous endoscopic gastrostomy (PEG) tube placement was in a 1980 by Ponsky, Gauderer and Izant. PEG tube insertion was initially reported in pediatric patients, subsequently popularized in adults and later reintroduced for use in children by pediatric gastroenterologists. Although initially developed by surgeons, it is now performed at an equal or greater frequency by adult and pediatric gastroenterologists. Despite many similarities in the indications and some technical aspects of the procedure between children and adults, there are also significant differences in the indications, limitations and technical aspects of the procedure.

Indications

PEG tubes are appropriate in any pediatric patient who requires a gastrostomy tube and does not require a simultaneous open abdominal procedure. PEGs can be placed for medication administration, feeding administration, gastric decompression or a combination of these. Patients undergoing a simultaneous fundoplication, pyloroplasty or pyloromyotomy are unlikely to derive additional benefit from placement of a PEG tube versus a surgical gastrostomy. PEG tube placement does not interfere with subsequent fundoplication, pyloroplasty or pyloromyotomy.

Benefits of PEG tube insertion compared to a surgical gastrostomy include reduced procedure time and cost, smaller incision, shorter length of stay, decreased incidence of postoperative gastroesophageal reflux (GER), and a decreased incidence of postoperative complications including wound infection, wound dehiscence, bowel obstruction, pain, atelectasis and impaired mobility.

Contraindications

There are only a few absolute contraindications to PEG placement. PEG tubes should not be attempted if there are patient factors that interfere with successful transillumination of the gastric wall, or with identification of the indentation performed during the procedure, or if there is suspicion that the anterior gastric wall is not opposed to the abdominal wall such as in the case of an intervening colon or other abdominal organ. If the anterior gastric wall cannot be opposed to the anterior abdominal wall due to ascites or similar conditions, PEG placement may not be feasible. As with any endoscopic procedure, the patient should be medically stable, airway protection and management is imperative and the endoscopist should be willing to abort the procedure if the procedure is not progressing as anticipated.

PEG tubes may be more difficult to place or may not be possible to place, must be placed with increased caution, may require additional pre-procedure evaluation and may also require extra care in patients with the following conditions: ascites or those on peritoneal dialysis, scoliosis or spine abnormalities, small-size, ventriculoperitoneal shunts, prior abdominal surgery, especially gastric surgery, congenital abnormalities such as situs inversus, hepatomegaly, splenomegaly or other abdominal masses, small laryngeal or tracheal size, tracheal compromise or ventilatory issues. The presence of a VP shunt or use of peritoneal dialysis prior to PEG placement is associated with a particularly poor outcome and high complication rate following PEG placement, especially infectious complications including fungal peritonitis. The presence of gastric ulceration or gastric varices precludes PEG placement.

Decision to proceed with PEG and preprocedure evaluation

The pre-procedure evaluation in most centers has evolved with time and may vary with indication and vary between centers. For example, in a well-nourished neurologically impaired child who is having a PEG tube placed for medication administration only, a preoperative evaluation for reflux may not be indicated. In the same child, who has severe vomiting and failure to thrive, additional testing including 24–48 hour pH or impedance probe testing, modified barium swallow and motility testing may be indicated preoperatively to determine if a simultaneous anti-reflux procedure is indicated. Open gastrostomy is associated with a significantly increased risk of severe postoperative GER compared to PEG insertion. (Odds ratio 6–7:1) Potential contributing factors include alteration of the angle of His, and reduced LES pressure by an open gastrostomy. In our center, the standard evaluation prior to PEG includes an Upper GI X-ray to exclude malrotation and to identify if part of the stomach is located below the rib cage. In an adult series from Taiwan, preprocedure PEG site marking by air insufflation and KUB the day prior to PEG insertion, has been reported as a method to identify the optimal PEG position. Using that technique, the optimal PEG position was in the left upper quadrant in approximately 60% of patients. To date, use of that technique has not been reported in children.

In patients who are having PEGs placed for feeding, we prefer if medically possible, to do a trial of outpatient nasogastric (NG) feedings for approximately ten days prior to placement of the PEG tube. Patients who are intolerant of NG feeds can undergo additional evaluation for an antireflux procedure. Patients who tolerate the feedings generally gain weight and improve their nutritional status prior to the operative procedure. Three important considerations are: PEG tubes do not prevent aspiration in a patient with oral pharyngeal dysphagia who continues oral feedings, if the stomach is completely under the rib cage a PEG is unlikely to be successfully placed, and like NG tubes, PEG tubes can be pulled out.

Technique

Personnel

In most pediatric centers, two physicians perform PEGs; one performs the endoscopic and the other the abdominal portion of the procedure, including catheter insertion. In our center, two pediatric gastroenterologists do this. In some centers, the procedure may be performed in conjunction with a pediatric surgeon or with an interventional radiologist. Insertion of a PEG tube is an advanced endoscopic procedure, with a higher rate of associated complications and the performing physicians must be able to recognize if the procedure is proceeding in a nonstandard fashion, and be able to make rapid adjustments or terminate the procedure if necessary.

Patient preparation

Patients should be NPO prior to the procedure. Administration of preoperative antibiotics with good coverage for skin flora and two additional peri-/postoperative doses has been shown to decrease the incidence of postoperative wound infections. The abdomen should be prepared and draped as for a standard operative procedure. Due to the lack of anticipated patient cooperation in pediatric patients, the type of pull technique that we utilize, and the need for airway protection, we generally perform this procedure utilizing a general anesthetic or sedation provided by a pediatric intensivist, although some centers utilize conscious or "deep" sedation. Deep sedation has been reported to be successful even in children with underlying congenital heart disease. Ideally, the patient is positioned in the supine position for the procedure.

Technique

Working as a team, the endoscopist will pass the appropriate-sized endoscope to fill the greater curvature of the stomach without intubating the pylorus. Excessive air insufflation (insufflation which significantly flattens the gastric rugae or results in visible abdominal distension) should be avoided as this may distend the small bowel loops, and interfere with the gastric indentation. The other physician, who is "sterile" throughout the procedure, will then perform finger indentation to identify an impression along the anterior gastric wall, preferably away from the gastric cardia and located near the junction of the gastric body and the antrum. (Figure 6.16) The indentation should be perpendicular to the anterior gastric wall to avoid entering the stomach inferiorly, which may increase the risk of entering the colon or its mesentery. The indentation should also be away from the costal margin as tubes placed too close to the ribs can be associated with significant pain.

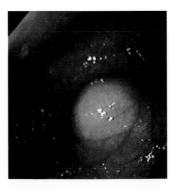

Figure 6.16 Finger indentation of the anterior gastric wall prior to trocar.

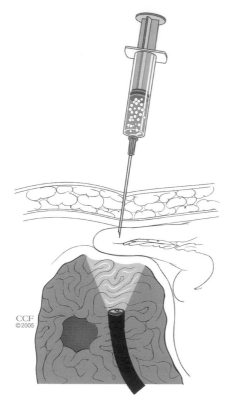

CCF
©2005

Figure 6.17 Schematic representation of the safe tract technique. In this case, a loop of bowel is present between the anterior gastric wall and the anterior abdominal wall. On occasion, this can be identified during the procedure by noting air bubbles in the syringe, *without* the endoscopist seeing the cannula in the gastric lumen. The trocar should be removed and repositioned to an alternate site, or the procedure should be converted to an open gastrostomy.

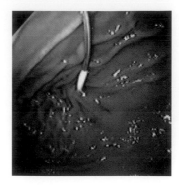

Figure 6.18 Placement of the blue guidewire through the catheter. A sufficient length of guidewire should be passed through the catheter to grasp with the endoscopic forceps.

After identification of a good impression, the sterile physician will inset a 25G or 21G needle attached to a syringe usually filled with 1% lidocaine solution to test the tract identified by the gastric indentation. This needle should pass into the stomach under the direct vision of the endoscopist in the same length as the anticipated internal length of the PEG tube. Failure to see passage of the needle into the stomach when it is inserted to its hub suggests that repositioning of the PEG site is necessary or that there is an intervening organ such as colon or bowel mesentery. One per cent lidocaine is injected with needle withdrawal. Some endoscopists will watch for bubbling of air in the syringe which is pulled back slightly during

needle insertion. This is known as the "safe tract" technique (Figure 6.17). Visualized air bubbling prior to the endoscopist seeing the needle in the stomach may indicate an intervening loop of bowel, which can result in complications as described below.

After a good site is identified, the sterile physician will make a small incision in the anterior abdominal wall at the site of catheter insertion. This is usually transverse and should be through the skin and large enough to allow passage of the PEG tube, but not large enough to require suturing. On occasion, this incision will need to be extended during the pull aspect of the PEG, if not initially large enough to allow the catheter to be pulled through the anterior abdominal wall. Too small an incision and, therefore, too tight a catheter increases the risk of postoperative wound infection and development of granulation tissue.

Under direct endoscopic vision, the sterile physician will then repeat the angiocatheter insertion using the same technique although usually with a larger size (14G) cannula/catheter, that will accommodate passage of the guidewire. As soon as the catheter is visualized in the stomach, the endoscopist passes biopsy forceps or a snare through the biopsy port in order to grasp the guidewire, which the sterile physician is simultaneously passing via the cannula through the anterior abdominal wall. (Figure 6.18) Preferential use of forceps versus a snare is at the discretion of the endoscopist. The sterile physician should hold the catheter carefully at all times until the endoscopist secures the guidewire. Once the guidewire is secured, the procedure can almost always be safely completed, but accidental dislodgement of the cannula prior to guidewire insertion can result in a free perforation or other complications. For smaller endoscopes with a 2.0 mm channel, guide wires are grasped utilizing small forceps. Small sized alligator forceps are also available. For standard endoscopes with a 2.8 mm channel, the guidewire can be grasped using standard forceps, foreign body forceps such as alligator or rat tooth forceps or a polypectomy snare. Some endoscopists elect to position an open snare around the expected entrance of the cannula into the stomach to facilitate grasping of the guidewire.

On occasion, a portion of the cannula is seen in the stomach but not enough that the endoscopist feels comfortable with the length of the cannula in the stomach, or the cannula may be seen coming up through the lower esophageal sphincter into the esophagus in very small patients, or across to the posterior gastric wall. The endoscopist can use very gentle endoscopic traction to reduce tenting of the gastric wall on the cannula, which will allow advancement of the cannula safely into the stomach without through and through placement. Additional air insufflation, immediately prior to catheter puncture, may also help if the gastric indentation is not optimal.

After the endoscopist grasps the guidewire, the guidewire and endoscope are withdrawn through the esophagus and out of the mouth. After withdrawal, the endoscopist will attach the PEG catheter to the guidewire. If using a looped guidewire, it is optimally attached at the very tip of the loop. The endoscopist will then guide the well-lubricated catheter down the patient's mouth and into the esophagus, while the sterile physician is pulling the catheter gently through the anterior abdominal wall. There may be some resistance when the guidewire catheter knot reaches the abdominal wall. In this case, slightly extending the incision may facilitate passage through the wall, and circular rotation of the guidewire, with steady traction by the sterile physician, will facilitate this maneuver. In the off-chance that the guidewire breaks as it is coming through the abdominal wall, hemostats can be used to bring the guidewire and catheter through the abdominal wall. Excessive traction should be avoided especially in small, malnourished or immunocompromised patients, as there have been reports of catheters being pulled entirely through the abdominal wall.

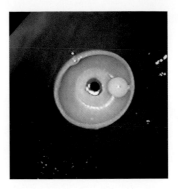

Figure 6.19 Internal view of a PEG tube along the anterior gastric wall. The particular tube used has a nondeflatable internal disc, which acts as the internal bolster.

The endoscopist will verify the position of the PEG tube and the length to the skin (Figure 6.19). If excessive length to the skin is present (i.e. 5–6 cm in a small child) the endoscopist should consider that something might be trapped between the stomach and the anterior abdominal wall. Most PEG tube lengths will be similar to standard gastrostomy button lengths, which pediatric gastroenterologists are used to estimating. If endoscopic biopsies are required, they are usually obtained at this point of the procedure after the PEG tube is secure.

An external bumper secures the PEG, leaving adequate room (usually at least 1 cm) between the external bolster and the skin to allow for swelling in the immediate perioperative period. The incision is dressed with antibiotic ointment, and additional intravenous antibiotics are administered in the postoperative period, usually for two additional doses. The tubes can generally be used within 6–24 hours. Early initiation of post-PEG feedings is not associated with an increased complication rate but may be associated with higher gastric residual volumes. Typically, we initiate feedings with a clear liquid such as a balanced electrolyte solution prior to initiation of formula feedings. Feedings are advanced, based on the individual patient's tolerance.

Consideration should be given to aborting the procedure if any of the following are identified or occur: failure to identify a good gastric impression, excess angiocatheter length without seeing the tip in the stomach, air bubbling in the needle syringe without seeing the tip in the stomach, gastric varices or significant ulceration, identification of fecal matter at any point during the procedure.

Laparoscopic assisted PEG (lap PEG)

This modification of the traditional PEG procedure is performed by a team usually consisting of a pediatric surgeon and a pediatric gastroenterologist. This technique may offer advantages in cases where identification of an ideal location of the PEG is anticipated to be difficult. This may include patients with prior abdominal surgery where adhesions are anticipated or in patients with a VP shunt. Air insufflation of the stomach may be performed prior to CO_2 insufflation of the abdomen to avoid abdominal overdistension. Utilization of the lap PEG allows the surgeon to take down adhesions and identify any intervening organs such as the colon, prior to PEG insertion. Once the abdomen is cleared, and an ideal location is identified, the PEG portion of the procedure proceeds as described earlier.

Post procedure management

Generally, we do not change catheters within 6 weeks of the procedure, and preferably wait at least 2 months after placement, to allow for tract maturation, although percutaneous replacement of PEG tubes following accidental dislodgement has been reported within a couple of weeks of placement. Because traction removal of catheters may be uncomfortable for children, and traumatic to the tract, and because we use a catheter with an internal bumper equivalent, we prefer to change them under anesthesia. We re-endoscope the patient at the time of catheter change, and cut and retrieve the catheter. The internal aspect of the catheter, once cut, is usually retrieved using alligator forceps or a small snare. Removal with the long axis of the cut PEG tube parallel to the axis of the esophagus rather than perpendicular is preferred, especially in smaller patients or with larger PEG tubes. Cutting the PEG tube as close to the skin as possible, thereby leaving a shorter internal portion to be retrieved, facilitates removal. We do not cut the bumper and allow it to pass, as intestinal obstruction, impaction, perforation and migration into the esophagus with subsequent tracheoesophageal fistula and other complications have been reported with cut and un-retrieved bumpers.

We also endoscopically visualize placement of the new gastrostomy button at the time of initial conversion from a PEG tube. If the button is placed in the tract but is not visualized in the stomach, there may be a false tract or a portion of the colon or small bowel may have been trapped between the PEG tube and the abdominal wall, and the "g-tube" button may be located in the colon, small bowel or mesentery. Surgical consultation is appropriate at this point.

Complications

Complications of PEG placement can be minor, major, early or late. New and unusual complications continue to be reported. Rates in the literature vary but are generally in the range of 5–30%. Some are preventable with appropriate antibiotic prophylaxis, good endoscopic/percutaneous technique, and recognition by the physicians performing the procedure that things are not going well, with a decision to abort the procedure and proceed with an open gastrostomy. Sometimes, as with percutaneous liver biopsy, complications are unavoidable due to patient anatomy or underlying disease and the possibility of these complications should be discussed with parents prior to the endoscopic procedure.

Reported minor complications which can become major complications include: cellulitis, uncomplicated pneumoperitoneum, tube defects/disconnection, GER, granulation tissue at insertion site, and pain at the insertion site.

Reported major complications include: gastrocolic fistula, gastroileal fistula, gastro-colo-ileal cutaneous fistula, intrahepatic placement, duodenal hematoma, complicated pneumoperitoneum, aspiration, peritonitis, catheter complications including migration, buried bumper syndrome (Figures 6.20–22), partial gastric separation, catheter/ bumper impaction if not retrieved, intussusception secondary to catheter migration, VP Shunt infection, gastric or bowel perforation, gastric or bowel volvulus and death.

Late complications include: gastrocolic fistula, gastroileal fistula, catheter migration/buried bumper syndrome/partial gastric separation, gastric ulceration, cellulitis, fasciitis, gastric or bowel perforation, catheter migration or other catheter related complications, bronchoesophageal fistula (following removal), and aortic perforation (following cut and pass technique).

PEG tubes in children are not associated with a higher rate of subsequent revision, when com-

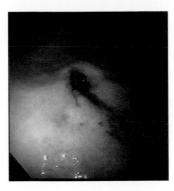

Figure 6.20 Buried bumper syndrome. The gastrostomy bumper is no longer in the stomach, but the impression of the bumper is seen within the abdominal wall. (Courtesy of George Gershman, MD)

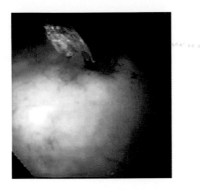

Figure 6.21 The gastrostomy tube is buried in the abdominal wall, although the stoma remains open. This was confirmed by injection of small amount of saline.

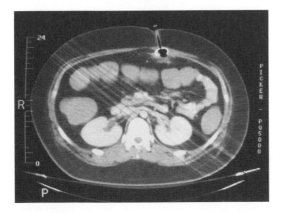

Figure 6.22 CT scan of the abdomen showing the extra-gastric location of a gastrostomy tube in a patient with buried bumper syndrome. (Courtesy of George Gershman, MD)

pared to surgically placed open gastrostomy tubes, if tube revisions due to unrecognized bowel perforation at initial PEG placement are excluded.

Once enteral access is no longer required, the gastrostomy tube or button can be removed and the gastrostomy site can be allowed to close on its own. Typically, this occurs over a period of several weeks. In some cases, a chronic gastrocutaneous fistula remains patent. This appears to occur in 5–30% of cases depending on the series.

Identified risk factors for chronic patent gastrocutaneous fistula include longer duration of gastrostomy use. In this circumstance we have utilized either endoscopic clipping, fibrin glue injection or surgical closure to close the g-tube site.

New uses of the PEG technique

Innovative pediatric and adult gastroenterologists and surgeons have further modified the techniques of PEG. Utilizing modifications of the PEG technique, tubes can be placed directly in the jejunum (DPEJ or PEJ) for feeding and in the cecum (PEC) for antegrade colonic enemas. The DPEJ technique currently has limited applicability in young children due to equipment and size limitations but has been reported in a small series of pediatric patients. If larger series confirm earlier reported success with PECs, this is likely to become an increasingly reported technique in children with neurologic abnormalities and developmental abnormalities resulting in chronic constipation.

Conclusions

PEGs are being increasingly utilized in pediatric patients. Placement of a PEG tube does not increase the incidence of postoperative gastro-esophageal reflux and does not interfere with subsequent gastric surgery. PEG placement is an advanced endoscopic procedure associated with a higher rate of complications than standard esophagogastroduodenoscopy. Placement of PEGs in children, requires modification of the technique used in adults due to size and anatomic considerations and also due to different anticipated duration of use. The key points of the safe technique of the PEG placement are summarized in Table 6.1.

Table 6.1 Tricks of the trade

1. This a procedure that is best done quickly. Once the endoscopic portion of the procedure starts, it is usually accomplished by an experienced team within approximately 10 minutes. Longer procedures are associated with excessive air insufflation which make identifying the gastric impression more difficult and may increase the risk of distending the small bowel or colon with air and, therefore, interposing a loop of bowel between the stomach and the anterior gastric wall, with its resultant complications.

2. If things aren't going well in terms of positioning, the PEG tube should not be placed. There may be something – liver, bowel, mesentery etc., between the trocar and the anterior gastric wall. Unless the liver has been punctured these complications are usually self-limited if the angiocatheter/ trocar is removed and the PEG is not placed.

3. If significant bleeding occurs, or stool is visualized, at any point surgical consultation is appropriate.

4. When faced with a patient with atypical anatomy (cardiac surgery patients; patients with a scoliosis etc.,) the PEG may require placement in a nonstandard position. (i.e. right side of the abdomen in a patient with situs inversus) The endoscopic technique should be similar to standard procedure. Avoid location selection by formulas (i.e. 1/3 the distance between . . .) Pick the location that is best based on the individual patient's anatomy.

Nasojejunal and gastrojejunal tube placement

A nasoduodenal or a Nasojejunal tube feeding is commonly used in children with severe gastro-esophageal reflux as a bridge nutritional therapy before surgery or nutritional support for critically ill children with various conditions in intensive care units.

An enteral tube may be placed endoscopically if other options such as spontaneous passage or installation under fluoroscopy with the use of a radiopaque guide wire have failed.

After the appropriate tube is chosen, it should be prepared by placing one silk suture at the tip. The patient is sedated and put in the left lateral decubitus position. First, the tube should be inserted into the stomach via the nose, followed by the endoscope. The tube may be found either conveniently positioned along the greater curvature of the stomach pointing to the antrum or coiled in the gastric body. In the second scenario, it is pulled back until the tip is visible. The tube with an internal guidewire can be advanced forward if it is not coiled. The smooth surface of the antrum and lack of mucosal folds simplifies grasping of the silk string. Regular biopsy forceps are preferable to use for grasping because it

usually eliminates sticking of the suture to the grasper and accidental dislodgement of the tube from the duodenum or jejunum back to the stomach during withdrawal of the forceps. Significant friction between the scope and the feeding tube creates a passive engagement of the nasoduodenal or nasojejunal tube when the shaft is advanced towards the pylorus. Therefore, the external part of the tube should be secured to prevent excessive insertion and coiling of the tube in the stomach.

Once the regular forceps grasp the silk suture, it is dragged through the biopsy channel to align the feeding tube with the tip of the scope. The shaft of the endoscope is maneuvered through the pylorus into the distal duodenum or proximal jejunum in a standard fashion. Then, the forceps are pushed forward a few centimeters while the shaft is simultaneously pulled back the same distance. These "exchange" sequences are repeated until the tip of the scope is drawn back to the antrum. A view of the forceps and the tube engaging through the pylorus is reassuring that the exchange procedure has been performed successfully. After that, the biopsy forceps are opened to release the string attached to the tube and pulled back into the stomach and closed before complete removal. Finally, the shaft is pulled out using the side-to-side gentle rolling technique to decrease friction and accidental dragging of the feeding tube back into the stomach. The position of the tube along the lesser curvature is ideal (Figure 6.23).

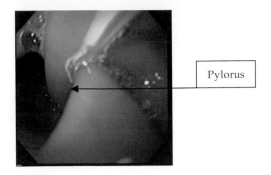

Pylorus

Figure 6.23 Nasojejunal tube. The adequate position of the tube is achieved: the distal part of the tube is in the duodenum while the rest of the tube is properly positioned in the stomach.

Simple postprocedure flat abdominal film or fluoroscopy confirms the appropriate position of the feeding tube.

A similar technique can be used for the placement of the gastroduodenenal or gastrojejunal feeding tube in children with an established gastrostomy. The only difference is the introduction of the feeding tube into the stomach through the gastrostomy.

Alternatively, nasojejunal intubation can be performed with the so-called over-the-wire method. First, a pediatric gastroduodenoscope or colonoscope is inserted into the distal duodenum or the proximal jejunum. Then, a Teflon-coated guidewire is placed in the biopsy channel and advanced a few centimeters beyond the tip of the scope. The next step involves synchronous withdrawal of the shaft and insertion of the guidewire until the endoscope is withdrawn completely. A soft lubricated tube is advanced into the oropharynx through the nose and blindly removed from the mouth using the index finger or with the help of a plastic grasper. After that, a guidewire is inserted into the tube and rerouted through the nose.

After insertion of the guidewire, the protective tube is removed. The final stage of the procedure is performed under fluoroscopy. A lubricated nasojejunal tube is advanced along the guidewire into the distal duodenum or proximal jejunum, after which the position of the guidewire and the enteral tube is adjusted under fluoroscopy.

📖 FURTHER READING

Abd El-Hamid N, Taylor RM, Marinello D, *et al.* (2008) Aetiology and management of extrahepatic portal vein obstruction in children: King's College Hospital experience. *Journal of Pediatric Gastroenterology & Nutrition*, **47**, 630–634.

Almendinger N, Hallisey MJ, Markowitz SK, *et al.* (1996) Balloon dilatation of the esophageal strictures in children. *Journal of Pediatric Surgery*, **31**, 334–336.

American Society for Gastrointestinal Endoscopy. ASGE guide-line, the role of endoscopy in acute non-variceal upper-GI hemorrhage. (2004) *Gastrointestinal Endoscopy*, **60**, 497–504.

Arana A, Hauser B, Hachimi-Idrissi, *et al.* (2001) Management of ingested foreign bodies in childhood and review of the literature. *European Journal of Pediatrics*, **160**, 468–472.

Avitsland TL, Kristensen C, Emblem R, *et al.* (2006) Percutaneous endoscopic gastrostomy in children: a safe technique with major symptom relief and high parental satisfaction. *Journal of Pediatric Gastroenterology & Nutrition*, **43**(5), 624–628.

Boyle JT, Cohen S, Watkins JB. (1981) Successful treatment of achalasia in childhood by pneumatic dilatation. *Journal of Pediatrics*, **99**, 35–40.

Berquist WE, Byrne WJ, Ament ME, *et al.* (1983) Achalasia: diagnosis, management, and clinical course in 16 children. *Pediatrics*, **71**, 798–805.

British Society of Gastroenterology Endoscopy Committee. (2002) Non-variceal upper gastrointestinal haemorrhage: guidelines. *Gut*, **51**(Supp IV), iv1–iv6.

Chaer RA, Rekkas D, Trevino J, *et al.* (2003) Intrahepatic placement of a PEG tube. *Gastrointestinal Endoscopy*, **57**(6), 763–765.

Chang WK, McClave SA, Yu CY, *et al.* (2007) Positioning a safe gastric puncture point before percutaneous endoscopic gastrostomy. *International Journal of Clinical Practice*, **61**(7), 1121–1125.

Charoniti I, Theodoropoulu A, Vardas E, *et al.* (2007) Combination of adrenaline injection and detachable snare application as hemostatic preventive measures before polypectomy of large colonic polyps in children. *Digestive Diseases and Sciences*, **52**, 3381–3382.

Duche M, Habes D, Roulleau P, *et al.* (2008) Prophylactic endoscopic sclerotherapy of large esophageal varices in infants with biliary atresia. *Gastrointestinal Endoscopy*, **67**, 732–737.

Ebina K, Kato S, Abukawa D, *et al.* (1997) Endoscopic hemostasis of bleeding duodenal ulcer in a child with Henoch-Schonlein purpura. *Journal of Pediatrics*, **131**, 934–936.

Ferguson CB, Mitchell RM. (2006) Non-variceal upper gastrointestinal bleeding. *Ulster Medical Journal*, **75**(1), 32–39.

Fortunato JE, Troy AL, Cuffari C, *et al.* (2010) Outcome after percutaneous endoscopic gastrostomy in children and young adults. *Journal of Pediatric Gastroenterology & Nutrition*, **50**(4), 390–393.

Fox VL, Carr-Locke DL, Karrer FM, *et al.* (1995) Endoscopic ligation of esophageal varices in children. *Journal of Pediatric Gastroenterology & Nutrition*, **20**, 202–208.

George DE, Dokler M. (2002) Percutaneous Endoscopic Gastrostomy in Children. *Techniques in Gastrointestinal Endoscopy*, **4**(4), 201–206.

Gershman G, Ament ME, Vargas J. (1997) Frequency and medical management of esophageal perforation after pneumatic dilatation in achalasia. *Journal of Pediatric Gastroenterology & Nutrition*, **25**, 548–553.

Gharpure V, Meert KL, Sarnaik AP, *et al.* (2000) Indicators of postpyloric feeding tube placement in children. *Critical Care Medicine*, **28**, 2962–2966.

Gun F, Salman T, Abbasoglu L, *et al.* (2003) Safety-pin ingestion in children: a cultural fact. *Pediatric Surgery International*, **19**, 482–484.

Hammond PD, Moore DJ, Davidson GP, *et al.* (1997) Tandem balloon dilatation for childhood achalasia. *Pediatric Radiology*, **27**, 609–613.

Hassall E, Berquist WE, Ament ME, *et al.* (1989) Sclerotherapy for extrahepatic portal hypertension in childhood. *Journal of Pediatrics*, **115**, 69–74.

Jacobson K, Phang M, *et al.* (2005) Endoscopic hemostasis in a neonate with a bleeding duodenal ulcer. *Journal of Pediatric Gastroenterology & Nutrition*, **41**, 244–246.

Jensen DM, Matchicado GA. (2002) Principles, technical guidelines, and results of arterial hemostasis with coagulation probes. In: Classen M, Tytgart GNJ, Lightdale C, (Eds) *Gastroenterological Endoscopy*. pp. 274–283, Thieme, Stuttgart.

Kay MH, Wyllie R. (2005) Pediatric foreign bodies and their management. *Current Gastroenterology Reports*, **7**, 212–218.

Kay MH, Wyllie R. (2007) Therapeutic endoscopy for nonvariceal gastrointestinal bleeding. *Journal of Pediatric Gastroenterology & Nutrition*, **45**, 157–171.

Khan S, Orenstein SR, Di Lorenzo C, *et al.* (2003) Eosinophilic esophagitis: Strictures, impactions, dysphagia. *Digestive Diseases and Sciences*, **48**, 22–29.

Khan K, Scharzemberg SJ, Sharp H, *et al.* (2003) Argon plasma coagulation: clinical experience in pediatric patients. *Gastrointestinal Endoscopy*, **57**, 110–112.

Kirby DF, Delegge MH, Fleming C. (1995) American Gastroenterological Association technical review on tube feeding for enteral nutrition. *Gastroenterology*, **108**, 1282–1301.

Lang T, Hummer HP, Behrens R. (2001) Balloon dilatation is preferable to bougienage in children with esophageal atresia. *Endoscopy*, **33**, 329–335.

Lan LCL, Wong KKY, Lin SCL, *et al.* (2003) Endoscopic balloon dilatation of esophageal strictures in infants and children: 17 years' experience and a literature review. *Journal of Pediatric Surgery*, **38**, 1712–1715.

Lee YL, Oh JM, Park SE, *et al.* (2003) Successful treatment of a gastric Dieulafoy's lesion with a hemoclip in a newborn infant. *Gastrointestinal Endoscopy*, **57**, 4356.

Levy H. (1998) Nasogastric and nasoenteric feeding tubes. *Gastrointestinal Endoscopic Clinics of North America*, **8**, 529–549.

Livovitz T, Schmitz BF. (1992) Ingestion of cylindrical and button batteries: an analysis of 2382 cases. *Pediatrics*, **89**, 747–757.

Lyons KA, Brilli RJ, Wieman RA, *et al.* (2002) Continuation of transpyloric feeding during feeding of mechanical ventilation and tracheal extubation in children: a randomized controlled trial. *Journal or Parenteral and Enteral Nutrition*, **26**, 209–213.

McCarter TL, Condon SC, Aguilar RC, *et al.* (1998) Randomized prospective trial of early versus delayed feeding after percutaneous endoscopic gastrostomy placement. [see comment]. *American Journal of Gastroenterology*, **93**(3), 419–421.

Maves MD, Carithers JS, Birck HG. (1984) Esophageal burns secondary to disk battery ingestion. *Annals of Otology Rhinology & Laryngology*, **93**, 364–369.

Mayberry JF, Mayell MJ. (1988) Epidemiological study of achalasia in children. *Gut*, **29**, 90–93.

Meert KL, Daphtary KM, Metheny NA. (2004) Gastric vs small-bowel feeding in critically ill children receiving mechanical ventilation. *Chest*, **126**, 872–878.

Moore FA, Feliciano DV, Andrassy RJ, *et al.* (1992) Early enteral feeding, compared with parenteral, reduces postoperative septic complications: the results of meta-analysis. *Annals of Surgery*, **216**, 172–183.

Mougenot JF. (2009) Endoscopic therapy for variceal and non-variceal bleeding. *Archives of French Pediatrics*, **16**, 805–7 French.

Myers NA, Jolley SG, Taylor R. (1994) Achalasia of the cardia in children: a world survey. *Journal of Pediatric Surgery*, **29**, 1375–1379.

Olives JP. (2000) Ingested foreign bodies. *Journal of Pediatric Gastroenterology & Nutrition*, **31**[supple], s188.

Panigrahi H, Shreeve DR, Tan WC *et al.* (2002) Role of antibiotic prophylaxis for wound infection in percutaneous endoscopic gastrostomy (PEG): result of a prospective double-blind randomized trial. *Journal of Hospital Infection*, **50**(4), 312–315.

Patrick PG, Marulendra S, Kirby DF, *et al.* (1997) Endoscopic nasogastric-jejunal feeding tube placement in critically ill patients. *Gastrointestinal Endoscopy*, **45**, 72–76.

Pineiro-Carrero VM, Sullivan CA, Rogers PL. (2001) Etiology and treatment of achalasia in the pediatric age group. *Gastrointestinal Endoscopy Clinics of North America*, **11**(2), 387–408.

Pobiel RS, Bisset GS III, Pobiel MS. (1994) Nasojejunal feeding tube placement in children: four years cumulative experience. *Radiology*, **190**, 127–129.

Podas T, Eaden J, Mayberry M, *et al.* (1998) Achalasia: a critical review of epidemiological studies. *American Journal of Gastroenterology*, **93**, 2345–2347.

Raval MV, Campbell BT, Phillips JD. (2004) Case of missing penny: thoracoscopic removal of a mediastinal coin. *Journal of Pediatric Surgery*, **39**, 1758–1760.

Rivet C, Robles-Medranda C, Durmotier J, *et al.* (2009) Endoscopic treatment of gastroesophageal varices in young infants with cyanoacrylate glue: a pilot study. *Gastrointestinal Endoscopy*, **69**, 1034–1038.

Sandgren K, Malmfors G. (1998) Balloon dilatation of esophageal strictures in children. *European Journal of Pediatric Surgery*, **8**, 9–11.

Schrag SP, Sharma R, Jaik NP, *et al.* (2007) Complications related to percutaneous endoscopic gastrostomy (PEG) tubes. A comprehensive clinical review. *Journal of Gastrointestinal & Liver Diseases*, **16**(4), 407–418.

Segal D, Michaud L, Guimber D, *et al.* (2001) Late-onset complications of percutaneous endoscopic gastrostomy in children. *Journal of Pediatric Gastroenterology & Nutrition*, **33**(4), 495–500.

Sharieff GQ, Brousseau TJ, Bradshaw JA, *et al.* (2003) Acute esophageal coin ingestions: is immediate removal necessary? *Pediatric Radiology*, **33**, 859–863.

Stark SP, Sharpe JN, Larson GM. (1991) Endoscopically placed nasoenteral feeding tubes: indications and technique. *The American Journal of Surgery*, **4**, 203–205.

Strong RM, Condon SC, Solinger MR, *et al.* (1992) Equal aspiration rates from postpylorus and intragastric-placed small-bore nasoenteric feeding tubes: a randomized, prospective study. *Journal of Parenteral and Enteral Nutrition*, **16**, 59–63.

Srinivasan R, Fisher RS. (2000) Early initiation of post-PEG feeding: do published recommendations affect clinical practice? *Digestive Diseases & Sciences*, **45**(10), 2065–2068.

Tanaka J, Yamashita M, Yamashita M, *et al.* (1998) Esophageal electrochemical burns due to button type lithium batteries in dogs. *Veterinary & Human Toxicology*, **40**, 193–196.

Taylor AL, Carroll TA, Jakubowski J, *et al.* (2001) Percutaneous endoscopic gastrostomy in patients with ventriculoperitoneal shunts. *British Journal of Surgery*, **88**(5), 724–727.

Tsoi KKF, Chiu PWY, Sung JJ. (2009) Endoscopy for upper gastrointestinal bleeding: is routine second-look necessary? *National Reviews of Gastroenterology & Hepatology*, **6**, 717–722.

Vervloessem D, van Leersum F, Boer D, *et al.* (2009) Percutaneous endoscopic gastrostomy (PEG) in children is not a minor procedure: risk factors for major complications. *Seminars in Pediatric Surgery*, **18**(2), 93–97.

Virnig DJ, Frech EJ, DeLegge MH, *et al.* (2008) Direct percutaneous endoscopic jejunostomy: a case series in pediatric patients. *Gastrointestinal Endoscopy*, **67**(6), 984–987.

Yardeny D, Yardeny H, Coran AG, *et al.* (2004) Severe esophageal damage due to button battery ingestion: can it be prevented? *Pediatric Surgery International*, **20**, 496–501.

Wyllie R. (2004) Changing the tube: a pediatrician's guide. *Current Opinions in Pediatrics*, **16**(5), 542–544.

Zargar SA, Lavid G, Khan BA, *et al.* (2002) Endoscopic ligation compared with sclerotherapy for bleeding esophageal varices in children with extrahepatic portal venous obstruction. *Hepatology*, **36**, 666–72.

7

Pediatric colonoscopy

George Gershman

KEY POINTS

- Modern colonoscopy is a procedure which combines examination of the entire colon and the terminal ileum, i.e. can be also named as ileocolonoscopy.
- Pediatric colonoscopy is a safe and high yield procedure if performed by a well trained pediatrics gastroenterologist.
- Pediatric colonoscopy requires an adequate sedation or general anesthesia.

- The good knowledge of embryology, gross and endoscopic anatomy of the large intestine are essential components of effective training.
- The cornerstone of colonoscopy is a prevention of loop formation by torque steering technique and maneuvers which allow an early recognition and elimination of the intestinal loops and proper steering along the colon and the terminal ileum.

Indications for colonoscopy

Traditionally, the indications for colonoscopy are classified based upon the goal of procedure: diagnostic or therapeutic. Over the last decade, a new concept of high-volume low-yield indications has been introduced in adult practice, as colonoscopy has been used as a part of a large-scale screening program for the early diagnosis of colon cancer. A low incidence of this disease in a pediatric population virtually eliminates the need for screening colonoscopy, except for a small group of children with suspected familial adenomatous polyposis or other rare forms of polyposis.

The indications for diagnostic pediatric colonoscopy are focused primarily on clinical symptoms: "red flags" and additional clues of serious pathology of the large intestine and the terminal ileum obtained from radiological and other diagnostic procedures or laboratory tests

(Table 7.1). In addition, surveillance colonoscopy is indicated for teenagers and young adults with 10 or more years' history of inflammatory bowel disease.

Colonoscopy is not indicated for patients with:

1. Acute self-limiting diarrhea.
2. Functional abdominal pain.
3. Irritable bowel syndrome.
4. Constipation with or without fecal impaction.

However, a colonoscopy is reasonable in children with acute onset of colitis and negative cultures for bacterial pathogens and parasites.

Diagnostic colonoscopy is absolutely contraindicated in anyone with fulminant colitis or toxic megacolon, suspected perforated viscous and recent intestinal resection (Table 7.2).

The diagnostic yield of a colonoscopy is low in children with chronic abdominal pain unless other symptoms, such as weight loss, unexplained fever, short stature, chronic diarrhea, presence of rectal fissure or abscess, signs of chronic anemia,

Practical Pediatric Gastrointestinal Endoscopy, Second Edition. George Gershman, Mike Thomson, Marvin Ament.
© 2012 Blackwell Publishing Ltd. Published 2012 by Blackwell Publishing Ltd.

Table 7.1 Indications for colonoscopy

Indications for diagnostic colonoscopy

Lower gastrointestinal bleeding
- Hematochezia
- Fecal occult blood

Unexplained chronic diarrhea

Suspected or established inflammatory bowel disease
- Diagnosis
- Extent of involvement and severity
- Unsatisfactory response to treatment
- Conformation of histological remission
- Surveillance for colorectal cancer in chronic inflammatory bowel disease

Clinical signs of Pseudomembranous colitis but negative results of confirmatory tests

Abnormal CT scan

Family history of polyps or polyposis syndrome

Cancer surveillance
- Ten or more years history of pancolitis
- Polyposis syndromes

Abdominal pain and chronic diarrhea in patients with HIV and other types of immunodeficiency disorders

Clinical signs of post-transplantation lymphoproliferative disorder
Clinical signs of Graft-versus-host disease

Acute or chronic diarrhea in children after small bowel transplantation without evidences or acute rejection

Intraoperative colonoscopy e.g. in children with recurrent intussusception

Indications for therapeutic colonoscopy
- Polypectomy
- Treatment of bleeding angiodysplasia
- Percutaneous colonoscopic cecostomy
- Decompression of acute megacolon (Ogilvie's syndrome) or colonic volvulus
- Balloon dilation of strictures

low serum albumin, elevated ESR or CRP point toward chronic inflammatory bowel disease or other rare disease of the large intestine.

Preparation for colonoscopy

The goal of the bowel cleaning is to create the best condition for visual assessment of the colon and successful intubation of the cecum and the terminal ileum. Small amounts of liquid stool are usually present in the colon, but can be aspirated easily, and do not complicate the procedure. However, a moderate quantity of liquid and hard stool promotes excessive insufflations and stretching of the colon, due to difficulties navigating the scope using the torque screw technique. It may induce pain and agitation and increase demand for additional doses of sedatives and an unjustified deeper level of anesthesia. Elevated intra-abdominal pressure may further

Table 7.2 Contraindications to Colonoscopy

Peritonitis
Conditions with a high risk of preparation • Fulminant colitis • Toxic megacolon • Recent surgical anastomoses
Inability to visualize mucosa • Poor bowel preparation • Massive gastrointestinal bleeding
Associated medical problems • Sepsis • Absolute neutropenia • Respiratory and cardiovascular distress

compromise respiration especially in young children, leading to hypoxia and bradicardia. Finally, an attempt to complete the colonoscopy, despite an inadequately prepared colon, carries an increased risk of perforation. Thus, the colonoscopy should be aborted if the colon is not adequately prepared.

Preparing infants and small children for colonoscopy can be challenging. The major obstacles related to the preparation for a colonoscopy in children are a large volume of laxatives and a restrictive diet. In recent years, a few new products have been tested. The first one is an electrolytes free solution of polyethylene glycol: PEG 3350 (MiraLax, Braintree Lab, Braintree, Mass). This has been used in one or four days preparation regimens. The proposed instruction for a one-day preparation cycle is adjusted to the patient's age.

The PEG 3350 solution is prepared as a mixture of 238 g of polyethylene glycol if purchased over the counter or 255 g if obtained by prescription with 1.9 L of water or commercially available electrolyte solution (e.g. Gatorade 2).

For older children, the suggested volume of PEG 3350 solution is 1.9 L. For children under 2 years of age, the PEG 3350 mixture is recommended to drink until 2 consecutive clear stools.

Children are allowed a regular breakfast and lunch the day before the procedure.

The four days regimen is based on the consumption of PEG 3350 solution (mixture of 17 g per 8 oz of preferred liquid). The recommended dose of PEG 3350 is 1.5 g/kg up to 100 g per day. A clear liquid diet is implemented for the day prior to the colonoscopy.

Both methods produced similar results: adequate preparation was achieved in 93 to 89%, respectively. Nausea and vomiting was reported more frequently with the four days regimen.

Another cleansing regimen consists of sodium picosulfate (stimulant laxative), combined with magnesium oxide and citric acid magnesium (Pico-Salax, Ferring Pharmaceutical Inc., Canada) and liquid diet. Each sachet of Pico-Salax contains 10 mg of sodium picosulphate, 3.5 g of magnesium oxide and 12 g of citric acid. Magnesium oxide and citric acid form magnesium citrate when dissolved in water. According to the manufacture's guidelines, doses of laxatives (per day) are calculated based on the patient's age: ¼ sachet for children from 1 to 6 years of age, ½ sachet per day for children 6 to 12 years of age and 1 sachet for older children from 12 to 18 years of age, for two consecutive days. A liquid diet is recommended during the preparation cycle.

Current data did not reveal a significant difference between Pico-Salax, Magnesium Citrate and PEG 3350 regimens.

Although it is debatable, we do not use anything to cleanse the colon of infants less than 4 months old. It is quite easy to irrigate and aspirate the small amount of liquid and semi-liquid stool during the procedure.

In infants between 4 and 12 months of age, satisfactory results of colonic cleansing could be achieved using a liquid diet and milk of magnesia (1 ml/kg per dose twice a day) for two consecutive days prior to the procedure.

Magnesium citrate can be used in toddlers and older children preparing for colonoscopy. The dose per day is calculated based on patient weight: 2 ounces for children between 10 to 15 kg, 3 ounces for children between 16 and 20 kg, 4 to 5 ounces for children between 21 to 35 kg, and 8 to 10 ounces in children whose weight is more than 35 kg. The other simple way to calculate the dose of magnesium citrate is one ounce per year of age up to 10 ounces. The daily dose is divided in two portions and given for two consecutive days before colonoscopy. It is best given cold and over ice, or mixed with lemon-lime type soft drinks. A combination of picolax ans senokot is also effective given 18 hours and 6 hours pre-procedure.

The night before the colonoscopy, a glycerin suppository can be used to enhance evacuation of the colon.

If a large volume lavage method is chosen, the patient is allowed to eat and drink up until the afternoon of the day before the procedure. The patient is then asked to fast overnight. A lavage solution contains a non-absorbable agent such as polyethylene glycol and electrolytes. Flavored solutions are available.

The cleansing agent (5 to 10 ml/kg up to 250 ml per dose) is given by mouth every ten minutes until the rectal effluent is clear.

There are some adolescents and teenagers who will accomplish this preparation readily. However, hospitalization for 24–48 hours may be necessary for uncooperative patients.

In recent years, serious side-effects of oral Sodium Phosphate colonic lavage in adults have been reported. Among those, were cases of fatal hyperphosphatemia with hypocalcemia, hypokal cemia, dehydration and acute nephrocalcinosis with renal failure.

Limited data related to the oral use of Sodium Phosphate in children and teenagers did not duplicate these side-effects although transient symptomatic hyperphosphotemia and hypocal-cemia in teenagers was reported. In 2007, the major manufacturer of Sodium Phosphate (CB Fleet Co, Lynchburg, VA) had advice against the use of this form of preparation for colonoscopy in children less than 18 years of age. In addition, oral Sodium Phosphate causes nonspecific erosions and histological changes complicating interpreta-tion of endoscopy and biopsy.

Currently, we would not recommend Sodium Phosphate for colonic cleansing in children and teenagers.

Enemas are not routinely used for children, especially those with suspected inflammatory bowel disease as they cause erythema, edema and petechiae of rectal and distal sigmoid mucosa complicating interpretation of endoscopic finding.

Equipment

Different types of slim colonoscopes less than 12 mm are commercially available (Table 7.3).

All of these have an adjustable stiffness mecha-nism and large (3.2 mm and 3.8 mm) biopsy channels, allowing application of all types of accessories, including standard and jumbo biopsy

Table 7.3 Important technical specifications of new slim colonoscopes

	Working Length (mm)	Insertion Tube Diameter (mm)	Biopsy Channel Diameter (mm)
Olympus Co			
PCF-160L	1680	11.5	3.2
PCF-Q180 AL/I*	1680	11.5	3.2
PCF-H180AL/I*	1680	11.8	3.2
Fujinon Co			
EC-450 LS5*	1690	11.1	3.2
EC-250 LP5	1690	11.1	3.2
EC-550 LS5*	1690	11.5	3.8
EC-250 LP5	1690	11.5	3.8
Pentax Co			
EC-3470 FK	1500	11.6	3.8
EC-3470 LK	1700	11.6	3.8
EC-3490Li HD**	1700	11.6	3.8

*High-resolution image and narrow band system.

**High-resolution image system with 2X close focus digital zoom.

forceps, snares, needles, and laser probes. These instruments are optimal for children two years and older.

Colonoscopes specifically designed for infants and toddlers do not exist. Instead, pediatric upper GI video endoscopes can be used. It is more difficult to telescope the sigmoid colon with these instruments, but their smaller diameter prevents excessive stretching of the bowel, especially in infants.

Informed consent and pre procedure preparation

Specific indications, risks and benefits of the colonoscopy are the subject of a detailed discussion with the family. This should leave parents comfortable and confident with the need and safety of the procedure before it is scheduled.

On the day of the procedure informed consent is obtained. The child and parents or guardian, are invited to the pre-procedure area.

In this area, the patient changes clothes and is prepared for intravenous line placement.

In order to minimize the discomfort of a venepuncture, EMLA® cream is applied to one or two potential intravenous sites 60 minutes before the procedure. EMLA® cream should be used with caution in infants because of reports of methemoglobinemia.

Infusion of age-appropriate solution is started once the venous excess is established and secured. The patient is then transferred to the procedure area where all necessary preparations for sedations or general anesthesia are taken care of.

Sedation for Colonoscopy

Pediatric colonoscopy is routinely performed under sedation or general anesthesia. Usually, an anxious and scared child does not allow even digital rectal exam or proper positioning on the bed until deeply sedated. The definition of deep sedation includes:

- patient is responsive only to painful stimuli
- spontaneous breathing
- presence of deep tendon reflexes.

General anesthesia with medication such as Ketamine® or Propofol® is not principally different from deep sedation, but is usually conducted by a pediatric anesthesiologist. In some institutions, pediatric gastroenterologists are certified for deep sedation. The logistics of choice usually depend on the specific policy of the hospital, the availability of an anesthesiologist and the economics of a particular medical practice.

The advantage of general anesthesia with Propofol® is fast induction time, minimal side-effects and short stay in recovery rooms, which is attractive for pediatric gastroenterologists, especially in private practice. It may also decrease the turnover time of each procedure and increase potential revenue. On the other hand, the higher cost of routine colonoscopy under general anesthesia may not be covered by all in North America.

The goal of any sedation for colonoscopy in children is maximal elimination of anxiety and pain during the procedure with minimal risk of complication.

Anxiety is relatively easy to overcome in the majority of children by an appropriate dose of tranquilizers.

However, the pain control and deepness of sedation is a more complex and controversial issue. It is important to realize, that pain during colonoscopy is always related to stretching and distention of the colon, and the degree of pain and discomfort can be reduced by proper technique of colonoscopy. The rule of thumb is: the dose of analgesics and other medications for sedation is inversely related to the skill of the endoscopist.

It is also important to accept that a moaning child under deep sedation is equal to a screaming non-sedated patient. It is typical for a less experienced endoscopist to apply more force to the twisted colon and ignore the warning signs (patient discomfort) and request additional doses of sedatives. This will lead to excessive and even critical stretching of the colon and an unacceptable risk of complications. It is incorrect practice to give an extra dose of sedatives in order to make some progress with bowel intubation. It is good practice, however, to hold intubation and make some adjustments to reduce the loop before further advancement. It is important to accept that not all colonoscopies can be completed, and it is wiser to abort the procedure rather than increase the risk of complications.

The relaxed patient is placed in the left lateral decubitus position. The parents are asked to leave the room once the child is fully sedated.

Embryology of the colon

Abnormal rotation and fixation of the embryonic colon is probably the major reason for a "difficult" colon and incomplete colonoscopy.

The rotation of the primitive large intestine begins when the embryo is only 10 mm long.

It occurs as a result of elongation of the intestinal tube, separation of the yolk stalk and stepwise herniation of the duodenojejunal loop into the umbilical cord.

A counterclockwise rotation around the superior mesenteric artery is the main mechanism of "packaging" the growing intestine in preparation for its return back to the abdomen. At a stage of a 25 mm embryo, almost the entire intestine is within the umbilical cord. When the embryo grows to 40 mm in length, there is enough space in the abdomen to accommodate the small and large intestine.

Additional counterclockwise rotation is again crucial for proper relocation of the intestine into the peritoneal cavity. As a result, the cecum swings to the right hypochondric area above the superior mesenteric artery. At the end of the rotation, the cecum migrates down to the right iliac fossa.

Finally, the mesentery of the descending and ascending colon fuses with the posterior peritoneum and disappears being pushed back by heavy loops of the small bowel. Under normal circumstances, the cecum also does not have a mesentery because it is an out pouching of the antimesenteric aspect of the ascending colon. Its incomplete posterior fixation allows some mobility of the cecum, which does not create any problems for endoscopists, unless the patient has a mobile cecum.

The rectum is derived from the cloacae and fuses with the sigmoid colon by the eighth week of gestation and has some limited mobility. Thus, as a result of a normal rotation, the colon acquires two zones of full fixation: the descending and ascending colon, as well as two areas of partial fixation: the cecum, and rectum. In addition, the mobility of the splenic and hepatic flexure is somewhat limited by a phrenocolic and extension of the hepatorenal ligaments respectively. Only the sigmoid and transverse colons possess their own mesentery and are fully mobile.

It is not surprising, that they became a target of various endoscopic maneuvers preventing or minimizing stretching of these vulnerable segments of the intestine. It is easy to imagine that abnormal rotation or fixation of the embryonic colon can multiply difficulties in telescoping of an unusually mobile bowel.

As a rule, this is a total surprise for the endoscopist. Some of the anomalies can be suspected during a procedure, for example, fixation of the cecum in the right hypochondrium. The intrinsic propensity of the embryonic colon to counterclockwise rotation from the left iliac fossa to the right one gives an important clue to the concept of a torque steering technique of a colonoscopy.

In general, counterclockwise rotation of an endoscope creates some deviations of the sigmoid colon to the right flank of the abdomen. The degree of sigmoid stretching is proportional to the length and plasticity of the attached mesentery and amount of force applied to the colonoscope to push it forward or rotate it counterclockwise. Thus, stretching and looping of the sigmoid colon should be anticipated during counterclockwise rotation of the endoscope. In contrast, clockwise rotations of the endoscope move the colon to the left and help to plicate the sigmoid colon and minimize stretching and loop formation.

Endoscopic Anatomy

The anal canal is less than 2 cm in a newborn, reaching an adult length of 3 cm by 4 years of age. It is normally closed due to a tonic contraction of the anal sphincter. If it is constantly open or if sphincter tone is substantially decreased, spina bifida, trauma or sexual abuse should be ruled out (Figure 7.1). It is important to remember that the axis of the anal canal is pointed anteriorly. Proper insertion of the colonoscope will minimize discomfort eliminating excessive stretching of the anus and prevent imbedding of the tip into the rectal mucosa.

The squamo-columnar junction or pectinate (dentate) line demarcates a proximal edge of the anal canal (Figure 7.2). Few longitudinal folds (the columns of Morgani) run within the anal canal and terminate at anal papillae (Figure 7.3). Occasionally, anal papillae may be quite prominent, cone-like grayish structures. The rectum becomes enlarged and fusiformed between the upper edge of the columns of Morgani and the recto sigmoid junction. This part of the rectum is called an ampulla. It is marked by three semi-lunar folds referred to as valves of Houston (Figure 7.4). There are two such folds on the left and one on the right lateral wall. The ampulla narrows at the level of recto-sigmoid junction, which is distanced from the anal verge by 9 cm in neonates and 15 cm in children 10 years and older. The rectal mucosa is smooth and transparent, which allows good visualization of submucosal veins (Figure 7.5).

Multiple small lymphoid follicles in the rectal mucosa are normally present in infants and

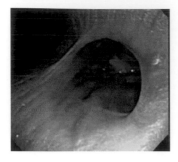

Figure 7.1 Unusually wide-open anus. This finding is suspicious for spina bifida, trauma, or sexual abuse.

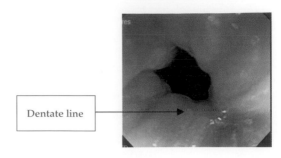

Figure 7.2 Squamocolumnar junction or dentate line.

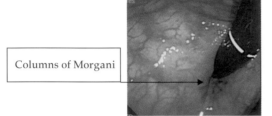

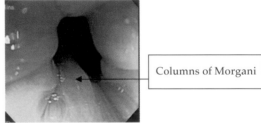

Figure 7.3 The longitudinal folds in the distal rectum (the columns of Morgani) and enlarged anal papilla. The u-turn maneuver in the rectum is useful for detailed observation of the distal rectum close to the anal canal.

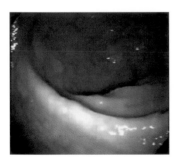

Figure 7.4 Semilunar folds of Houston in the rectum.

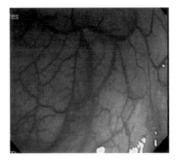

Figure 7.5 Typical vascular pattern of the normal rectum.

toddlers, but when excessive or surrounded by erythema may indicate an allergic colonopathy. The sigmoid colon is the most "unpredictable" part of the colon due to its long, "V"-shape mesocolon. Stretching during colonoscopy could double the length of the sigmoid colon. Therefore, an absolute length of the sigmoid colon is not important unless it is tremendously elongated.

The mobility and displacement of the sigmoid colon may be limited due to previous surgery, adhesions or shortening of the mesentery.

A relatively small sigmoid colon in infants and toddlers has some disadvantages for the endoscopist: First, it decreases the threshold for pain during stretching, and limits the application of standard pediatric colonoscopes, secondary to the relatively large radius of curvature.

Second, it makes it impossible to perform the alpha loop maneuver, leaving no choice but precise telescoping of the sigmoid colon without any room for even small technical mistakes. The normal sigmoid colon appears tubular because of the prominence of a circular muscle layer. The mucosa is less transparent than in the rectum. There are multiple circular folds throughout the sigmoid colon (Figure 7.6).

The taenia coli are not usually visible along the sigmoid colon except on the area adjacent to the sigmoid descending junction. The appearance of taenia coli in this area indicates significant stretching of the sigmoid colon.

During colonoscopy, the sigmoid colon becomes more spiral and twisted clockwise between the rectum and descending colon. The concave sacrum and a forward-projecting sacral promontory determine the initial anterior deviation of the sigmoid loop. At this stage of the procedure, a colonoscope can be palpated easily unless the sigmoid colon is extremely stretched.

In children, a palpable loop can be reduced or modified by the withdrawal maneuver performed by the endoscopist and coordinated pressure applied to the palpable loop by the assistant.

The transition zone between the sigmoid and descending colon is usually located at the level of the pelvic brim. It is artificially angled by the twisted and stretched sigmoid colon. The angle is sharper when the descending colon extends down below the pelvic brim due to an unusually low

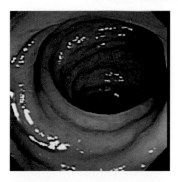

Figure 7.6 The sigmoid colon. The endoscopic markers of normal sigmoid colon are (i) rounded lumen, (ii) circular folds, and (iii) subtle vascular pattern.

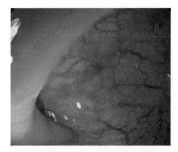

Figure 7.7 The angle is sharper when the descending colon extends down below the pelvic brim due to unusually low fixation and/or when the sigmoid colon was stretched out extensively.

fixation and/or when the sigmoid colon was stretched out extensively (Figure 7.7).

Once the endoscope is passed through the junction between the sigmoid and descending colon, the "surprises" are usually over unless the patient has a lax phrenicocolic ligament or persistent ascending mesocolon. Normally, the descending colon is relatively short, about 10 cm in infants and 20 cm in toddlers. It is slightly wider and more oval than the sigmoid colon (Figure 7.8).

It runs straight up toward the left hypochondrium to join the splenic flexure. The mucosa of the descending colon appears pink or slightly grayish. The stems of the vessels run along folds, i.e. perpendicular to the lumen. The small branches spread around and across the folds (Figure 7.9). It may help to verify the axis of the colon without a panoramic view of the lumen, when pulling back may induce untwisting and escaping the plicated bowel. The folds of the descending colon are spread more apart relative to the folds of the sigmoid colon. The teniae coli are usually not visible.

These minor endoscopic changes help to verify the position of the shaft in the descending colon during the advancing phase of colonoscopy.

The splenic flexure is marked by the bluish color of the transilluminated spleen (Figure 7.10).

This area should occupy the right part of the lumen if the colonoscope was positioned properly inside the sigmoid and descending colon. The same color spot can be seen occasionally when the tip of a colonoscope is trapped within a very large sigmoid loop. Thus, this color mark does not definitively prove that the splenic flexure has been reached. The splenic flexure is firmly attached to the diaphragm by the phrenocolic ligament at the level of 10th and 11th ribs. That could explain

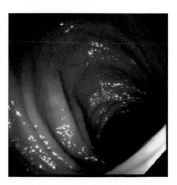

Figure 7.8 The descending colon. The descending colon is oval in shape.

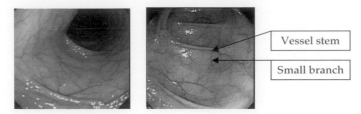

Figure 7.9 The vascular pattern of the descending colon. The stems of the vessels run along folds, i.e., parallel to the lumen. The small branches spread around and across the folds and along the lumen.

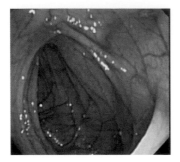

Figure 7.10 The splenic flexure. It is marked by bluish discoloration.

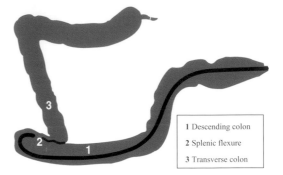

Figure 7.11 The relationship of the angle between the descending colon and the splenic flexure and the position of the patient during colonoscopy. The irregular configuration encountered at the splenic flexure and adjacent descending colon is created by the transverse colon, which is hanging down during colonoscopy when the patient is in the left lateral position.

occasional hiccups and transient hypoxia during exploration of the transverse colon due excessive pressure and irritation of the phrenic nerve especially in infants and young children.

The junction with the transverse colon is located along the upper aspect of the medial wall of the splenic flexure. It is "naturally" angled by the mobile transverse colon, which hangs down from the elevated splenic flexure. The junction is more sharply angled and even folded when the patient is in the left lateral position (Figure 7.11).

The transverse colon is relatively short in children. It is about 14 cm in newborns and 30 cm in 10-year-olds, which is a big help during pediatric colonoscopy. Relatively thin circular rather than the thicker longitudinal layers of the muscularis propria are responsible for the triangular shape of the transverse colon (Figure 7.12). The slope of the transverse colon is pointed toward the hepatic flexure, which is more voluminous than the adjacent colonic segments and has bluegrey color acquired from the neighboring liver (Figure 7.13). The folds are circular at both ends of the hepatic flexure. They are less prominent on the apex.

The junction with the ascending colon is located higher than the adjacent transverse colon. It points toward the right lobe of the liver and is

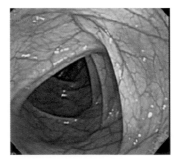

Figure 7.12 The transverse colon. The triangular shape is the endoscopic hallmark of the transverse colon.

sharply angled posteriorly (Figure 7.14). The ascending colon is a short, retroperitoneal and fixed segment of the right colon. It runs between the cecum anteriorly and the lower pole of the right kidney posteriorly. The lumen of the ascend-

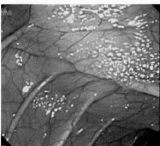

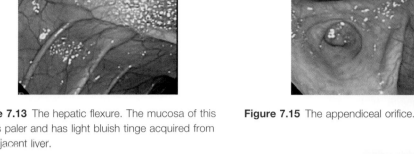

Figure 7.13 The hepatic flexure. The mucosa of this area is paler and has light bluish tinge acquired from the adjacent liver.

Figure 7.15 The appendiceal orifice.

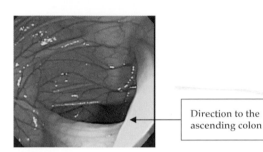

Direction to the ascending colon

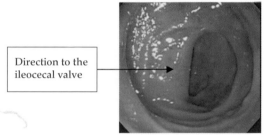

Direction to the ileocecal valve

Figure 7.16 The ileocecal valve. A focal widening of the circular fold in the cecum is the sign of the hiding ileocecal valve.

Figure 7.14 The hepatic flexure. It is dome-shaped. The junction between the hepatic flexure and the ascending colon is always hidden in the right upper corner of the screen behind the mucosal fold. Steering of the shaft counterclockwise, pulling it back, and elevation of the tip help to stretch the folded lumen. Subsequent clockwise rotation and deviation of the tip to the right and decompression of the colon facilitate exploration of the ascending colon.

ing colon is wide and constantly opened. It terminates as a "blind" pouch-cecum, which has two landmarks:

- appendiceal orifice; and
- ileo-cecal valve.

The appendiceal orifice is usually oval or rounded (Figure 7.15), and located at the intersection of the taenia coli.

The ileo-cecal valve is situated at the posterior medial aspect of the cecum. The orifice of the ileo-cecal valve is usually parallel to the axis of a colonoscope. That is why it is only partially seen as a focal widening of the circular fold (Figure 7.16).

In the newborn, the cecum has a cone shape with the appendix in the middle. Later on, the

cecum expands sideways by unequal enlargement of the haustra: a lateral sac becomes more spacious than the medial one. Thus, the cecum assumes an eccentric shape. The wall of the cecum is thinner than the rest of the colon. This should be borne in mind during polypectomy.

Torque steering technique

A special colonoscopy technique has been developed to overcome a high flexibility, elasticity and multiple angulations of the large intestine (the sigmoid colon in particular). The main principle of this technique often called the torque steering technique is a substitution for corkscrew maneuvering around an angled segment of the colon for pushing forward approach, which leads to a loop formation.

The elements of the technique are:

- Rotation around bent colon segments instead of pushing up against them.
- Slow rather than rapid start of each maneuver with a colonoscope.
- Frequent pulling back for shortening the sigmoid and transverse colon and

straightening of twisted segments of the large intestine.

- Prediction rather searching for the lumen.
- Pulling back when orientation is lost.
- Ascertainment of the correct axis of the colon before manipulations with a colonoscope (this is much more important for progress than search for a fully opened lumen).
- Substitution of clockwise or counterclockwise torque and up and down angulations for manipulations with the R/L knob.
- Avoidance of full angulations of the tip while advancing the scope. It will not slide along the colon.
- Anticipation of a spring effect of twisted colon and prevention of spontaneous untwisting of coiled segment by repeated clock and counterclockwise rotations.
- Programed rotation of the lumen: the colon usually moves in the opposite direction to the rotation of a shaft.
- Minimal insufflations: excessive air in the colon makes it ridged and elongated.
- Frequent air suction and infrequent suction of fluid.

Sharing "inherited" similarity, pediatric colonoscopy is not a traditional colonoscopy for a small patient. The most important difference between the techniques used during colonoscopy in adults and children is a low efficacy of an "Alpha" maneuver and a more detrimental effect of a loop formation for children, especially younger ones. The rule of thumb is: the younger the child the more difficult it will be to bypass the sigmoid-descending junction if a big loop occurs.

Handling a colonoscope.

There are two ways to perform a colonoscopy:

- With the endoscopist managing all manipulation with a control panel and the shaft with the left and right hand respectively (one person – single handed approach).
- By the endoscopist working with the control panel and the assistant handling the shaft according to the instruction of the endoscopist (two persons-double handed approach). It is generally accepted, that, one-person single-handed technique is the most effective way to conduct a colonoscopy. The benefits of this approach are:
  - Precise control of an entire colonoscope

- Coordinated activity of the left hand operated up/down control knob and the right hand rotated shaft.
  - Almost instantaneous response to a changing position of the colon.
  - Constant assessment and control of the bowel resistance.
  - An ability to prevent unwinding of the telescoped bowel.

A colonoscope is held similarly to an upper GI videoendoscope (*see* chapter 5).

Ensure a constant grip of the shaft by the right thumb, index and middle finger. The intensity of grip varies from light to firm with continuous rotation. A common mistake of the beginner is to lose hold of a shaft while attempting to use an R/L control knob. The unsecured shaft untwists immediately allowing the bowel to escape from the colonoscope and regain its natural elongated configuration and position. A three-finger rotation technique is the most effective way to torque a colonoscope for a full 360 degrees. An additional 180 degree rotation can be achieved by moving the wrist in clockwise or counterclockwise direction.

If continuous rotation is required, an assistant can hold the shaft while the endoscopist adjusts the grip. Alternatively, the endoscopist moves the control panel secured by the fourth and fifth fingers of the left arm under the shaft and anchors it tightly by the left index and middle fingers, then adjusting the grip of the right hand without "loosening" a telescoped bowel. A colonoscope should be maximally straightened to optimize transmission of rotating force from the control panel to the shaft. It can be achieved by keeping an optimal distance between the child and the endoscopist. One of the most common mistakes of the beginners is holding the shaft too close to the anus. Grasping a colonoscope at the level of 20 to 25 cm from the anus decreases the need for frequent changes of handgrip and facilitates an application of torque and control of rotation.

Position of the patient and insertion technique

Traditionally, colonoscopy is performed with the patient in the left decubitus position. The child's head is resting on a small firm pillow. The arms are relaxed along the torso; the left leg is stretched while the bended right leg is positioned across the left one. It protects the patient from accidentally rolling back or turning prone.

The insertion of the colonoscope into the rectum and control of the shaft is easier when the patient is in the left decubitus rather than the supine position.

There are three disadvantages of the left decubitus position:

- Less precise control of the sigmoid colon, which is easier to palpate and support by hand pressure when the patient is supine.
- The sigmoid colon tends to crumple down toward the left flank making the transition into the descending colon more angled and difficult to bypass.
- The transverse colon flops down and narrows the connection with the splenic flexure.

Thus, a procedure could be started with the child in the left decubitus position then the patient can be turned supine when the sigmoid-descending junction is approached. Alternatively, a supine position can be used from the beginning of colonoscopy in infants, toddlers and preschool children.

Insertion technique

Before insertion, the entire equipment and suction system should be checked for proper function. A gurney is lifted to the most comfortable height for the endoscopist. The distal 20 cm of the shaft is lubricated. A rectal exam prior to the procedure serves two purposes:

- lubrication of the anal canal, and
- reassurance that the patient has been adequately prepared and sedated.

If there are any doubts about the quality of bowel preparation, a rectal exam should be performed before sedation to avoid unnecessary exposure to medication.

The assistant gently lifts up the right buttock to expose the anus. The endoscopist grips the shaft at 20 to 30 cm marks, positions the tip into a gentle contact with the anus and aligns the bending portion of the shaft with the axis of the anal canal, which runs toward anterior abdominal wall. Insufflations of the anal canal and slight clockwise torque of the shaft facilitate sliding of the tip into a distal rectum with minimal pressure. This technique virtually eliminates any discomfort or accidental trauma of the distal rectum. Immediately after initial exploration of the rectum, a colonoscope is pulled back slightly and angled upwards to establish a panoramic view of the rectal ampula.

Any liquid stool can easily be aspirated to simplify the approach to the proximal rectum. Do not aspirate semi-formed stool at the beginning of colonoscopy to avoid clogging of the suction channel. After that, the colonoscope is advanced toward the rectosigmoid area. It is distant from dentate line for about 10 to 15 cm. This is the first but not the last time when the lumen may disappear.

Endoscopic clues of a hidden lumen

To reach the splenic flexure reasonably quickly, it is important to accept the concept that a constant search for a fully opened lumen is not a productive way to conduct a colonoscopy. It creates more problems than benefits for the endoscopist and the patient. First of all, it is not possible because many segments of the colon, especially the sigmoid colon, are sharply angulated. Second, a long opened upstream segment of the sigmoid colon indicates a big loop formation and should be avoided. Third, an extensive search for a fully open lumen leads to over-inflation of the colon, which makes it ridged and elongated. Distention of the colon induces discomfort and pain leading to over-sedation and increased risk of complications.

Instead, the endoscopist should not waste time searching for a full lumen but concentrate on the axis of the upstream colon and the way to approach it.

In general, intubation of the sigmoid colon creates clusters of sharply angled and bent segments, which have a saw-tooth pattern. It means that the axis between two adjacent colonic segments runs in opposite directions, e.g. if the visible segment climbs up diagonally from right to left to 11 o'clock, the following segment falls down in the opposite direction toward 5 o'clock.

Disappearance of the lumen can be explained by unequal shortening of the mesenteric and antimesenteric edges of the sigmoid colon during rotation, pulling back maneuvers, and positioning of the tip close to the mucosa with sudden loss of orientation.

Two strategies are useful in these circumstances:

- search for a hidden lumen and colonic axis using endoscopic clues.
- pulling the scope slowly and torquing it gently clockwise and counter-clockwise.

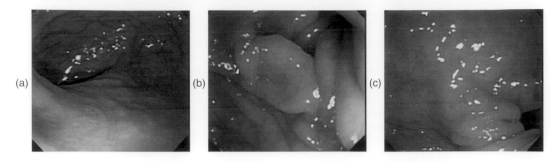

Figure 7.17 Common locations of the lumen. (a) The lumen is located at 9 o'clock; (b) the lumen is between 1 and 2 o'clock; (c) the lumen is located at 5 o'clock.

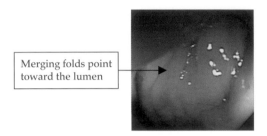

Merging folds point toward the lumen

Figure 7.18 Slightly depressed groove-like area and merging folds are the signs of the hidden lumen.

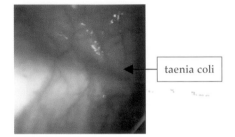

taenia coli

Figure 7.20 Prominent tenia coli. An appearance of the tenia while approaching the sigmoid–descending junction indicates the presence of the significant loop in the sigmoid colon.

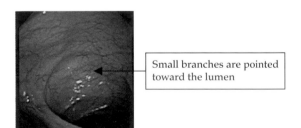

Small branches are pointed toward the lumen

Figure 7.19 The main submucosal veins and their branches. The main vessels are parallel to the circular folds. The small branches are pointed toward the lumen. This endoscopic clue may be useful when the tip of the scope is distant from the mucosa for at least 1 or 2 cm.

A narrowed slot-like or dimpled lumen of a twisted colon is usually located in three areas: between 10 and 12 o'clock, 1 and 3 o'clock or 4 and 6 o'clock (Figure 7.17).

Another clue to an obscure lumen is converging folds pointed to the slightly depressed, funnel-like area (Figure 7.18). It is useful to remember that the main submucosal vessels are parallel to the circular folds. However, their small branches usually spread around between the folds and can highlight the axis of the lumen (Figure 7.19).

When the tip is close to the sigmoid-descending junction a prominent longitudinal fold or the center of a convex fold indicates the direction of the colonic axis and the location of the next segment (Figure 7.20).

The following is a description of the corkscrew technique, which is particularly useful for sliding through the sharply angled segments of the sigmoid colon and sigmoid-descending junction:

• Orient the tip towards the narrowed lumen and advance the shaft forward slowly. If the lumen is located at 11 o'clock, rotate the shaft counterclockwise and angle the tip up. As soon as the edge of the lumen is approached, rotate the shaft clockwise and pull it back. If the lumen is located between 4 and 6 o'clock, rotate the shaft clockwise and pull it back. It will untwist the lumen and facilitate sliding of the tip into the proximal segment of the colon. If the next segment is open, advance the shaft forward a few centimeters. Rotate it clockwise and pull it back to telescope (shorten) the colon. Repeat this maneuver several times until the sigmoid-descending junction is reached. This technique is equally applicable to the rectosigmoid area and the junction between the splenic flexure and the transverse colon.

Exploration of the sigmoid colon and sigmoid-descending junction

The sigmoid colon is the most vulnerable part of the large intestine. It is not as long in children as in adults. However children, especially infants and toddlers, are less tolerant to stretching of the sigmoid colon. A relatively short mesentery is less elastic which decreases the threshold for pain.

Nevertheless, in deeply sedated infants and toddlers a less experienced endosocopist can create a huge loop which is not palpable through the abdominal wall because it occupies both lateral gutters and pushes up against the liver and left diaphragm.

This may create a false impression of a properly performed procedure without a significant loop. The clinical clues to this dangerous condition are sudden changes in oxygen saturation, hiccups, shallow breathing, and irritability of the patient followed by signs of respiratory distress. Immediate reduction of the loop and interruption of the procedure is mandatory until the child becomes stable.

During exploration of the sigmoid colon small loops are unavoidable, but easy reducible and considered a routine part of the procedure. However, formation of the larger loops should be prevented.

There are several clues to recognition of clinically significant loops:

- discomfort and pain
- long tubular segment of the bowel visualized ahead

- loss of the "one to one" relationship between pushing of the colonoscope and advancement in the colon
- paradoxical movement of the lumen away from the tip with attempts to advance the shaft
- increased stiffness of the angulations control and increased resistance to the shaft.

The elements of the most effective technique preventing a big loop are:

- corkscrew sliding around sharply angled colonic segments
- establishing an appropriate angle for corkscrew sliding maneuvers
- avoidance of forceful advancement (push through a significant resistance)
- frequent pulling back with simultaneous clockwise rotation of the shaft
- minimal insufflations
- trans-abdominal hand pressure support of the sigmoid colon
- changing of the patient's position.

A presence of a big loop is a sign of two possible scenarios:

- formation of a large "N" loop
- existence of a large "Alpha" or reverse "Alpha" loop.

For successful reduction of a sigmoid loop and advancement of the tip into descending colon proceed with the following:

First: turn the patient to the back to decrease the sharpness of the sigmoid-descending junction.

Second: in case of an "Alpha" loop scenario: pull the shaft back slowly and rotate it clockwise.

Third: reverse "Alpha" loop should be suspected if the lumen slips away from the tip. Stop withdrawing. Move the shaft to the initial position and then pull it back slowly with simultaneous vigorous counterclockwise rotation. Significant reduction of resistance and effective withdrawal of at least 20 to 30 cm of the shaft with a stable position of the tip is a sign of successful loop reduction.

Fourth, if "N" loop is suspected, rotate the shaft clockwise until the lumen opens up and the slightly grayish mucosa of the descending colon appears on the screen. Pull the shaft back slightly until the ridge of the next bent segment is reached; rotate the shaft clockwise and advance it forward until a reasonably long segment of the descending colon appears. At this point, the shaft has been advanced deeply into the descending colon and is stable enough to complete the reduction of the "N" loop by pulling the shaft back. During shortening and steering maneuvers, the bowel becomes twisted and creates enough force to untwist spontaneously and slip away from the shaft. The likelihood of this undesirable effect increases when the tip is very close to or inside the junction between the sigmoid and descending colon. All manipulations with the shaft should be made very carefully, slowly and sequentially. As mentioned above, the supine position reduces the sharp angle of the sigmoid-descending colon junction. Hand pressure stabilization of the sigmoid colon is very appropriate for the moment. The key for success is a vigorous clockwise rotation, which facilitates sliding of the tip into the descending colon. If an additional segment is located ahead at 11 o'clock, pull the shaft back slowly, elevate the tip up above the edge of the fold and rotate the shaft clockwise until a wide-open oval lumen of the descending colon appears. Then, advance the shaft and align the tip with the axis of the upstream segment.

The lumen of the descending colon is more oval, compared to the sigmoid colon. The folds are less frequent, the color is more grayish, and the vascular pattern is more prominent. Once the descending colon is reached, advance the shaft quickly toward the splenic flexure. It is one of the easiest steps of a colonoscopy because loops are reduced, the shaft is fully straightened and the descending colon is fixed in the retroperitoneum.

Splenic flexure and transverse colon

In order to untwist the external portion of the colonoscope, the shaft should be rotated counterclockwise. Attention should be given to the lumen of the bowel, to avoid laceration of the mucosa by the tip of the colonoscope. This maneuver facilitates an exploration of the splenic flexure.

To simplify the entrance into the transverse colon, pull the shaft back gently; rotate it counterclockwise, and angle it toward 11 o'clock. Initially, the lumen of the transverse colon appears as a slot along the line between 7 and 1 o'clock. An additional deflection in the same direction and counterclockwise rotation makes the lumen wider. At this point, rotate the shaft clockwise a quarter turn and bring the tip down slowly. It is necessary to turn the shaft counterclockwise again and elevate the tip up before pushing the shaft into the transverse colon. Exploration of the transverse colon does not require forceful advancement of

the colonoscope. In the absence of visible progress or in case of increasing resistance, pull the shaft back a few centimeters while keeping the lumen opened, then elevate the tip and push it forward applying clockwise torque simultaneously. Repeat this maneuver two or three times. If no significant progress has been made, rotate the patient into right lateral position, straighten the colonoscope by pulling it back, apply external pressure to stabilize the sigmoid colon and advance the shaft forward. Decreased resistance and progression of the tip forward indicate successful exploration of the transverse colon, which has a distinctive triangular lumen. At this point, the hepatic flexure can be reached almost momentarily by either pulling the shaft back with simultaneous counterclockwise rotation or pushing it gently forward.

A creation of so-called "gamma" loop is uncommon element of pediatric colonoscopy. The formation of this loop manifests by increasing resistance and paradoxical movement of the proximal transverse colon away from the tip with attempts to push the shaft forward. Successful reduction of a "gamma" loop can be challenging. First, rotate the patient onto their back, than pull the shaft back and rotate it counterclockwise. If the tip remains stable during the withdrawal phase of the maneuver, continue pulling back until the shaft is straightened. It is possible that after the initial counterclockwise rotation a clockwise torque should be applied.

Hepatic flexure, ascending colon and cecum

Exploration of the hepatic flexure may be challenging for beginners. It is important to remember that the axis of the hepatic flexure has a reverse gamma configuration. The entrance to the area is always located at an 11 o'clock position. A vigorous search in the wrong direction may induce pain secondary to pressure and distention of the bowel, small mucosal trauma or coiling of the colonoscope. The correct approach to the hepatic flexure consists of few steps:

1. Orientation. The transitional area between the transverse colon and the hepatic flexure often appears as a blind pouch. The right part of the pouch is convex with few circular folds creating an illusion of the lumen. The left wall of the pouch is short due to its rotation and the spiral configuration of the bowel.

Attention should be focused on the upper portion of this area.

2. Withdrawal. Pull the shaft back slowly and orient the tip to the 11 o'clock direction. Continue withdrawing and deflecting the tip in the same direction until the lumen starts to open up with an initial slot-like appearance.

3. Decompression. Decompress the bowel until the lumen begins to collapse.

4. Switching direction. Rotate the shaft clockwise and move the tip to the right and slightly down using the R/L knob.

5. Advancement. Advance the shaft forward and adjust the position by counterclockwise rotation and elevation of the tip enough to keep it in the center of the lumen.

6. Advance a colonoscope until the cecum is reached.

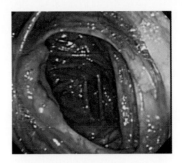

Figure 7.21 The ileocecal valve. It is usually located between the 9 and 11 o'clock position of the cecum.

Terminal ileum

The ileo-cecal valve is tucked behind the folds. It is usually located between the 9 and 11 o'clock positions (Figure 7.21). However, occasionally it might be found in the lower aspect of the cecum between 5 and 7 o'clock (Figure 7.22). The ileo-cecal valve appears as a lip-shaped thickening of the mucosal fold. An exploration of the terminal ileum begins with detection of the ileo-cecal valve by pulling the shaft away from the appendix orifice. Once the valve is located, the tip is moved forward closer to the appendix. The following steps should be adjusted to the actual position of the ileo-cecal valve. If it is located at 11 o'clock the endoscopist should:

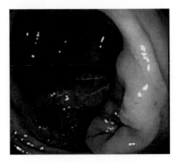

Figure 7.22 The less common position of the ileocecal valve. The ileocecal valve is at 5 o'clock position.

1. Decompress the cecum.
2. Orient the tip to 11 o'clock.
3. Slowly pull the shaft back until the tip slips into the terminal ileum.

When the ileo-cecal valve is between 5 or 7 o'clock, proceed with:

(1) Bend the tip down and to the right toward the target with simultaneous clockwise rotation, and;

(2) Pull the shaft back.

The so-called forceps maneuver can be also used. The scope is rotated to approach the valve at 6 o'clock position. The forceps are extended from the scope about 2 mm and then used as a quid wire to intubate the ileo-cecal, by tip deflection downward and opening up the valve lip which is the lower of the two. De-tenting by suction of the cecum can be helpful as can mebeverine iv injection to open the valve.

Successful exploration of the terminal ileum is manifested by the change in color and texture of the mucosa; while the cecum appears pink-grayish and smooth with prominent vessels, the mucosa of the terminal ileum is light pink or yellowish, velvet, with multiple small (less than 3 mm) lymphoid follicles (Figure 7.23).

Withdrawing

The withdrawing phase of colonoscopy is the best for detail assessment of the colonic mucosa. However, some stretching of the bowel during advancement of a colonoscope makes the circular folds more flat and easy to explore. It is useful for detection of small lesions such a sessile polyp.

Complications

Routine use of colonoscopy in children would be impossible without solid proof that the procedure is safe. It does not mean, however, that it is free from complications (*see* Table 7.4). This issue should be fully disclosed and explained to the parents or caretaker as a part of informed consent.

Complications associated with colonoscopy in children can be classified according to:

1. A necessity for hospitalization, and
2. An absence or presence of structural damage of the intestine and/or adjacent organs.

The incidence of minor complications is difficult to estimate. However, it is likely that this is under reported. First, it is unlikely that all minor complications are going to be counted. Second, some complications are clinically silent: serosal tears and small mesenteric hematomas have been accidentally discovered during unrelated surgery soon after colonoscopy in adults.

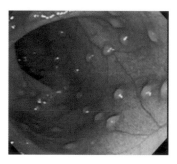

Figure 7.23 The terminal ileum. Velvet texture, yellowish tinge, and lymphoid follicles are the main endoscopic characteristics of the mucosa of the terminal ileum in children.

The reported frequency of serious complications related to pediatric colonoscopy is about 0.2 %, which is similar to the data from large-scale multi-center studies in adults. Perforation; a major complication associated with colonoscopy can occur due to four reasons:

• Excessive pressure created by advancing forward or forcefully withdrawing the shaft of a colonoscope.
• Embedding of the colonoscope into the bowel wall.
• Excessive air pressure.
• Inappropriate technique of polypectomy, hemostasis or balloon dilation of a benign stricture.

Three types of perforations related to diagnostic colonoscopy have been described. Shaft-induced perforations are the result of big loop formation. It is usually larger than expected and located on the antimesenteric wall.

Tip perforations are smaller and typically occur when the "sliding by" technique is used inappropriately or a tip is trapped in wide diverticula or imbedded into mucosa when orientation is lost.

Excessive air pressure perforation has been documented primarily with strictures of the left colon. Attempts to bypass the narrowed area create intermittent obstruction of the colon, accumulation of air in the upstream colon and increased hydrostatic pressure, which could reach a critical level of 81 mmHg for the cecum. This could explain the fact that the majority of air pressure related perforations have occurred in the cecum and even in the ileum after so-called uneventful colonoscopies.

Table 7.4. Complications associated with pediatric colonoscopy

	Minor complications: no needs for hospitalization	Major complications: requirements for hospitalization
Structural damage of the intestine or adjacent organs	Small, non-obstructing mucosal or submucosal hematomas, small mucosal lacerations, petechiae	Perforation. Bleeding requiring blood transfusion and endoscopic or surgical hemostasis; post polypectomy syndrome
Absence of structural damage	Transient abdominal pain, bloating, abdominal distention resolving after passing gas, mild dehydration secondary to bowel preparation.	Cardiovascular and respiratory distress, prolonged episode of hypoxia requiring resuscitation and or endotracheal intubation

Hydrostatic perforations have not been described in children.

Most large traumatic perforations are immediately obvious. The presenting symptoms include a sudden onset of irreducible abdominal distention, decreased resistance to insertion of a colonoscope, failure to insufflate the collapsed colon, visible organs of a peritoneal cavity and severe and progressively increasing abdominal pain. Immediate discontinuation of the procedure and request for plain abdominal films are mandatory. Closed perforations are less dramatic.

Almost 10% of patients with a perforated colon can initially be symptom free. In addition another 10 to 15% of patients may develop mild to moderate abdominal pain or discomfort. Absence of free air in the peritoneal cavity does not rule out perforation. High level of suspicion and careful post procedure observation are clues for early recognition of complications.

Persistent abdominal pain and/or low-grade fever should be considered as a sign of perforation until proven otherwise. Early diagnosis in these circumstances is absolutely crucial to prevent or decrease morbidity and mortality associated with perforation of the colon. Treatment of colonic perforation can be non-operative or surgical. Patients with a well-prepared colon and therefore decreased risk of significant contamination of the peritoneal cavity, absence of peritonitis and who are otherwise stable can be treated medically with bowel rest, broad-spectrum antibiotics and parenteral nutrition. Deterioration of a patient's condition, signs of peritoneal irritation, suspicion of a large spillage of intestinal contents into the peritoneal cavity mandates a surgical exploration. According to large-scale studies in adults, the frequency of colonic perforation after polypectomy is usually higher by two or three fold. It results from excessive thermal coagulation of the tissue either due to an inappropriate power setting and current mode (more often when a "blended" mode is used), cutting the large sessile polyp more than 2 cm without a piece-meal technique or accidental contact of the adjacent mucosa with the head of a excised polyp. These perforations are often small and subtle and cause late onset of abdominal pain a few hours after the procedure. Severity of pain usually increases with time. Fever is another common sign of deep tissue necrosis. The treatment of these complications (polypectomy syndrome) is similar to uncomplicated diverticulitis, i.e. aggressive treatment with broad-spectrum antibiotics, bowel rest and good hydration.

Bleeding after a diagnostic colonoscopy is quite rare and can be prevented by a thorough history and physical exam. The history should be focused on a family history of bleeding diathesis, frequent nasal bleeding, oozing from gums after the brushing of teeth and easy bruising without obvious trauma. A simple question about recent treatments with aspirin and or NSAIDs is an effective way to prevent bleeding secondary to platelets dysfunction.

Bleeding disorders are not a contraindication to pediatric colonoscopy. Even patients with moderate to severe hemophilia could undergo successful colonoscopy with biopsy or polypectomy after special preparations have been made by a pediatric hematologist. According to the American Society for Gastrointestinal Endoscopy (ASGE) colonoscopy and colonoscopic polypectomy are classified as a low-risk for bacteremia. In recent publications, a transient bacteremia has been reported in less than 4% of patients after an uneventful colonoscopy. The patients usually remain asymptomatic without requiring any medical treatment. If a patient becomes febrile, flat abdominal and cross-table films, blood culture and empirical treatment with broad-spectrum antibiotics are mandatory. Careful observation in a recovery room (until the child is fully awake and ready to leave), and next day telephone follow-up should be a routine part of the post-procedure protocol.

Common pathology

Rectal bleeding

Every child with hematochezia does not require colonoscopy. Careful history and physical examination are essential for diagnoses of an anal fissure, bacterial, or protozoal hematochezia.

However, colonoscopy is the procedure of choice in children with persistent or recurrent, unexplained hematochezia.

The role of the colonoscopy in patients with suspected or established inflammatory bowel disease is to define the extent of inflammation, obtain tissue samples, establish the specific diagnosis, and assess the efficacy of the therapy and mucosal healing and screening for malignancy.

Common findings in children with untreated ulcerative colitis include continuous and circumferential mucosal inflammation with diffuse

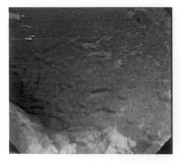 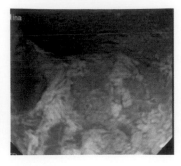 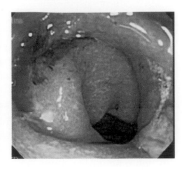

Figure 7.24 Ulcerative colitis. Diffuse inflammation is typical for ulcerative colitis: erythema, exudates, loss of vascular pattern.

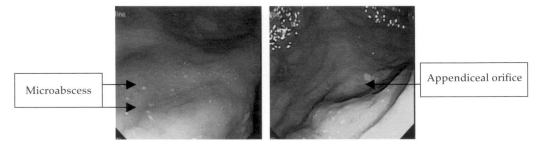

Microabscess

Appendiceal orifice

Figure 7.25 Rare case of "cecal patch" in a child with left-sided ulcerative colitis. Left picture: multiple micro abscess around the appendiceal orifice (close-up view); Right picture: appendiceal orifice.

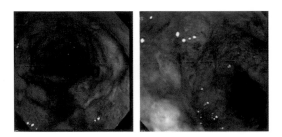

Figure 7.26 Severe form of ulcerative colitis. Large amount of pus, severe edema, loss of vascular pattern, and small ulcerations are seen.

erythema, edema, increased mucosal friability, a disappearance of vascular pattern, grayish exudates, erosions, or shallow ulcers (Figure 7.24). Rectal involvement is universal. An inflammation can be restricted to the rectum, the left or entire colon. A local inflammation surrounding the appendicial orifice's so-called "cecal patch" may co-exist with left-sided colitis (Figure 7.25). Signs of the "back-washed" ileitis consist of diffuse mild to moderate erythema, edema and petechiae within 5 to 10 cm of the ileum adjacent to the ileo-cecal valve. The severe form of ulcerative colitis presents endoscopically with some degree of narrowing and tubular appearance of the bowel due to severe edema and loss of circular folds; striking erythema, large amount of pus, and shallow ulcerations (Figure 7.26).

Deep ulcers are not typical for ulcerative colitis even with the severe form of the disease. A chronic and relapsing course of ulcerative colitis leads to unequal distribution of inflammation, appearance of pseudopolyps and attenuation of vascular pattern (Figure 7.27).

Colitis in patients with Crohn's disease is patchy with so-called "skip lesions" rather than diffuse or uniform. It could be mild or intense, and may involve the entire colon or just a part of it. Fifty per cent of patients with Crohn's colitis have rectal sparing. At least half of children with Crohn's disease have ileo-cecal involvement. An aphthoid ulcer is a common manifestation of Crohn's disease. It is a small 4–5 mm ulcer surrounded by a thin rim of erythema (Figure 7.28).

Aphthoid ulcers can be clustered in a few colonic segments or spread throughout the colon. Narrowing of the lumen, strictures, mucosal bridging and deep, stellate, longitudinal, and serpiginous ulcers (Figures 7.29, 7.30) reflect the intramural nature of inflammation.

Allergic proctocolitis is characterized by inflammatory alterations of the colon and rectum, secondary to an immune reaction triggered by the ingestion of foreign proteins. The prevalence and

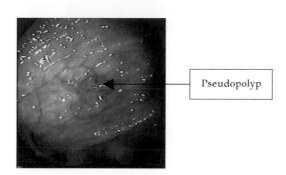

Figure 7.27 Pseudopolyp in a patient with long-standing ulcerative colitis.

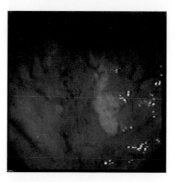

Figure 7.29 Deep longitudinal ulcers in a patient with Crohn's disease.

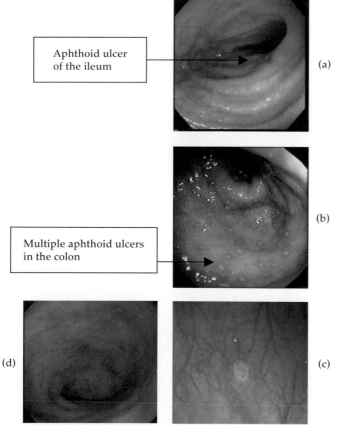

Figure 7.28 Aphthoid ulcer. It is small, shallow lesion with the rim of erythema. (a) Aphthoid ulcer of the ileum; (b) multiple aphthoid ulcers in the colon; (c) multiple aphthoid ulcers in the colon; (d) a close-up view of the aphthoid ulcer.

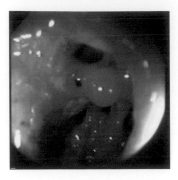

Figure 7.30 Mucosal bridging in the cecum in 14-year-old patient with Crohn's disease.

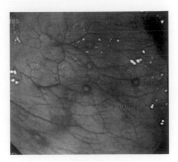

Figure 7.32 Small aphthoid-like lesions can be occasionally induced by bowel preparation.

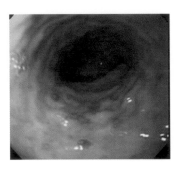

Figure 7.31 Allergic colitis. Multiple lymphoid follicles with rim of erythema: the "halo" sign and edema of the sigmoid colon.

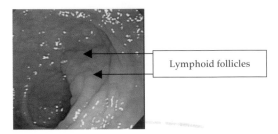

Lymphoid follicles

Figure 7.33 Numerous lymphoid follicles in the sigmoid colon.

natural history of allergic proctocolitis is unclear, although its frequency appears to be increasing even in infants who are exclusively breastfed. The most allergenic protein is μ-lactoglobulin. The clinical manifestations occur in the first weeks or months of life. The common symptoms are rectal bleeding frequently associated with diarrhea and mucus in stool. The endoscopic findings consist of patchy edema and erythema, nodular lymphoid hyperplasia and occasional erosions or superficial small ulcers. The most affected area is the sigmoid colon, although the rectum and descending colon could be involved (Figure 7.31).

It should be distinct from isolated petechiae or small ulcerations in the sigmoid or descending colon induced by bowel preparation (Figure 7.32).

Pseudopolyps, juvenile polyps and polyposis syndromes

Small lymphoid aggregates in the colon are common in infants and toddlers. They appear as light pink or yellowish polypoid or umbilical-like

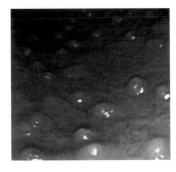

Figure 7.34 Multiple, enlarge (more than 3 mm) lymphoid follicles in the terminal ileum is the sign of intestinal lymphoid hyperplasia: a non-specific reaction of the intestinal immune system to the various food or bacterial/viral antigens.

structures less than 3 mm (Figure 7.33). The rectum and sigmoid colon are the most commonly involved. The clinical significance of these lesions in asymptomatic children is unknown.

Intestinal lymphoid hyperplasia of the terminal ileum is defined as presence of multiple lymphoid follicles more than 3 mm in size (Figure 7.34). It is a frequent finding in infants with abdominal pain

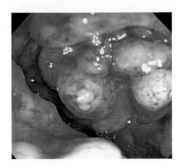

Figure 7.35 Six-year-old boy with recurrent ileocolonic intussusceptions. Intra-operative ileoscopy revealed highly enlarged (more than 4 mm) lymphoid follicles with multiple petechiae in the terminal ileum. Four week treatment with oral prednisone was successful with complete resolution of lymphoid nodular hyperplasia and recurrent abdominal pain.

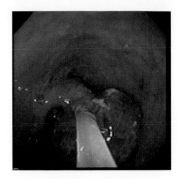

Figure 7.37 Pedunculated juvenile polyp.

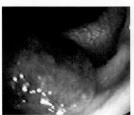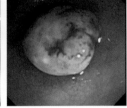

Figure 7.36 Sessile juvenile polyp.

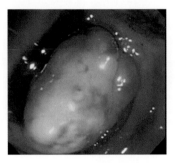

Figure 7.38 Large juvenile polyp in the descending colon.

and recurrent rectal bleeding due to food allergy or unrelated processes.

Occasionally, intestinal lymphoid hyperplasia could be the source of recurrent ileo-colonic intussusception (Figure 7.35).

Juvenile polyps are the most common type of polyps in children. They have distinctive cystic architecture, mucus-filled glands, prominent lamina propria, and dense infiltrations with inflammatory cells. They are most prevalent in children under 6 years of age. Recurrent painless rectal bleeding is a typical presenting symptom. Other manifestations include prolapsing rectal mass and an occasional presence of mucus in stool.

A typical juvenile polyp is about a 1 cm pedunculated structure. Polyps less than 1 cm are usually sessile and have a raspberry or smooth appearing "head" (Figure 7.36, 7.37). Although auto-amputation occurs frequently, some polyps grow longer, reaching a significant size of up to 3 or even 4 cm. A large juvenile polyp is usually located in the sigmoid colon. In rare cases, it might be found

in the descending or transverse colon (Figure 7.38). Such a polyp may induce an intermittent pain due to colonic intussusceptions. The appearance of pale light yellow-speckled mucosa, a so-called chicken skin mucosa, (Figure 7.39) should alert the endoscopist about an adjacent large juvenile polyp. The hallmark of "chicken skin" mucosa is an accumulation of lipid-laden macrophages in the lamina propria.

The co-existence of juvenile polyps in both sites of the colon has been documented in at least one-third of children. For this reason, a colonoscopy with polypectomy is the procedure of choice for children with recurrent painless rectal bleeding.

Rare pathology

Polyposis syndromes

Different types of hereditary polyposis syndromes can be revealed during a pediatric colonoscopy.

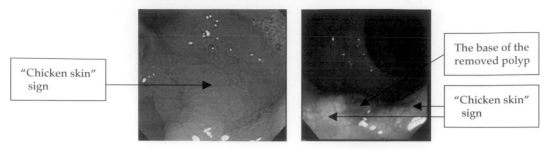

Figure 7.39 The "goose skin" sign. The mucosa around a large juvenile polyp has specific pattern induced by lipid-loaded macrophages.

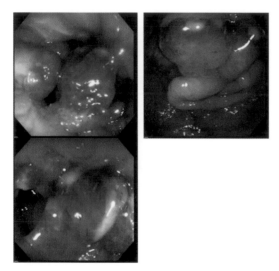

Figure 7.40 Juvenile polyposis. Multiple juvenile polyps in the rectum and the colon.

Diagnostic criteria for juvenile polyposis include the presence of 5 or more juvenile polyps in the colon (Figure 7.40). Surveillance colonoscopy is indicated due to an increased risk of colon cancer.

Peutz-Jeghers syndrome

Peutz-Jeghers syndrome is a unique form of hamartomatous polyposis associated with distinctive mucocutaneous pigmentation. It is caused by a germline mutation in the STK11 (LKB1) gene. The incidence of this condition is estimated to be between 1:50 000 to 1:200 000 live births. The polyps in patients with Peutz-Jeghers syndrome (PJS) display arborizing smooth-muscle proliferation distinguishing them from the polyps in other forms of juvenile polyposis syndromes.

The diagnostic criteria of Peutz-Jeghers syndrome are: two or more histologically confirmed PJ polyps, any number of PJ polyps or characteristic mucocutaneous pigmentation in patients with close relatives diagnosed with PJS, any number of polyps in individuals with characteristic mucocutaneous pigmentation.

Polyps occur more commonly in the small intestine. At least half of the patients have additional polyps in the colon and the stomach. Polyps in children with PJS vary from a few millimeters to more than 5 cm. They are usually subpedunculated and firmly anchored to the bowel wall by arborized smooth-muscle bundles preventing spontaneous amputation and predisposing to the small bowel intussusception. Surveillance protocols in PJS target two goals: detection and removal of the sizable polyps preventing intussusception and detection of cancers in early stage.

A base line EGD, colonoscopy and capsule endoscopy is indicated at the onset of clinical manifestation or at 8 years of age in asymptomatic children. All significant polyps (1 cm or bigger) should be removed. Children with significant polyps should be scheduled for a surveillance endoscopy every 3 years or sooner if symptoms occur. Double balloon enteroscopy is the procedure of choice for treatment of symptomatic children with the small bowel hamartomas.

Familial Adenomatous Polyposis

Familial Adenomatous **Polyposis** is a group of hereditary polyposis syndromes including autosomal dominant forms: Familial Adenomatous Polyposis (FAP), attenuated Familial Adenomatous Polyposis (AFAP), and autosomal recessive MYH-associated polyposis (MAP). Germline mutations of the adenomatous polyposis coli (APC) gene are present in 60 to 80% of classic FPC and 10 to 30% of AFPC patients respectively. Mutations of base excision repair (MYH) gene are likely to account for about 10, 20 and 25% of individuals with FPC, AFPC and MAP respectively.

Mutations associated with classical FAP inevitably lead to colorectal cancer before the age of 39 in affected individuals without colectomy.

There is some correlation between specific mutation and clinical phenotype.

Mutations between APC codons 1250 and 1464 cause severe polyposis, generally with >5000 polyps, and the recurrent codon 1309 mutation is associated with early onset and development of thousands of polyps.

Mutations linked with AFPC are responsible for different phenotypes as well: a late onset of polyps and cancer, a smaller number of polyps (less than 100 (average 30), a predisposition toward involvement of the proximal colon and extracolonic manifestations.

Most children with FAP do not have any gastrointestinal manifestation of polyposis. The exception is a group of young children without a family history of FAP. They tend to have an earlier onset of hematochezia. In this scenario, colonoscopy should not be delayed. Once the diagnosis of FAP is confirmed, upper GI endoscopy is reasonable for early detection of adenomatous polyps in the duodenum.

The main endoscopic feature of FPC in children is usually dozens or hundreds of small sessile polyps (Figure 7.41).

Multiple biopsies and polypectomies of the largest polyps are essential for diagnosis of adenomatous polyps and low or high-grade dysplasia.

Genetic testing and surveillance sigmoidoscopy for asymptomatic children with family history of FAP usually begins between 11 and 15 years of age. Once the patient is diagnosed with FAP a prophylactic colectomy should be planned.

According to recommendations of the American Society of Colon and Rectal Surgeons, for patients with mild disease and low cancer risk, prophylactic colectomy can be done in the mid-teen years (15–18 years). When severe disease is found, or if the patient is symptomatic, surgery is performed as soon as convenient after diagnosis.

Colon cancer

Sporadic adenocarcinoma of the colon in children is extremely rare. The presenting symptoms include progressive weight loss, changes of bowel movement habits, fatigue, anemia and intermittent rectal bleeding. Despite the warning signs, the diagnosis is typically delayed by a few months due to a low level of suspicion. Tumors are equally distributed between the left and right colon. During colonoscopy, adenocarcinomas appear as discolored masses (Figure 7.42). It is quite difficult to examine the entire lesion due to an almost

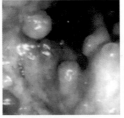
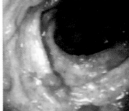

Figure 7.41 Multiple colon polyps in a 5-year-old-boy with FAP.

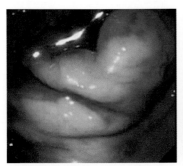
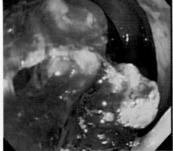
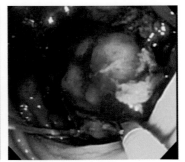

Figure 7.42 Adenocarcinoma of the right colon in 11-year-old boy with significant weight loss, anemia, and ascites. Colonoscopy revealed severe edema of the distal part of the ascending colon. Further exploration of the ascending colon showed ulcerated large tumor. The biopsy confirmed the diagnosis of mucinous adenocarcinoma.

complete obstruction of intestinal lumen and severe edema of the surrounding tissue. Usually, the tumor edge is firm and easily fragmented during biopsy. Most of tumors are mucinous adenocarcinoma.

Adenocarcinoma of the colon in ulcerative colitis

The determining factor of malignancy in patients with ulcerative colitis seems to be the severity of the original disease as well as the extent of mucosal involvement and the duration of colitis.

The cancer risk for patients with pancolitis is 3% in the first decade of disease and 1–2% per year thereafter. Patients with pancolitis should begin bi-yearly colonoscopies, ten years after the onset of the disease. Multiple biopsies taken at intervals of a few centimeters of each other are recommended. Any flat or elevated lesions should be additional targets. Chromoendoscopy has been found useful to increase the yield of finding high-grade dysplasia in adults. More recently confocal endo-microscopy has allowed greater accuracy in biopsy targeting.

Non-Hodgkin's lymphoma of the terminal ileum

Non-Hodgkin's lymphoma of the terminal ileum can be discovered during colonoscopy in children with intermittent abdominal pain and weight loss. Pain is usually a result of ileo-colonic intussusception. During the colonoscopy, irregular masses occupying the intestinal lumen could be found in the cecum or ascending colon (Figure 7.43). Care

should be taken to avoid deep embedding of the forceps into the tumor in order to prevent pealing of a large tissue fragment. Proper fixative solution is important for correct morphological and cytogenetic diagnosis.

Vascular malformation of the colon

Vascular malformation of the gastrointestinal tract is a rare finding in children. Two types of vascular malformation of the colon have been described in children: hemangiomas (Figure 7.44) and angiodysplasia (Figure 7.45). The hallmark of these lesions is lower GI bleeding, which could be life-threatening. Unlike adults, angiodyplastic lesions in children have a predisposition to the left side of the colon and rectum. Endoscopic hemostasis of bleeding angiodysplasis could be achieved using argon plasma coagulation.

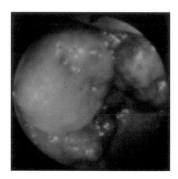

Figure 7.44 Large hemangioma of the sigmoid colon in a 3-year-old girl with recurrent episodes of low GI bleeding.

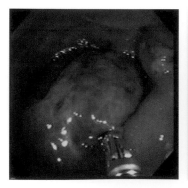 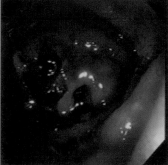 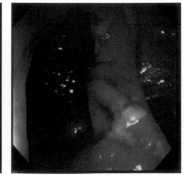

Figure 7.43 Non-Hodgkin's lymphoma of the ileum. The indications for a colonoscopy were intermittent severe right low quadrant pain, weight loss, and anemia. The intussusception was found in the descending colon. It was gently reduced after the tissue samples were cautiously obtained.

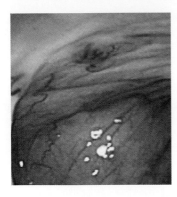

Figure 7.15 Angiodysplasia of the colon in a child with recurrent low GI bleeding. Tortuous, engorged small vessels are quite different from the normal colonic vasculature on the back ground of the image.

📖 FURTHER READING

Adamiak T, Altaf M, Jensen MK, *et al*. (2010) One-day bowel preparation with polyethylen glycol 3350: an effective regiment for colonoscopy in children. *Gastrointestinal Endoscopy*, **71**, 573–577.

Arain Z, Rossi TM. (1999) Gastrointestinal bleeding in children: an overview of conditions requiring non-operative management. *Seminars in Pediatric Surgery*, **8**, 172–180.

Atkinson RJ, Save V, Hunter JO. (2005) Colonic ulceration after sodium phosphate bowel preparation. *American Journal of Gastroenterology*, **100**, 2603–5.

Berkelhammer C, Caed D, Mesleh G, *et al*. (1997) Ileo-cecal intussusception of small-bowel lymphoma: diagnosis by colonoscopy. *Journal of Clinical Gastroenterology*, **25**, 358–361.

Begs AD, Latch ford AR, Vase HFA, *et al*. (2010) Peutz-Jeghers syndrome: a symptomatic review and recommendations for management. *Gut*, **59**, 975–986.

C.B. Fleet Company. Letter to US health care professionals (2006) Changes to professional labeling of Fleet® Phosphosoda®. Available at: http://www.phosphosoda.com/professional

Cotton PB, Williams C, Hawes RH, *et al*. (2008) *Practical Gastrointestinal Endoscopy. The Fundamentals*. (6th edn.) pp. 87–175, Blackwell Publishing, Oxford.

De La Torre L, Carrasco D, Nora MA, *et al*. (2002) Vascular malformations of the colon in children. *Journal of Pediatric Surgery*, **37**, 1177–1200.

Differentiating Ulcerative Colitis from Crohn's Disease in Children and Young Adults: report of a Working Group of the North American Society for Pediatric Gastroenterology, Hepatology, and Nutrition and the Crohn's and Colitis Foundation of America. (2007) *Journal of Pediatric Gastroenterolology & Nutrition*, **44**, 653–674.

Durno CA. (2007) Colonic polyps in children and adolescents. *Canadian Journal of Gastroenterology*, **21**, 233–239.

Elitsur Y, Teitelbaum LE, Rewalt M, *et al*. (2009) Clinical and endoscopic data in juvenile polyposis syndrome in preadolescent children. *Journal of Clinical Gastroenterology*, **43**, 734–736.

Farley DR, Bannon MP, Scott PZ, *et al*. (1997) Management of colonoscopic perforations. *Mayo Clinic Proceedings*, **72**, 729–733.

Garbay JR, Suc B, Rotman N, *et al*. (1996) Multicenter study of surgical complications of colonoscopy. *British Journal of Surgery*, **83**, 42–44.

Gershman G, Ament ME. (2007) *Practical Pediatric Gastrointestinal Endoscopy*. Blackwell Publishing, Oxford, UK.

Goldin E, Libson E. (1986) Intussusception in intestinal lymphoma: the role of colonoscopy. *Postgraduate Medical Journal*, **62**, 1139–1140.

Gupta SK, Fitzgerald JF, Croffie JM, *et al*. (2001) Experience with juvenile polyps in North American children: the need for pancolonoscopy. *American Journal of Gastroenterology*, **96**, 1695–1697.

Haens GD, Rutgeerts P. (2003) Endoscopy of inflammatory bowel diseases. In: Waye JD, Rex DK, Williams CB, (eds) *Colonoscopy. Principles and Practice*. pp. 573–581, Blackwell Publishing, Oxford.

Haubrich W. (1995) Anatomy of the colon. In: Haubrich W, Schaffner F, (eds) *Gastroenterology*, (Vol 2, 5th edn.). pp. 1573–1591, WB Saunders, Philadelphia, PA.

Hoppin A. (2000) Other neoplasms. In: Walker WA, Durie PB, Hamilton JR, *et al*, (eds) *Pediatric Gastrointestinal Disease: Pathophysiology, Diagnosis and Management*. (3rd edn) 2000; pp. 810–820, BC Decker, Hamilton (ON).

Hill DA, Furman WL, Billups CA, *et al*. (2007) Colorectal carcinoma in childhood: a clinicopathological review. *Journal of Clinical Oncology*, **25**, 5808–5814.

Huang SC, Erdman SH. (2009) Pediatric juvenile polyposis syndromes: an update. *Current Gastroenterology Reports*, **11**, 211–219.

Hyar W, Neale K, Fell J, *et al*. (2003) At what age should routine screening start in children at risk of familial adenomatous polyposis? *Journal of Pediatric Gastroenterology & Nutrition*, **31 (Suppl 2),** 135.

Iacono G, Ravello A, Di Prima L, *et al*. (2007) Colonic lymphoid nodular hyperplasia in children: relationship to food hypersensitivity. *Clinical Gastroenterology & Hepatology*, **5,** 361–366.

Iqbal CW, Askegard-Giesmann JR, Pham TH, *et al*. (2008) Pediatric endoscopic injuries: incidence, management, and outcomes. *Journal of Pediatric Surgery*, **43,** 911–915.

Iqbal CW, Chun YS, Farley, DR. (2005) Colonoscopic Perforations: A Retrospective Review. *Journal Gastrointestinal Surgery*, **9,** 1229–1236.

Jerkis S, Rosewich H, Scharf JG, *et al*. (2005) Colorectal cancer in two pre-teenage siblings with familial adenomatous polyposis. *European Journal of Pediatrics*, **1,** 306–310.

Ker TS, Wasseberg N, Bear, RW Jr. (2004) Colonoscopic perforation and bleeding of the colon can be treated safely without surgery. *American Journal of Surgery*, **70,** 922–944.

Kokkonen J, Kartunen TJ. (2002) Lymphonodular hyperplasia on the mucosa of the lower gastrointestinal tract in children: an indication of enhanced immune response? *Journal of Pediatric Gastroenterology & Nutrition*, **34,** 42–46.

Kravarusic D, Feigin E, Dlugy E, *et al*. (2007) Colorectal carcinoma in childhood: a retrospective multicenter study. *Journal of Pediatric Gastroenterology & Nutrition*, **44,** 209–211.

Nieuwenhuis MH, Matus-Vliegen LM, Slors FJ, *et al*. (2007) Genotype-phenotype correlations as a guide in management of Familial Adenomatous Polyposis. *Clinical Gastroenterology & Hepatology*, **5,** 374–378.

Pashankar DS, Uc A, Bishop WB. (2004) Polyethylene glycol 3350 without electrolytes: a new safe, effective and palatable bowel preparation for colonoscopy in children. *Journal of Pediatrics*, **144,** 358–362.

Ravelli A, Villanacci V, Chiappa S, *et al*. (2008) Dietary protein-induced proctocolitis in childhood. *American Journal of Gastroenterology*, **103,** 2605–2612.

Rothbaum RJ. (1996) Complications of pediatric colonoscopy. *Gastrointestinal Endoscopy Clinics of North America*, **6,** 445–459.

Reijchrt S, Bureš J, Široký M, *et al*. (2004) A prospective, observational study of colonic mucosal abnormalities associated with orally administered sodium phosphate for colon cleansing before colonoscopy. *Gastrointestinal Endoscopy*, **59,** 651–654.

Snyder J, Bratton B. (2002) Antimicrobial prophylaxis for gastrointestinal procedures: current practice in North American academic pediatric programs. *Journal of Pediatric Gastroenterology & Nutrition*, **35,** 564–569.

Safder S, Demintieva Y, Rewalt M, *et al*. (2008) Stool consistency and stool frequency are excellent clinical markers for adequate colon preparation after polyethylene glycol 3350 cleaning protocol: a prospective clinical study in children. *Gastrointestinal Endoscopy*, **68,** 1131–1135.

Saoul R, Wolff R, Seligman H, *et al*. (2001) Symptoms of hyperphosphotemia, hypocalcemia, and hypomagnesemia in an adolescent after the oral administration of sodium phosphate in preparation for a colonoscopy. *Gastrointestinal Endoscopy*, **53,** 650–652.

Thomson M, Murphy MS.(2006) In: Winter HS, Murphy MS, Mougenot JF, *et al*. (eds) *Pediatric Gastrointestinal Endoscopy*. pp. 81–91, BC Decker, Hamilton, Ontario.

Troncone R, Descepolo V. (2009) Colon and food allergy. *Journal of Pediatric Gastroenterology & Nutrition*, **48(Suppl 2),** s89–s91.

Radhakrishnan CN, Bruce J. (2003) Colorectal cancer in children without any predisposing factors. A report of eight cases and review of the literature. *European Journal of Pediatric Surgery*, **13,** 66–68.

Snyder WH. (1969) The embryology of alimentary tract with special emphasis on the colon and rectum. In: Turell R, (ed) *Diseases of Colon and Anorectum*, (Vol 1, 2nd edn). pp. 3–19, WB Saunders; Philadelphia, PA.

Valentin J, (ed) (2003) *Alimentary system. In: Annals of the ICRP: Basic Anatomical and Physiological Data for Use in Radiological Protection, Reference Values*. pp.109–117, Pergamon, Oxford.

Vastyan AM, Walker J, Pinter AB, *et al*. (2001) Colorectal carcinoma in children and adolescents – a report of seven cases. *European Journal of Surgery*, **11,** 338–341.

Vasudevan SA, Patel JC, Wesson DE, *et al*. (2006) Severe dysplasia in children with familial adenomatous polyposis: rare or simply overlooked? *Journal of Pediatric Surgery*, **41,** 658–661.

Weaver LT. (1992) Anatomy and embryology. In: Walker WA, Durie PB, Hamilton JR, *et al*.

Pediatric Gastrointestinal Disease: Pathophysiology, Diagnosis, and Management. (1st edn). pp. 195–216, Mosby, St. Louis.

Wexner SD, Beck DE, Baron TH, *et al.* (2006) A consensus document on bowel preparation before colonoscopy: Prepared by a Task Force from the American Society of Colon and Rectal Surgeons (ASCRS), the American Society of Gastrointestinal Endoscopy (ASGE) and Endoscopic Surgeons (SAGES). *Gastrointestinal Endoscopy,* **63,** 894–909.

Williams C, Nicholls S. (1994) Endoscopic features of chronic inflammatory bowel disease in child-hood. *Baillieres Clinical Gastroenterology,* **8,** 121–131.

Xanthakov SA, Schwimmer JB, Melin-Aldana H, *et al.* (2005) Prevalence and outcome of allergic colitis in healthy infants with rectal bleeding: a prospective cohort study. *Journal of Pediatric Gastroenterology & Nutrition,* **41,** 16–22.

Zwas FR, Cirillo NW, El-Serag HB, *et al.* (1996) Colonic mucosal abnormalities associated with oral phosphate solution. *Gastrointestinal Endoscopy,* **43,** 463–466.

8

Polypectomy

George Gershman

 KEY POINTS

- Knowledge of the principles of electro-surgery is an essential component of safe polypectomy technique.
- Knowledge of snare designs and choosing the appropriate snare are essential parts of a successful polypectomy.
- Navigation of the scope to an optimal position and a clean environment create an optimal condition for a safe polypectomy.

- The size and the shape of the polyp dictates the choice of the proper technique.
- Short distances (less than 2 cm) between the tip of the snare and a polyp, minimal opening of the metal loop and simultaneous advancement of the snare toward the polyp, along with tightening of the loop are the key elements of the technique.
- Polypectomy of a large polyp requires additional training in the piece-meal technique.

Basic principles of electrosurgery

The cornerstone of electric cutting and coagulation of living tissue is the heating of the restricted area by radio-frequency alternating current (RF) without stimulation of nerves and muscles. When current alternates up to a million times per second it does not stimulate muscle and nerve membranes long enough to induce depolarization before the next alternation occurs. Cutting is produced by rapid and strong heating, which creates evaporation of intra-and extracellular fluids.

Coagulation is initiated when the speed and degree of tissue heating is slower and less intense, leading to cellular desiccation. Specific effects of different types of RF currents and heat-related tissue destruction are illustrated in Figures 8.1 and 8.2.

Several factors regulate the degree of tissue heating:

- Voltage (V) is the force required to push current through the tissue. The higher the voltage, the deeper the thermal tissue destruction.
- Tissue resistance (R) or impedance (for alternating current) is the force generated by tissue to resist electrical flow. It is directly proportional to the amount of tissue electrolytes.

Resistance increases dramatically during tissue heating and desiccation. Normal tissue resistance is not uniform; it is lowest along blood vessels and highest at the level of the skin.

- Time (T) is an essential factor of energy (E) regulation, which can be expressed as:

$$\mathbf{E} \text{ (in joules)} = \mathbf{P} \text{ (power in watts)} \times \mathbf{T}$$

Tissue heating increases with time, although the process is quite complex:

Practical Pediatric Gastrointestinal Endoscopy, Second Edition. George Gershman, Mike Thomson, Marvin Ament.
© 2012 Blackwell Publishing Ltd. Published 2012 by Blackwell Publishing Ltd.

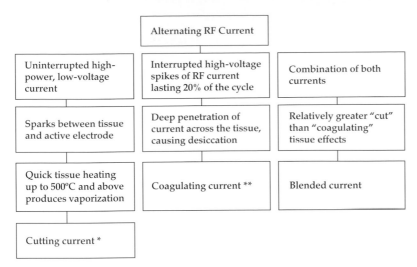

* Low-voltage current penetrates less through desiccation tissue and has limited ability to induce deep tissue heating.

** Spikes of high-voltage coagulating current allow a deeper spread through desiccated tissue and induce more tissue destruction.

Figure 8.1 Different types of alternating RF currents and specific tissue response.

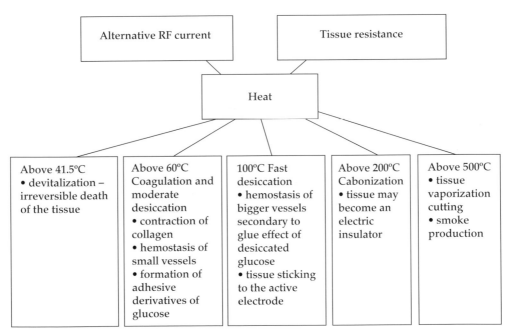

Figure 8.2 Temperature-related tissue destruction always induced by RF current.

- Heating produces water loss and increases resistance.
- Increasing resistance shifts the distribution of current from the lowest resistance pathway.
- Fluctuation of the resistance affects the power output produced by the generator.

- Some of the released heat is removed from high-temperature areas by blood flow.

The cooling effect of bloodflow explains why the same energy applied to the tissue generates less destruction if delivered slowly.

• Current density is a measure of RF current (I) which flows through a specific cross-section area (a):

$$\frac{I}{a} = \frac{I}{\pi r^2}$$

The amount of heat generated in tissue is directly proportional to power density (P) expressed as a square value of current density multiplied by resistance:

$$P = \left(\frac{I}{a}\right)^2 \Re = \frac{I^2}{\pi r^2} \times \Re$$

This important equation implies that power density is an inverted relationship with the square of the cross-sectional area (πr^2). It means that even a small tightening of the loop produces a profound effect on tissue heating. This can be illustrated by the polypectomy of a one centimeter polyp.

If a snare decreases the diameter of a polyp in half, the cross-sectional area at the level of the loop will be only $0.2\,cm^2$. It is 4 times less than a cross-sectional area at the base of a polyp and about 500 times less than a cross-sectional area of skin under a $10\,cm \times 10\,cm$ plate of the "return" electrode.

If $0.2\,A$ electric current is applied through the snare it produces a current density of $1\,A/cm^2$, $0.25\,A/cm^2$ and $0.002\,A/cm^2$ at the level of the loop, polyp bases and skin level respectively.

The fall of the power density, i.e. power actually delivered to the tissue and generated heat, is even more dramatic: from $1\,A/cm^2 \times R$ at the level of the loop, to $0.06\,A/cm^2 \times R$ and $0.000004\,A/cm^2 \times R$ at the base of the polyp and skin under the "return" electrode respectively. Narrowing of a cross-sectional area by a closing snare produces the most significant effect on heat production compared with increasing the power setting and time of electric current application. It also allows one to perform a polypectomy at a lower power using a coagulating mode safely.

The law of current density is vital for polypectomy. Narrowing of a cross-sectional area is the most important safety technique, which produces a coagulation of the core vessels of the polyps before cutting, restricts the area of maximal tissue heating around the loop, and limits tissue destruction of the deep bowel wall layers.

Snare loops

Commercially available snares vary by size, configuration of the loop, design, and mechanical characteristics of the handles and wire thickness. Reusable snares often lose their mechanical properties and can peel and break at the tip. Disposable snares are more durable and predictable. The thickness of the wire loop and handle "behavior" can significantly affect the results of polypectomy. Snares with thick wire loops have two important advantages:

1. A decreased risk of snapping a polyp without adequate coagulation and
2. A large surface contact with tissue resulting in better coagulation.

A standard snare with an opening diameter of 2.5 cm can be used for different size polyps. A special small or "mini" snare (1 cm loop) has been designed for polyps less than 1 cm. It is important for endoscopists to find an "optimal" snare for routine practice in order to avoid any unexpected "surprises" during cutting or coagulation.

A chosen snare should be fully open and then closed to the point when just the tip of a wire loop is outside of outer sheath. Marking of the so-called closing point on the handle of the snare (Figure 8.3) serves two important safety features:

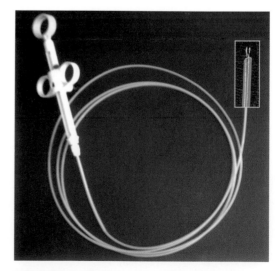

Figure 8.3 Snare preparation before polypectomy: marking of so-called closing point on the handle of the snare.

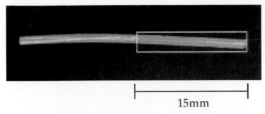

|—————————| 15mm |—————————|

Figure 8.4 Squeezing pressure. A 15 mm retraction of the wire into the plastic sheath provide an optimal narrowing of the polyp base or the stalk for adequate constriction of the blood vessels and generation of an appropriate power density.

1. Protects from premature cutting of a small sessile or pedunculated polyp without adequate coagulation and
2. Alerts the endoscopist of a partial polyp's head entrapment or underestimation of the stalk size.

It is very important to check how far the tip of a wire loop is retracted into the outer plastic sheath when a snare is fully closed. The distance of 15 mm reassures an adequate squeezing pressure (Figure 8.4). If the stalk of a large polyp is not squeezed adequately, it compromises the coagulation of core vessels for two reasons:

- Blood vessels remain open and bloodflow continues producing a cooling effect but more importantly
- A cross-sectional area is not narrow enough to concentrate the current flow to an appropriate power density to coagulate core vessels.

Closure of a snare loop with excessive pressure can induce premature cutting before coagulation. Both conditions could lead to significant bleeding.

The Routine Polypectomy

Polypectomy is the most common therapeutic procedure in pediatric GI Endoscopy. It can be simple or more complex depending on the size or location of the polyp and personal experience. No matter how easy the procedure appears to the endoscopist, it is always wise to follow a simple rule: safety before action.

Safety Routine

It is always useful to routinely inspect the snare and generator as well as prepare the hemostatic equipment such as detachable loops, metal clips, and needle for epinephrine injection. The polypectomy snare should be checked for smooth opening, thickness of the wire (a thin snare predisposes to a premature cut of a small polyp before appropriate coagulation), adequate squeezing pressure, and closing point. It is extremely important to test the generator to find a minimal power setting, which is necessary to induce whitening and swelling of the tissue inside a wire loop. It should be done at least once by adjusting the power output according to the effect of short (2–3 seconds) burst of coagulating current until a visible effect is achieved. The generator setting should be inspected routinely before the procedure to avoid an accidentally high power setting. A foot pedal should be conveniently positioned in front of the endoscopist. A teaching session with the assistant or technician is important for safe and optimal manipulations with a snare during opening or closure.

Safety conditions and techniques

A good bowel preparation is essential not only for optimal viewing and positioning of the loop around a polyp stalk or base, but also to avoid an accidental burning or coagulation of normal mucosa. A large amount of liquid or solid stool increases the chance of missing a small or even a good size polyp. An obscure view often leads to excessive use of air and bowel stretching, which makes the bowel wall thinner.

Sudden patient irritability, unexpected waking or movements complicate the polypectomy, especially during a snare closure and should be prevented by adequate sedation. The technique of polypectomy consists of three important elements:

1. Navigation of the scope to an optimal position, angle and distance to a polyp;
2. Placement of a wire loop around a polyp, and
3. Cutting.

A six o'clock position is an ideal for polypectomy. The location of a polyp between 4 and 5 or 7 and 8 o'clock is suboptimal. Polypectomy is very difficult and somewhat unsafe if a polyp is located on the upper aspect of a lumen between 9 and 3 o'clock.

An ideal 6 o'clock position could be created by clock- or counterclockwise rotation of the shaft and downward deflection of the tip. Careful assessment of the stalk size and location of a polyp is obligatory before polypectomy. It can be done by rotation, advancement of a scope beyond a polyp and pulling the shaft backwards. Once an optimal position and clear view of the polyp is achieved, the scope is moved toward the polyp base. An ideal distance from the tip of the scope to the polyp is 1–2 cm unless the polyp is hiding beyond a fold. In this case, the tip should be positioned just above the fold and pressed down to reveal the polyp. The same effect can be achieved by a closed snare.

All manipulations with a snare should be done slowly.

It is opened just enough to embrace a polyp. Full opening of a snare makes the wire loop floppy and less controllable.

Snaring a sessile polyp at the 6 o'clock position is easy if the wire loop is horizontal to the polyp. Simple downward tip deflection is necessary to encircle the polyp. If an opened wire loop creates an angle at the base of the polyp, the shaft of the scope should be rotated toward a polyp until it is captured. The technique is modified if a sessile polyp is located between 4 and 5 o'clock or 7 and 8 o'clock and previous attempts to establish an ideal 6 o'clock position have failed. The shaft is slightly rotated away from the polyp. The snare is opened more than usual making it less rigid and advanced toward the polyp (Figure 8.5). Once the polyp is inside the loop, the scope is rotated slowly toward the polyp to align the plane of the snare with the axis of a bowel lumen. Then, the snare is closed slowly and moved forward until it reaches the base of the polyp. At this moment, the snare should be completely closed (Figure 8.6).

Occasionally, a backward snaring is more effective, especially if the polyp is more than 1.5 cm in length. An open loop is pointed down towards the area where a polyp head touches the bowel wall. When the snare is advanced, tissue resistance creates a bowing effect and induces a loop opening. As a result, the loop slides between the mucosa and the polyp head. An additional clockwise rotation of the tip using both knobs swings a

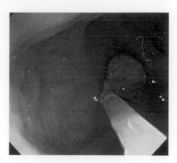

Figure 8.5 The snare is placed around the polyp.

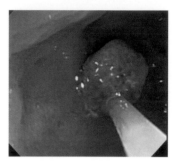

Figure 8.6 The snare is closed tight but not enough to amputate the polyp.

wire loop under the polyp head. If the position of the snare is satisfactory, the snare is slowly closed tight enough for polypectomy.

If a polyp is facing away from the tip, the snare is advanced and opened slowly until the tip of the wire is beyond the polyp's head. The tip of the scope is deflected down slightly to move the wire loop below the polyp. After this, the snare is pulled back until the head of the polyp is inside the loop and the wire is just under the polyp head. The snare is closed slowly and advanced toward to the polyp to prevent sliding of the wire along the stalk.

Advancement of the snare towards the polyp during wire loop closure is a key element to polyp snaring. It secures a polyp within the loop and allows precise navigation of the snare. Capturing a small polyp with a standard snare may be challenging. A slight decompression of the bowel may elevate the polyp above a wire loop and facilitate a capture.

The technique of polypectomy is different when applied to small polyps less than 5 mm, broad-base polyps more than 15 mm, or pedunculated polyps more than 20 mm. Diminutive or small sessile polyps less than 5 mm can be removed safely by cold biopsy forceps (hot biopsy forceps should be avoided as these may be associate with perforation).

Two helpful hints:

1. If a polyp is located on the edge of a fold, position the tip of the colonoscope within a distance of 2 cm from the polyp, open the forceps and place the open cusps perpendicular to the fold just above the polyp and close it. Avoid pushing the forceps up against mucosa as it will stretch tissue and result in suboptimal sampling.

2. If a small polyp is between the folds, try to position the snare with cusps opened horizontally and just enough to outline the polyp. Advance the forceps forward slightly to cover the polyp and close the forceps slowly. An alternative technique consists of
   - Opening the forceps with cusps vertical to the folds
   - Positioning the lower cusp just below the polyp to avoid grasping normal mucosa
   - Closing a snare.

A large sessile polyp is rare in children except in patients with Peutz-Jegher's syndrome. Polyps more than 2.5–3 cm are usually located in the small intestine, primarily in the jejunum. If the size of a polyp is between 10 and 15 mm a single cut polypectomy may be safe if advancement of a snare with the captured polyp does not produce synchronous movements of the underlying wall. This indicates that the submucosa and muscularis propria are not trapped within the wire loop.

Piece-meal technique entails piece-by-piece removal of a large broad-base polyp more than 15 mm. A submucosal injection of saline, hypertonic saline, or epinephrine (1:10 000) solution before polypectomy decreases the risk of the transmural burns.

Injection at the site proximal to the polyp is performed first if possible, followed by injection at the distal edge and both sides of a polyp. Injection of 3 to 10 cc of a chosen solution in three to four sites is usually adequate to create a liquid "cushion" under the polyp. The needle should be oriented tangentially to minimize a risk of transmural injection.

Once again, a broad-base polyp more than 15 mm should be removed in pieces to minimize the risk of perforation. The risk of bleeding is not high as blood vessels in such polyps are much smaller than in large pedunculated polyps.

The piece-meal technique consists of placement of a wire loop diagonally across a polyp and removing the polyp in few pieces. The remaining central area is cut at the end. Excessive closing pressure should be avoided because it may compromise initiation of cutting, due to lack of electrical arc from the active electrode to the tissue. In addition, decreased wire-tissue contact area increases the current density, which may induce excessive desiccation and cease current flow.

Polypectomy of pedunculated polyps more than 2 cm may be challenging. Attention should be paid to proper positioning of the wire loop at the narrowest portion of the stalk right below a polyp head. Thick blood vessels in the middle of the stalk require slow desiccation for complete coagulation and hemostasis before the final cut. Occlusion of a thick stock with Endo-loop® just before manipulations with the snare is effective way to prevent immediate and delayed bleeding after polypectomy.

Clipping devices should be available for immediate action. Do remember that epinephrine injection will only cause vasospasm and apparent hemostasis for 20 minutes or so. It is quite difficult to avoid direct contact of a large pedunculated polyp with normal mucosa during polypectomy. However, attempts should be made to keep a snared polyp close to the center of the bowel lumen to minimize thermal destruction of adjacent tissue. Careful inspection of a long stalk should precede any manipulations with the snare. The location of the polyp base and position of the long stalk are crucial for optimal approach to the polyp. The snare is advanced forward to the lowest point of the polyp head and opened slowly until the loop is big enough to embrace the polyp.

Further manipulation with the snare should be coordinated with either right or left torque of the shaft toward the 6 o'clock direction. Backward snaring may be useful. A reduction of a polyp size by piece-meal technique with prior injection of epinephrine solution (1:10 000) into the stalk below the polypectomy site is the last option to complete the procedure.

After successful capture and adequate tightening of the wire loop, a polyp less than 10 mm is removed using a low power coagulating current (15–18 W) continuously for 2–3 seconds and slow closure of a snare after whitening and tissue swelling has occurred. A modified technique is applied to sessile polyps less than 15 mm or large pedunculated polyps with a small pseudo stalk. Injection of saline or epinephrine (1:10 000) solution underneath the polyp head protects deep tissue from desiccation and decreases mobility of the polyp. This simplifies the placement of the wire loop without trapping a part of the polyp head. A slightly longer duration of coagulation (2–3 cycles) may be necessary for adequate coagulation of blood vessels.

A blended current up to 20–25W may be reasonable for the polypectomy of a broad-base polyp using a piece-meal technique. Lower power setting (10 to 15 watts) is preferable for polypectomy of the polyps in the right side colon or the small bowel.

Different electro-surgical generators have two different setting systems – a dial type with a scale from 0–10. Usually, a setting point between 2 ½ and 3 are equivalent to a low power of 15–20W; – a numeric type system when displayed numbers represent current power in watts.

An endoscopist should become familiar with the particular electrosurgical generator available to his or her practice to avoid an application of excessively high power above 30W, which could lead to a transmural tissue necrosis.

A polypectomy can be performed during colonic intubation or the withdrawal phase of a colonoscopy. The decision is made based on size of the polyp. It is wise to remove a small sessile or pedunculated polyp as soon as it is discovered to eliminate the chance of missing this polyp later on. Removal of a large polyp is more convenient after the entire colon has been inspected, except in the case when the position of a polyp is ideal for polypectomy. Careful examination of the colon, especially behind the folds, can be accomplished by circumferential rotation of the tip and the shaft, aspiration of excessive fluid and repeat insertion of the scope for a few segments if the bowel quickly slipped away from the tip.

After polypectomy, polyps less than 10 mm can be easily sucked into a biopsy channel and eventually into a filtered polyp suction trap. Water irrigation and proper orientation of a suction nostril at the tip of a scope facilitates the recovery process.

During polypectomy, attention should be paid to observing the direction in which the polyp falls. The first place to look for a hidden polyp is in a pool of fluid. If the polyp is not discovered, flush some water and watch where it flows: backflow indicates that the polyp is distal to the tip of a scope.

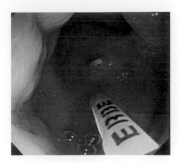

Figure 8.7 APC is useful tool of hemostasis. Bleeding after polypectomy can be successfully controlled by argon plasma probe.

Nylon polyp retrieval nets or metal baskets can be used for removal of multiple polyps. Grasping of a large polyp using the snare is the most reliable way to bring it to the rectum. Manual assistance for the recovery of a specimen may be necessary to squeeze a large polyp more than 3 cm through the anus.

Complications

Three types of complications can occur after polypectomy. The most common one is bleeding. In contrast to adults, a delayed bleeding within 2 weeks after the procedure is quite rare.

Immediate onset of bleeding is more common, although the incidence of this complication is less than 1% in infants and children. This may reflect a smaller size, the number of polyps and the absence of co-morbid conditions such as hypertension, atherosclerosis etc. A slow oozing from the polypypectomy site is easy to control by injection of epinephrine solution (1:10 000) or bipolar or argon plasma coagulation (Figure 8.7).

The risk of arterial bleeding always exists immediately after polypectomy of a large pedunculated polyp due to incomplete coagulation of thick vessels. Endoscopic hemostasis should be prompt before a large amount of blood and clots make the bleeding vessel invisible. A temporary hemostasis can be achieved almost immediately by resnaring and tightening of the stalk. After a few minutes, the wire loop should be replaced by the Endo loop® for permanent hemostasis. In addition, injection of epinephrine below the Endo loop® can augment a hemostatic effect.

FURTHER READING

Cappell MS, Abdullah M. (2000) Management of gastrointestinal bleeding induced by gastrointestinal endoscopy. *Gastrointestinal Endoscopy Clinics of North America*, **29,** 125–167.

Charotini I, Theodoropaulou A, Vardas E, *et al.* (2007) Combination of adrenaline injection and detachable snare application as haemostatic preventive measure before polypectomy of large polyps in children. *Digestive Diseases and Sciences*, **52,** 338–339.

Cotton PB, Williams C, Hawes RH, *et al.* (2008) *Practical Gastrointestinal Endoscopy. The Fundamentals.* (6th edn). pp. 182–201, Blackwell Publishing, Oxford.

Gershman G, Ament ME. (2007) *Practical Pediatric Gastrointestinal Endoscopy.* Blackwell Publishing, Oxford, UK.

Mougenot JF, Vargas J. (2006) Colonoscopic polypectomy and endoscopic mucosal resection. In: Winter HS, Murphy MS, Mougenot JF, *et al*, (eds) *Pediatric Gastrointestinal Endoscopy*. pp. 163–181, BC Decker, Hamilton, Ontario.

Tappero G, Gaia E, DeFiuli P, *et al.* (1992) Cold snare excision of small colorectal polyps. *Gastrointestinal Endoscopy*, **38,** 310–313.

Waye JD. (1997) New methods of polypectomy. *Gastrointestinal Endoscopy Clinics of North America*, **7,** 413–422.

Way JD. (2001) Endoscopic mucosal resection of colon polyps. *Gastrointestinal Endoscopy Clinics of North America*, **11,** 537–548.

9

Chromoendoscopy

Alberto Ravelli, MD

KEY POINTS

- Chromoendoscopy facilitates the optimal mucosal sampling, for example, in children with Barrett's esophagus, celiac sprue, polyposis syndromes and long history of inflammatory bowel disease.
- Technique of mucosal staining is simple and adds only few minutes to the routine endoscopic procedure.

- Interpretation of the stained mucosa is required the knowledge of a positive or negative techniques of chromoendoscopy.
- It is an essential part of enhanced magnification endoscopy or magnification chromoendoscopy.

Indications

Esophageal disorders

One potential indication of chromoendoscopy in the pediatric esophagus is intestinal metaplasia, i.e. Barrett's esophagus. If this condition is suspected, the main aim of chromoendoscopy is to help increase the diagnostic yield of endoscopic biopsies. Positive staining with methylene blue could also be used to identify endoscopically invisible intestinal metaplasia of the cardia region which may exist in patients with GERD. However, it is questionable if methylene blue staining should be applied to all patients with longstanding GERD who undergo upper endoscopy, since intestinal metaplasia can also be found in asymptomatic individuals and the advantage of methylene blue staining over random biopsy is controversial. In adult patients with short-segment Barrett's esophagus, the sensitivity of methylene blue staining for the detection of intestinal metaplasia varies from 60 to 98%, but is generally higher than that of random biopsies. Abnormal

methylene blue staining can also be helpful in delineating dysplastic or malignant areas for endoscopic treatment such as mucosal resection or photodynamic therapy. If mucosectomy is planned, a minimum amount of methylene blue injected with saline into the underlying submucosa which stain it blue, thereby facilitating an accurate removal of the mucosal lesion. In patients who have undergone mucosal ablation, chromoendoscopy could also help distinguish the regenerating squamous epithelium from residual Barrett's mucosa. Lugol's solution has also been used in follow-up endoscopic examination of young patients who have been treated for Barrett's esophagus or dysplasia, in order to promptly detect remnants of unstained Barrett's epithelium.

Studies in adults have shown that chromoendoscopy with Lugol's solution is superior to conventional endoscopy for the detection of severe dysplasia and early squamous cell carcinoma of the esophagus. In a Chinese population with a high esophageal cancer rate, chromoendoscopy with Lugol's solution showed a sensitivity of 62 to 96% and a specificity of 63%. However, esopha-

Practical Pediatric Gastrointestinal Endoscopy, Second Edition. George Gershman, Mike Thomson, Marvin Ament.
© 2012 Blackwell Publishing Ltd. Published 2012 by Blackwell Publishing Ltd.

geal dysplasia and cancer are extremely uncommon in pediatric patients and it should be kept in mind that Lugol's solution can also stain an inflamed esophageal mucosa, namely reflux esophagitis. Other staining techniques such as indigo carmine and acetic acid have been proposed in association with magnification endoscopy to detect Barrett's esophagus and dysplasia. Staining with toluidine blue has been reported to have a very high (98%) sensitivity for Barrett's esophagus, but cannot distinguish between gastric and intestinal metaplasia.

Although studies in adults have shown promising results, so far there are insufficient data supporting a routine use of chromoendoscopy for detecting Barrett's esophagus and dysplasia in children.

Helicobacter pylori infection and related disorders

To date, there are no clear-cut indications for the use of chromoendoscopy to detect specific gastric disorders in clinical practice. At least two reactive dyes, however, deserve attention and may prove useful in the near future. Congo red stains acid-secreting mucosa and has been used in adult patients to detect gastric atrophy, which appears as an area of negative staining on the dark blue/black background of the normal mucosa of the gastric fundus and body. Phenol red turns from yellow to red in the presence of alkaline pH, such as that related to the hydrolysis of urea by urease-producing *H. pylori*, and has been used to map the extent of *H. pylori* colonization in the stomach. Both these staining techniques could, therefore, find an application in pediatric patients with long-standing or refractory *Helicobacter pylori* infection.

Celiac Disease

Gluten-sensitive enteropathy (celiac disease) usually result in endoscopically visible changes of the duodenal mucosa, including a "mosaic" pattern, loss or indentation (scalloping) of Kerckring's folds and a visible vascular pattern. Chromoendoscopy with methylene blue emphasizes the mosaic pattern, although it does not seem to increase the diagnostic yield of endoscopy, at least when performed by experienced gastroenterologists. In one study, indigo carmine scattering combined with magnification endoscopy proved superior to standard endoscopy for the detection of small bowel enteropathy, mainly because it was able to distinguish between total and partial villous atrophy. However, since the diagnosis of celiac disease is established by histology and not by endoscopy, duodenal biopsies should be taken whenever celiac disease is suspected, irrespective of the endoscopic appearance of the duodenal mucosa. Therefore, the major contribution of chromoendoscopy in celiac disease is to allow for better targeting – and consequently some sparing – of duodenal biopsies.

Polyposis syndromes

Chromoendoscopy may be very useful to detect smaller lesions in the duodenum of patients with familial adenomatous polyposis (FAP). Small flat duodenal adenomas may, in fact, go unnoticed during standard endoscopy and even capsule endoscopy, but can be identified as negative-staining lesions when an absorptive dye such as methylene blue is sprayed onto the mucosa. In *colonic polyposis*, the main aim of chromoendoscopy is the same as in the duodenum, i.e. to increase the detection rate by facilitating the identification of small flat polyps, especially adenomas. The preferred dye for the detection of colonic polyps is indigo carmine, a contrast stain that pools in areas of mucosal irregularity and often gives a three-dimensional effect, which is particularly useful for the detection of small protruding lesions. Needless to say, magnification endoscopy and high-resolution endoscopy can add to the accuracy of the technique. In adult studies, left-sided or total colonic indigo carmine staining significantly increased the detection rate of small flat or depressed adenomas. Chromoendoscopy can also help distinguish between hyperplastic and adenomatous polyps, as they produce different staining patterns. In a recent multicenter study, more than 90% of colonic polyps were correctly classified according to the staining pattern, and for adenomatous polyposis, the sensitivity and specificity were 82% and the negative predictive value was 88%.

Inflammatory Bowel Disease

In inflammatory bowel disease (IBD), the greatest potential for chromoendoscopy is the ability to detect dysplasia or cancer early in patients with long-standing ulcerative colitis. Colonic dysplasia and colitis-related colon cancer may also, occasionally, be a problem in pediatric patients, as in the case of ulcerative colitis presenting before 10 years of age, especially if associated with sclerosing cholangitis. In a randomized controlled trial on 174 patients with long-standing ulcerative colitis, total colonic methylene blue staining was clearly superior to conventional surveillance endoscopy with biopsy for the detection of early neoplasia (32 versus 10 overall intraepithelial lesions; 24 versus 8 low-grade and 24 versus 10 in flat mucosa).

Other indications

In the duodenal bulb, methylene blue spray can help identify areas of gastric metaplasia, which is a marker of inflammation such as that related to *H. pylori* infection. Methylene blue was also used to identify the minor papilla in patients with pancreas divisum.

Application technique

Equipment

Special reusable spray catheters such as those used for ERCP (e.g. Olympus PW-5L1) are preferable. The biopsy channel of all modern pediatric videoendoscopes allows the passage of such catheters (Figure 9.1). It is also convenient to use a new biopsy channel cap in order to minimize the leakage of dye. Endoscopists and support staff with less experience in chromoendoscopy should be particularly careful, as most dyes can produce a fairly persistent staining of skin and clothing. Depending on the specific indication and need, different type of stains can be used, i.e. stains that are absorbed by the mucosa (vital stains), stains that produce contrast (reactive stains), and stains for tattooing of the mucosa (Table 9.1).

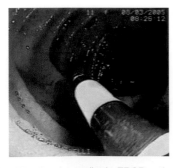

Figure 9.1 The tip of a pediatric ERCP catheter pushed through the biopsy channel is seen in the distal duodenum, prior to dye spraying.

Methylene blue

Methylene blue is actively absorbed by the intestinal epithelium and does not stain non-absorptive tissues such as the normal esophageal or gastric mucosa. Optimal staining requires washing of the mucosa with a mucolytic agent such as N-acetylcysteine prior to spraying a 0.25–0.5% solution of the dye, and subsequent washing with water. The absorptive intestinal epithelium – including metaplastic epithelium as in Barrett's esophagus – is stained blue, whereas the non-absorptive epithelium – such as ectopic gastric metaplasia – is delineated as an area of negative staining against a blue-stained background. The presence of dysplasia or early malignancy within Barrett's epithelium results in inhomogeneous staining, as a consequence of the differential absorption of methylene blue from cells that are depleted of goblet cells and have less cytoplasm. Methylene blue is generally considered to be safe. However, it has been reported that, once photosensitized by white light, methylene blue may induce oxidative damage of the DNA and although it does not usually stain the dysplastic intestinal epithelium, there is concern that it may increase the risk of carcinogenesis in patients with Barrett's esophagus. The parents of patients in whom methylene blue staining is being used should be warned that their child's urine and stool might temporarily acquire a green-bluish color.

Lugol's solution

Lugol's solution contains iodine, which has a special affinity for the glycogen contained in squamous epithelia. For this reason, it is most commonly used in the esophagus, where the normal squamous epithelium is stained green/brown to dark brown or black. Malignancy, dysplasia, metaplasia or even simple inflammation is associated with glycogen depletion and the affected mucosa will thus appear as an unstained area on a dark stained background. Severe allergic reactions to iodine have been reported, so allergy to iodine should be carefully excluded in patients who are undergoing chromoendoscopy with Lugol's solution.

Toluidine blue

Toluidine blue is a basic dye that binds to the nuclear DNA of epithelial cells, and can, therefore, be used to identify tissues with an increased DNA

Table 9.1 Types of staining

Dye (%)	Staining mechanism	Color	Main clinical application(s)
Methylene blue (0.5%)	Absorption into intestinal epithelial cells	Blue	Intestinal metaplasia in esophagus (Barrett's) Intestinal metaplasia in stomach Gastric metaplasia in duodenum *(negative staining)* Celiac disease
Lugol's solution (1%–5%)	Binding to glycogen-containing cells	Dark green/brown or black	Squamous esophageal cancer *(negative staining)* Residual post-ablation Barrett's *(negative staining)* Esophagitis *(negative staining)*
Toluidine blue (1%)	Binding to nuclear DNA of malignant cells	Blue	Squamous esophageal cancer
Indigo carmine (0.1%–0.5%)	Pools in mucosal crevices and pits	Indigo (blue-violet)	Small, flat or superficial polyps Barrett's esophagus Dysplasia or cancer in ulcerative colitis
Congo red (0.3%–0.5%)	Stains acid-producing mucosa (pH <3)	Turns red to dark blue/black	Mapping of acid-secreting mucosa Gastric cancer, gastric atrophy and intestinal metaplasia *(negative staining)*
Phenol red (0.1%)	Stains alkalinized mucosa	Turns yellow to red	Mapping of *H. pylori*-infected mucosa Gastric metaplasia *(negative staining)*
India ink (1%)	Staining of mucosa at site of injection	Black (permanent)	Site of endoscopically removed polyp

(From: Kiesslich R, Neurath MF. (2004) Surveillance colonoscopy in ulcerative colitis: magnifying chromoendoscopy in the spotlight. *Gut*, **53**, 165–167, with permission.)

synthesis such as malignancy. Toluidine blue staining has mainly been used in the endoscopic screening for malignant gastric ulcers and early squamous esophageal cancers in at-risk populations, e.g. heavy alcohol drinkers and smokers.

Indigo carmin

Indigo carmine is the most widely used contrast stain, and is especially useful to identify and define the margins of neoplastic lesions. Indigo carmine, in fact, typically pools in areas of mucosal irregularity, which are stained indigo (blue/violet) color. After washing, pits, grooves and edges of the lesion are highlighted and this may produce a three-dimensional effect, which is particularly useful for the detection of small superficial lesions. Indigo carmine at a concentration of 0.1–0.5% is usually sprayed onto the gut mucosa, but may also be given orally in a capsule. Although mostly utilized to identify small superficial polyps, indigo carmine has been applied in several other conditions such as Barrett's esophagus, gastric cancer, sprue, and ulcerative colitis.

Congo red

Congo red reacts to an acidic pH by changing from red to dark blue or black. Its major application is the identification and mapping of non-secretory gastric mucosa such as that of gastric atrophy, intestinal metaplasia and gastric cancer, which will appear red in contrast to blue/black secretory areas. A stimulation of acid production with pentagastrin is therefore necessary before staining.

Phenol red

Phenol red is also a reactive dye, but unlike Congo red it reacts to an alkaline pH by changing from yellow to red. Patients should undergo pre-treatment with a proton pump inhibitor and an anti-cholinergic, plus the local application of a mucolytic. Once 0.1% phenol red and 5% urea have been sprayed onto the gastric mucosa of *H. pylori*-infected individuals, the alkalinized mucosa is stained red whereas areas of intestinal metaplasia in the stomach will stain negative.

Acetic acid

Acetic acid is a newcomer to GI chromoendoscopy. Preliminary studies suggest that acetic acid stain may help identify Barrett's esophagus as well as duodenal atrophy in celiac disease, by delineating the features of the metaplastic or atrophic intestinal epithelium.

India ink

When injected into the mucosa, 1% India ink produces a permanent black staining. India ink can be injected superficially into the mucosa to mark the site where a worrisome polyp has been endoscopically removed, or it can be injected deeper to mark a lesion that has to be removed surgically.

Patient's sedation

As the main aim of chromoendoscopy is to allow for the visualization of small and fine features of the gut mucosa, the whole procedure can be rendered completely useless if the patient is restless or agitated. Therefore, unless the patient is fully cooperative – which is the exception rather than the rule in pediatric endoscopy – an adequate sedation is mandatory to maintain the patient still throughout the procedure. Conscious sedation with midazolam 0.05–0.01 mg/kg i.v. may not be sufficient in infants or very anxious children, where deep sedation with propofol or a brief general anesthesia may be necessary.

Preparation of the mucosa

There is no doubt that chromoendoscopy gives better results when the gut mucosa to be examined is cleared from mucus (and blood, bile or food debris, if present). So, whenever possible, the mucosa should be washed prior to staining. A better washing is obtained if forceful pressure is applied with a syringe either through the spray catheter or directly into the biopsy channel. If absorptive dyes such as methylene blue or Lugol's solution are to be used, the mucosa should be washed with a few ml of 10% N-acetylcysteine to adequately remove mucus. Once the tissue has been stained, a wash with water or saline can remove the excess, non-absorbed dye. If the vision is disturbed by bubbles or foam, a small volume of an antifoam preparation (e.g. simethicone 10–20 drops) can be added to the wash. A spasmolytic drug such as hyoscine N-butylbromide can be administered i.v. to reduce peristalsis or smooth muscle spasm and maximize visualization of the mucosal area of interest. As mentioned above, when a pH-sensitive dye is used, acid secretion should be either stimulated or suppressed, depending on the dye being used.

Staining technique

The technique for staining is fairly simple. Once the gut area of interest has been reached and adequately washed (see above), the endoscope and the tip of the catheter should be directed towards the mucosa with a combination of clockwise and counterclockwise rotation movements, and the dye should be sprayed onto the mucosa while the tip of the endoscope is gently and slowly withdrawn. The only exception is India ink staining which is, in fact, a permanent tattoo of the mucosa and as such requires injection into the mucosa or submucosa. Once satisfactory images are obtained, it is always advisable to take photographs of the stained mucosa, in order to compare staining features with the histological abnormalities, to assess interobserver variability and also to monitor the improvement of the staining technique over time. Recently, guidelines have been proposed for optimal chromoendoscopy in ulcerative colitis (Table 9.2), but most of these guidelines do apply to chromoendoscopy in general.

Table 9.2 "Surface" guidelines for chromoendoscopy in ulcerative colitis
1. **S**trict patient selection patients with histologically proven ulcerative colitis and at least 8 years' duration in clinical remission; avoid patients with active disease
2. **U**nmask the mucosal surface excellent bowel preparation; remove mucus and remaining fluid in the colon when necessary
3. **R**educe peristaltic waves when drawing back the endoscope, a spasmolytic agent should be used if necessary
4. **F**ull length staining of the colon in ulcerative colitis, perform pan-chromoendoscopy rather than local staining
5. **A**ugmented detection with dyes vital staining with 0.4% indigo carmine or 0.1% methylene blue should be used to unmask flat lesions more frequently than with conventional colonoscopy
6. **C**rypt architecture analysis using magnification endoscopy, all lesions should be analyzed according to the pit pattern classification; whereas pit pattern types I-II suggest the presence of non-malignant lesions, staining patterns III-IV suggest the presence of intraepithelial neoplasias and carcinomas
7. **E**ndoscopic targeted biopsies perform targeted biopsies of all mucosal alterations, particularly of circumscribed lesions with staining patterns indicative of intraepithelial neoplasias and carcinomas, i.e. pit patterns III–IV.
(From: Kiesslich R, Neurath MF. (2004) Surveillance colonoscopy in ulcerative colitis: magnifying chromoendoscopy in the spotlight. *Gut*, 53, 165–167, with permission).

Recognition of the lesions

Barrett's esophagus and related disorders

Methylene blue is absorbed by the intestinal epithelium, so it has been used for the endoscopic detection of the intestinal metaplasia typical of Barrett's esophagus, especially when the diagnosis is uncertain as it may be in short-segment Barrett's. The staining is usually homogeneous but in short-segment Barrett's it may be somewhat patchy due to the presence of non-intestinal columnar cells. More importantly, in Barrett's esophagus, the pattern of methylene blue staining is irregular and heterogeneous if dysplasia or cancer is present (Figure 9.2). Heterogeneously stained or light blue/unstained areas should be biopsied with particular care in search of high-grade dysplasia and early adenocarcinoma. If Lugol's solution is used, Barrett's epithelium, dysplasia or carcinoma will appear as areas of negative staining on the dark green/brown stained background of the normal squamous epithelium.

Helicobacter pylori infection and related disorders

In patients with long-lasting *H. pylori infection*, chromoendoscopy with Congo red will demonstrate gastric atrophy as an area of negative staining on the dark blue/black background of the normal mucosa of the gastric fundus and body. Chromoendoscopy with phenol red will define the extent of *H. pylori* colonization in the stomach by producing a yellow staining throughout the affected gastric mucosa, which is alkalinized by urease.

– Celiac Disease

Staining with methylene blue, even without preparation of the duodenal mucosa, makes the typical mosaic pattern more prominent and crisp, emphasizing the coarse, "cobblestone" appearance of the celiac mucosa that may not be evident at standard endoscopy (Figure 9.3). Immersion chromoendoscopy – i.e. 1% methylene blue spray

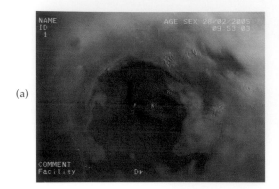

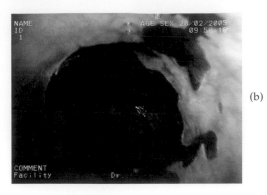

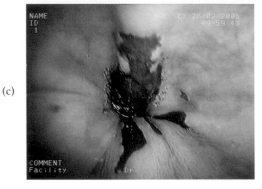

Figure 9.2 Endoscopic view of Barrett's esophagus: (a) plain close view; (b) close view after 0.1% methylene blue staining; (c) with the endoscope slightly withdrawn, a small area of negative staining can be seen in the uppermost part of the lesion (top); biopsy of this area showed moderate grade dysplasia.

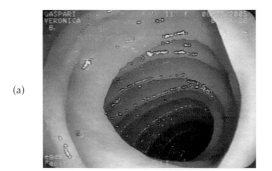

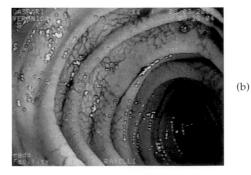

Figure 9.3 Endoscopic view of the distal duodenum in a patient with celiac disease and total villous atrophy. (a) A very mild scalloping of Kerckring's folds can be seen, but there is no clear evidence of mucosal atrophy; (b) Even without preparation of the mucosa, the mosaic pattern typical of gluten-sensitive enteropathy is clearly seen following methylene blue spray.

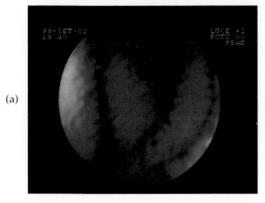 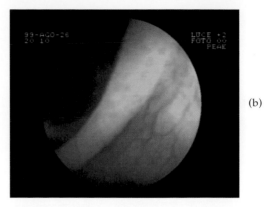

(a) (b)

Figure 9.4 Immersion chromoendoscopy after methylene blue spray, without preparation of the mucosa. Unlike the normal duodenum, where villi are clearly seen along the mucosal folds (a), in patients with celiac disease and total villous atrophy duodenal folds appear flat and "denudated" and the typical cobblestone or mosaic pattern of the mucosa is highlighted (b).

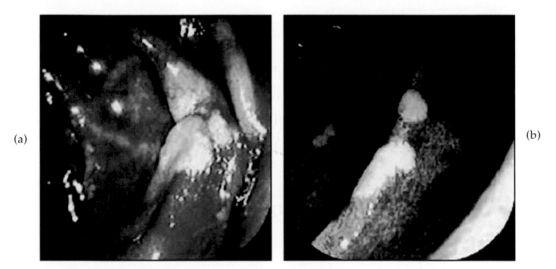

(a) (b)

Figure 9.5 In a patient with familial adenomatous polyposis coli, flat (a) or minimally raised (b) duodenal adenomas stand out as small areas of negative staining following methylene blue spray (From: Weinstein W. Tissue sampling, specimen handling, and chromoendoscopy. In: Ginsberg GG, Kochman ML, Norton ID, Gostout CJ (Eds), *Clinical Gastrointestinal Endoscopy,* Elsevier Science 2005;59–75, with permission).

combined with magnification obtained by immersion of the endoscope tip – can amplify the difference between the mosaic pattern due to villous atrophy and the normal duodenal mucosa where villi can be clearly seen along the duodenal folds (Figure 9.4).

Polyposis syndromes

In patients with familial adenomatous polyposis (FAP), small flat duodenal adenomas will be easily identified as negative-staining plaques following methylene blue spray (Figure 9.5). In colonic polyposis, indigo carmine staining can help identify small superficial lesions such as flat or depressed adenomas. Indigo carmine and methylene blue can also differentiate hyperplastic (i.e. non-neoplastic) polyps from adenomatous (i.e. neoplastic) polyps, as the former are characterized by a regular pitted pattern (Figure 9.5), whereas a grooved or sulcus pattern is typical of adenomatous polyps (Figure 9.6).

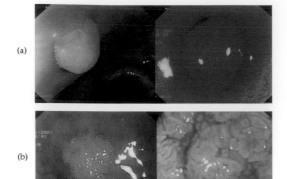

(a)

(b)

Figure 9.6 Colonic polyps before and after chromoendoscopy: (top) hyperplastic polyp showing a regular pitted pattern, and (bottom) neoplastic polyp showing a sulciform pattern. *(From: Kiesslich R, Neurath MF. Surveillance colonoscopy in ulcerative colitis: magnifying chromoendoscopy in the spotlight. Gut 2004;53:165–7, with permission).*

Inflammatory Bowel Disease (IBD)

In patients with long-standing ulcerative colitis, colonic dysplasia will appear as an area of negative-staining following methylene blue spray. If an early cancer is present within a metaplastic area, the staining will appear inhomogeneous and subsequent carmine red staining could be helpful to outline the margins of the lesion. As in colonic polyposis syndromes, methylene blue and indigo carmine staining can help discriminate between hyperplastic and neoplastic lesions (Figure 9.6).

 FURTHER READING

Acosta MM, Boyce HW Jr. (1998) Chromo-endoscopy: where is it useful? *Journal of Clinical Gastroenterology*, **27**, 13–20.

Bernstein CN. (1999) The color of dysplasia in ulcerative colitis. *Gastroenterology*, **124**, 1135–1138.

Canto MI. (1999) Staining in gastrointestinal endoscopy: the basics. *Endoscopy*, **31**, 479–486.

Da Costa R, Wilson BC, Marcon NE. (2003) Photodiagnostic techniques for the endoscopic detection of premalignant gastrointestinal lesions. *Diagnostic Endoscopy*, **15**, 153–173.

Canto MI, Yoshida T, Gossner L. (2002) Chromo-scopy of intestinal metaplasia in Barrett's esophagus. *Endoscopy*, **34**, 330–336.

Eisen GM, Kim CY, Fleischer DE, *et al.* (2002) High-resolution chromoendoscopy for classifying colonic polyps: A multicenter study. *Gastrointestinal Endoscopy*, **55**, 687–694.

Kiesslich R, Mergener K, Naumann C, *et al.* (2003) Value of chromoendoscopy and magnification endoscopy in the evaluation of duodenal abnormalities: a prospective, randomized comparison. *Endoscopy*, **35**, 559–563.

Kiesslich R, Neurath MF. (2004) Surveillance colonoscopy in ulcerative colitis: magnifying chromoendoscopy in the spotlight. *Gut*, **53**, 165–167.

Siegel LM, Stevens PD, Lightdale CJ, *et al.* (1997) Combined magnification endoscopy with chromoendoscopy in the evaluation of patients with suspected malabsorption. *Gastrointestinal Endoscopy*, **46**, 226–230.

Weinstein W. (2005) Tissue sampling, specimen handling, and chromoendoscopy. In: Ginsberg GG, Kochman ML, Norton ID, Gostout CJ (eds.). *Clinical Gastrointestinal Endoscopy*. pp. 59–75, Elsevier Science.

Part Three

Advanced Pediatric
Endoscopy
Techniques

10

Endoscopic hemostasis of variceal bleeding with polymeric glue:
indications, preparation, instruments and technique and complications of N-butyl-2-cyanoacrylate injection

Mike Thomson

 KEY POINTS

- The most important issue is prevention of introduction of the glue into the endoscope biopsy channel which leads to irreparable damage to the instrument.
- To avoid endoscopic glue damage, the tip of the injection catheter should be cut with scissors and retrograde removal of the remainder of the catheter then safely undertaken.
- Gastric fundal varices are amenable to the use of glue and this is the standard now for their treatment.

- Embolization of the glue has been reported.
- The glue is now provided in a single vial for ease of administration.
- Safe and effective use of glue for fundal varices is well reported in children, and can be aided by endo-ultrasound for site identification and confirmation of successful obliteration of the varices.

Practical Pediatric Gastrointestinal Endoscopy, Second Edition. George Gershman, Mike Thomson, Marvin Ament.
© 2012 Blackwell Publishing Ltd. Published 2012 by Blackwell Publishing Ltd.

This technique has gained popularity due, in the main, to the higher incidence of complications emanating from band ligation of fundal varices. This will often lead to hemorrhage which can be uncontrollable, or significant ulceration at the site of banding. Equally, the injection of sclerosant such as ethanolamine is complicated by lack of sufficient speed of action such that hemorrhage will result.

It should be pointed out, however, that some groups continue to employ banding of fundal varices with success, but will employ strict post-banding 'nil-by-mouth' regimes for up to one week subsequently. (Mortada, personal communication)

It is generally held, nevertheless, that injection of a tissue glue such as N-butyl-2-cyanoacrylate for fundal varices is the optimum method endoscopically for dealing with the difficult clinical situation represented by gastric varices. Usually, these will be dealt with prior to esophageal variceal banding in view of the proximal site of blood flow of gastric versus esophageal variceal site. Equally it may be felt, especially in the very young child, that a surgical solution might be preferable such as a REX shunt or a tranjugular intrahepatic porto-systemic shunt (TIPSS).

This is an effective technique both in achieving hemostasis immediately and in the prevention of late bleeding, and is well documented in the adult literature. Longer term efficacy is also recognized in adult GI experience. In one retrospective study recently published, 31 patients received histoacryl for gastric variceal bleeding. Seventy-four per cent of patients had alcohol-related liver disease and 58% were actively bleeding during the procedure with 100% hemostasis rates achieved. Two patients developed pyrexia within 24 hours of injection settling with antibiotics. No other complications were encountered. Mean overall follow-up was 35 months, with mean follow-up of survivors, 57 months. Forty-eight per cent of patients had endoscopic ultrasound assessment of varices during follow-up with no effect on rebleeding rates. Thirteen per cent required subsequent transjugular intrahepatic portosystemic shunt placement. Gastric variceal rebleeding rate was 10% at 1 year and 16% in total. One- and two-year mortality was 23% and 35%, respectively.

Acute injection in esophageal variceal bleeding has recently been receiving attention. One study prospectively performed glue injection in 133 adult cirrhotic patients: 52 patients were actively bleeding at endoscopy and 81 showed stigmata of recent hemorrhage. Initial hemostasis was achieved in 49/52 active bleeders (94.2% [95% CI 85.1–98.5]). Overall, early recurrent bleeding occurred in 7 patients (5.2% [95% CI 2.3–10.1]). No major procedure-related complication was recorded. At 6 weeks, death occurred in 11 patients, with an overall bleeding-related mortality of 8.2% [95% CI 5.8–15.3]. Mortality was higher in active (15.4% [95% CI 6.9–28.1]) than non-active bleeders (3.7% [95% CI 0.8–10.4], OR 4.7 [95% CI 1.05–28.7], $p = 0.02$). Of those surviving the first bleeding episode, 112 patients subsequently underwent ligation. No technical difficulties were encountered in performing the banding procedure which was successfully completed in all cases.

In children, the use of the glue injection technique has been utilized in infants in whom the diameter of the esophagus may preclude introduction of the banding devices, and in pilot studies does seem effective and safe in the short-term, with rebleeding rate of 3/8 young children under 2 years old within 12 weeks.

Preparation and technique

A standard upper GI endoscope is used with a 2.8 mm biopsy channel. Endoultrasound (radial or linear) can be used prior to injection (Figure 10.1) in order to firstly identify varices with blood flow

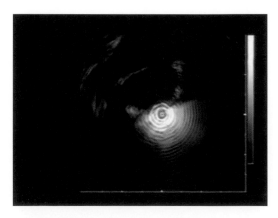

Figure 10.1 Endoultrasound of a fundal varix can assist in needle placement and can allow the operator to ensure adequate variceal obliteration.

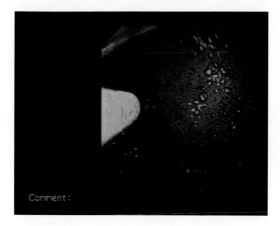

Comment:

Figure 10.2 Firm injection into the varix of the glue with close cooperation of endoscopist and needle operator is essential.

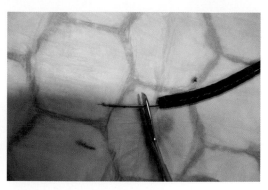

Figure 10.4 The glue-contaminated 5–10 cm of catheter is cut with scissors prior to catheter withdrawal through the endoscope in order to prevent the inevitable and irrevocable damage by glue to the biopsy channel of the endoscope.

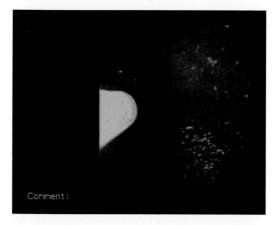

Comment:

Figure 10.3 Subsequent to glue injection hemostasis is assured and the needle is withdrawn into its sheath.

Standard technique is well described in the literature and is as follows:

1. Dilution of 0.5 mL of N-butyl-2-cyanoacrylate with 0.8 mL of Lipiodol – pre-mixed solution in an ampoule with blue dye is now standard however (Histoacryl®);
2. Limiting the volume of mixture to 1.0 mL per injection to minimize the risk of embolism;
3. Repeating intravariceal injections of 1.0 mL each until hemostasis is achieved;
4. Obliteration of all tributaries of the FV;
5. Repeat endoscopy 4 days after the initial treatment to confirm complete obliteration of all visible varices and repeat N-butyl-2-cyanoacrylate injection if necessary to accomplish complete obliteration.

amenable to injection, and then to identify successful injection of glue into the varix. Otherwise, direct vision and presumption of success is used, such that a bulge is produced in the varix and hemostasis is assured. (Figure 10.2) The needle operator must work closely with the endoscopist to ensure no leakage of glue occurs, that the needle is withdrawn into the catheter, and that hemostasis is observed before the next varix is injected. (Figure 10.3) The number of varices does not seem to matter in terms of a single endoscopy, as long as hemostasis is not a problem, which it rarely is.

At the end of the procedure, the needle catheter is NOT withdrawn into the endoscope biopsy channel, thereby avoiding any glue entering the inside of the endoscope. The endoscope is withdrawn from the patient with the needle housed in the catheter but with the catheter still protruding from the tip of the endoscope. The catheter can then be flushed and the tip further extended from the endoscope, and finally the distal 5 cm of the catheter is cut off with scissors. (Figure 10.4) It is at this point only that the remainder of the catheter can be pulled out through the biopsy channel i.e., at NO time should the catheter be withdrawn once it is first placed through the biopsy channel until the procedure is finished, and the glue-contaminated catheter tip is cut off and discarded. Strict adherence to this rule will prevent the unfortunate ruining of an endoscope by biopsy channel blockage, and an experienced endoscopy assistant is recommended.

Complications

Embolization is a potential risk, and if a right to left intra-cardiac communication such as an atrial or ventricular septal defect is present, then systemic rather than pulmonary embolization may be a risk.

Local hemorrhage can occur but is short-lived and will usually spontaneously stop, but apart from this, and with careful technique, with or without endoultrasound, local complications are limited – hence this is a relatively safe technique which can be repeated, and is usually successful in variceal obliteration.

However, glue extrusion does occur and Wang's paper has highlighted this recently. The instantaneous hemostatic rate was 96.2%. Early rebleeding after injection in 9/148 cases (6.2%) was estimated from rejection of adhesive. Late rebleeding occurred in 12 patients (8.1%) at 2–18 months. The glue cast was extruded into the lumen within one month in 86.1% of patients and eliminated within one year. Light erosion was seen at the injection position and mucosal edema in the second week. The glue casts were extruded in 18 patients (12.1%) after one week and in 64 patients (42.8%) after two weeks. All kinds of glue clumping shapes and colors on endoscopic examination were observed in 127 patients (86.1%) within one month, including punctiform, globular, pillar and variform. Forty one patients (27.9%) had glue extrusion after 3 months, and 28 patients (28.9%) after six months. The extrusion time was not related to the injection volume of histocryl. Obliteration was seen in 70.2% (104 cases) endoscopically. The main complication was rebleeding resulting from extrusion. The prognosis of the patients depended on the severity of the underlying liver disease.

One report of pyogenic portal vein complication is recently noted by Chang.

The major limitation of injecting this glue is not embolization or local complication for the child, but damage to the biopsy channel of the endoscope itself. If **any** glue were to leak from the injecting endoscopic needle (which is the same as a standard injecting needle) then this will be blocked, thus rendering the endoscope totally unusable. This dictates that the operator employs great care when performing this procedure.

Thrombin

Acute injection of thrombin into gastric varices is described in small series but is generally not common practice. In adult patients who have undergone thrombin injections, hemostasis in the acute setting has been successful in up to 92% of cases. Patients usually receive 1 to 4 sessions of thrombin, with a mean total dose of approximately 10 mL for variceal eradication. Dry thrombin for reconstitution can be kept in the endoscopy unit in the fridge for acute use and technique is identical to other injection techniques.

In summary then, there is little reported literature describing pediatric experience of glue injection for esophagogastric varices, but extrapolating from adult practice would seem reasonable, given that this is now regarded as a well-established technique. The caveat of extreme care to be taken when injecting cannot be over-emphasized.

📖 FURTHER READING

Al-Ali J, Pawlowska M, Coss A, et al. (2010) Endoscopic management of gastric variceal bleeding with cyanoacrylate glue injection: safety and efficacy in a Canadian population. *Canadian Journal of Gastroenterology*, **10,** 593–596.

Chang CJ, Shiau YT, Chen TL, et al. (2008) Pyogenic portal vein thrombosis as a reservoir of persistent septicemia after cyanoacrylate injection for bleeding gastric varices. *Digestion*, **78(2–3),** 139–143.

Cheng LF, Wang ZQ, Li CZ, et al. (2007) Treatment of gastric varices by endoscopic sclerotherapy using butyl cyanoacrylate: 10 years' experience of 635 cases. *Chinese Medicine Journal (Engl)*, **120(23),** 2081–2085.

Cipolletta L, Zambelli A, Bianco MA, et al. (2009) Acrylate glue injection for acutely bleeding oesophageal varices: A prospective cohort study. *Digestive Liver Disease*, **41(10),** 729–734.

Marion-Audibert AM, Schoeffler M, Wallet F, et al. (2008) Acute fatal pulmonary embolism during cyanoacrylate injection in gastric varices.

Gastroenterology Clinical Biology, **32(11)**, 926–30.

Rajoriya N, Forrest EH, Gray J, *et al.* (2011) Long-term follow-up of endoscopic Histoacryl glue injection for the management of gastric variceal bleeding. *Quarterly Journal of Mathematics*, Sep **104(1)**, 41–47.

Ramesh J, Limdi JK, Sharma V, *et al.* (2008) The use of thrombin injections in the management of bleeding gastric varices: a single-center experience. *Gastrointestinal Endoscopy*, **68(5)**, 877–882.

Rivet C, Robles-Medranda C, Dumortier J, *et al.* (2009) Endoscopic treatment of gastroesophageal varices in young infants with cyanoacrylate glue: A pilot study. *Gastrointestinal Endoscopy*, **69(6)**, 1034–1038.

Romero-Castro R, Pellicer-Bautista FJ, Jimenez-Saenz M, *et al.* (2007) EUS-guided injection of cyanoacrylate in perforating feeding veins in gastric varices: results in 5 cases. *Gastrointestinal Endoscopy*, **66(2)**, 402–407.

Seewald S, Ang TL, Imazu H, *et al.* (2008) A standardized injection technique and regimen ensures success and safety of N-butyl-2-cyanoacrylate injection for the treatment of gastric fundal varices (with videos). *Gastrointestinal Endoscopy*, **68(3)**, 447–454.

Yan-Mei Wang, Liu-Fang Cheng, Nan Li, *et al.* (2009) Study of glue extrusion after endoscopic N-butyl-2-cyanoacrylate injection on gastric variceal bleeding. *World Journal of Gastroenterology*, **15(39)**, 4945–4951.

11

Endoscopic treatment of benign esophageal strictures with removable or biodegradable stents

Yvan Vandenplas, Bruno Hauser, Thierry Devreker, Daniel Urbain, Hendrik Reynaert, Antonio Quiros

---

 KEY POINTS

- Esophageal stenting is a feasible alternative for children with recurrent esophageal stricture unresponsive to standard therapy.

- Retrievable, fully covers self-expendable metal and especially biodegradable stents have potential to become a standard therapy for children with refractory esophageal strictures.

- Esophageal stenting should be performed in specialized pediatric centers under general anesthesia by experience pediatric or adult gastroenterologists.

- Despite lack of convincing evidence, esophageal stenting is a reasonable choice for some children with refractory esophageal stricture facing surgery.

- Further research is necessary for development of uniform recommendations related to different aspects of this advanced procedure in children.

Introduction

In contrast to pediatric gastroenterologists, adult colleges have accumulated substantial experience with different types of esophageal stents. The main indication for esophageal stenting in adults is palliative therapy in patients with unresectable esophageal cancer. Esophageal stents also have been used for the management of benign esophageal strictures, fistulas, esophageal perforation and anastomotic leaks. In children, esophageal stents gained some ground in treatment of refractory or recurrent esophageal strictures following caustic ingestion or repaired esophageal atresia. A role for esophageal stenting as an alternative treatment of foreign body or procedure-related esophageal perforation or anastomotic leak in pediatric patients is the subject of future research.

Conventional treatment of esophageal strictures in children

Endoscopic balloon dilatation or bougienage are the two standard modalities often used as an initial therapy for children with esophageal strictures. The technique of endoscopic balloon dilatation is described in Chapter 6 of this book.

Savary-Miller dilatators are more frequently used in older children with a technique similar to that used in adults. The preventive role of steroids in children with high risk of esophageal stricture (mainly caustic injury) is still debatable. High doses of methylprednosolone ($1 g/1/73 m^2$) have been advocated to reduce the frequency and severity of strictures. However, early treatment (within 24 hours after ingestion of the caustic product) versus delayed treatment, or short versus long treatment (less than or more than 21 days) was reported to make no difference. Topical application of mitomycin C has been used with some success (about 66%) to prevent recurrence of the stricture or scar formation. Colonic interposition or gastric pull-up is reserved for severe and relapsing cases such as long strictures after ingestion of corrosive agents. The long-term outcome after the surgical reconstruction of the esophagus is associated with various complications requiring additional therapy and even reconstructive surgery in some patients.

Esophageal stent: the new approach to refractory or relapsing benign esophageal strictures

The development of removable stents stimulated an application of these devices for treatment of benign esophageal strictures and other conditions unrelated to the esophageal malignancy. Various types of esophageal stents are commercially available. They differ in stent material, design, luminal diameter, radial force exerted, flexibility, degree of shortening after placement and extent of coverage. In order to achieve the best results, it is impor-

tant to weigh the benefits against the shortcomings and complications associated with various stents. Currently, self-expandable plastic stents (SEPS) and self-expanding metal stents (SEMS) mostly made from nitinol (alloy of nickel and titanium), dominate the market.

Self-Expandable Metal Stents

At first, expandable stents were made from stainless steel and were uncovered. Despite many imperfections, these stents had several advantages over plastic prostheses: a very small (3 mm) diameter before deployment, expansion up to 16 mm[9] and flexibility, which simplified the technique and made it less traumatic. The newer stents are made of nitinol and have a diameter up to 23 mm after expansion. Nitinol is a biocompatible alloy with shape memory and high elasticity. Nitinol stents are flexible, kink-resistant, and exert a persistent radial outward force, which make them very attractive to manage malignant strictures.

Although the palliation for dysphagia caused by esophageal cancer was not superior to plastic prosthesis, the complication rate of SEMS was significantly lower compared to plastic devices. Major complications associated with SEMS include hemorrhage, aspiration, perforation, food impaction, and migration, sometimes causing bowel obstruction. Minor complications include chest pain or sore throat, nausea, fever, and reflux. Stents that are close to the upper esophageal sphincter induce a high degree of intolerance due to pain and globus sensation, as well as an increased risk of complications such as tracheoesophageal fistula and aspiration pneumonia. Therefore, a stent should be placed at least 2 cm below the upper esophageal sphincter.

The big disadvantage of uncovered metal stent is obstruction caused by tumor growth through the metal mesh.

Covered SEMS were developed to overcome this problem. In fact, these stents were only covered from the inside, allowing the uncovered external part to embed and anchor into the mucosa. However, these stents have a higher incidence of migration compare to uncovered stents.

Experience with SEMS in benign strictures is by far less rewarding than in malignancy. Several limitations of SEMS preclude their routine use in benign esophageal strictures. The most important one is difficulty removing the stent because of tissue embedment that occurs through the uncovered surface. Traumatic removal results in complications such as bleeding and the development of new strictures at the site of injury caused by granulation tissue. Moreover, SEMS placed for benign disease are associated with significant other complications such as high migration rates, fistula, erosion into vital structures, and even death. Based on the high complication rate, **partially covered SEMS cannot be recommended for patients with benign esophageal stricture**.

Self- Expandable Plastic Stents

This type of stent (Figure 11.1) is made from polyester netting embedded in a silicone membrane. A proximal flare improves stent fixation and prevents migration. Silicone reinforced ends of the stent help resist tissue damage and development of granulations. The diameter of the delivery device is 12–14 mm, which makes dilatation of the stricture before stent insertion mandatory. Similar to SEMS, the plastic stent should cover the entire length of the structure with an additional 1–2 cm above and below. Retrieval and repositioning of this fully covered stent can be done with a foreign body forceps or a standard polypectomy snare.

The steps of the procedure are, an endoscopic assessment of the length of the stricture and balloon dilatation to the size appropriate to accommodate the delivery system, placement of a stiff guidewire into the stomach, removal of the endoscope and positioning of the stent across the stricture using a delivery system under fluoroscopy and actual deployment of the stent.

Over the last decade, SEPS have been found ground in treatment of benign recurrent or refractory esophageal strictures. The main advantage of SEPS over the older types of SEMS in the field of benign esophageal disorders is elimination of the hyperplastic granulomatous reaction induced by the uncovered ends of the metal stents. Additional benefits are low risk of granulation tissue embedding into the stent and new stricture develop-

ment, safe process of SEPS removal and lower cost. Until now, there have been no large randomized control studies (RCTs) evaluating the role of SEPS in benign esophageal strictures, but there are several case studies. Initial results were promising with sustain relief of dysphagia in a high number of patients (up to 95%). However, subsequent data was conflicting. Although, a recent pooled-data analysis from 10 studies including 130 patients who were treated with SEPS for benign refractory esophageal strictures showed a favorable risk/benefit ratio. Sixty-eight of 130 (52%) adult patients were symptom-free without the need for further endoscopic dilatations during median follow-up after SEPS procedure. The success rate appeared to be statistically higher in patients with strictures in the mid-or low-esophagus than in those with strictures in the upper esophagus (54% versus 33%) and in patients with stricture equal or longer than 2 cm rather than shorter strictures (49% versus 28%). Early stent migration occurred in 19 (23%) patients. Twelve patients (9%) experienced complications including three cases of perforation, three cases of bleeding, two cases of tracheal compression and two cases of inability to remove the stent. This study supports the idea that SEPS could be a valuable alternative to repeat endoscopic dilatation for patients with refractory esophageal.

In the pediatric population, the biggest limitation of SERS is the size of current delivery devices and need for a stiff guidewire. The procedure is associated with radiation exposure and use of general anesthesia with endo-tracheal intubation for airway protection.

Fully covered, retrievable SEMS

Fully covered retrievable SEMS (Figure 11.2) have been developed and approved for malignant disease, but also show promise for the treatment of benign esophageal disorders. The stent is composed of a nitinol wire covered with polyurethane.

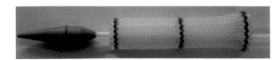

Figure 11.1 Self expendable plastic stent (Polyflex, Boston Scientific Co. Natic, MA, USA) with delivery device. The stent is made from polyester netting embedded in a silicone membrane. A proximal flare improves stent fixation and prevents migration.

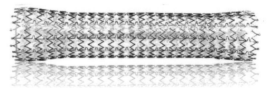

Figure 11.2 Fully covered self expandable metal stent (Alimaxx-E Inc, Charlotte, NC, USA).

Nylon loops are woven into the ends. Grasping the stent by the biopsy forceps will stretch and narrow it down and makes the retrieval process easier and less traumatic. A specific stent retrieval system has been designed. The data from small series indicated varied relief of dysphagia in most patients with benign esophageal strictures. However, stent migration was recorded in almost 80% of the patients during 8 weeks, and new or recurrent strictures were seen in about half of them. An additional complication is folding of the stent if it was too wide. A folded stent can be replaced with a smaller one. Nitinol stents will expand when heated and continue to expand through the first 2 days after deployment, mandating a strict liquid room temperature diet for the first 48 hours. The risk of distal migration increases with time in parallel to softening of the stricture and decreasing of inflammation. Repositioning of the original stent or replacement with the larger size is feasible.

Biodegradable stents

A recent evolution of stent technology led to the development of biodegradable stents (Figure 11.3). These types of stent are made from degradable synthetic material. In Europe, biodegradable stents are manufactured from commercially available polydioxanone absorbable surgical suture ((ELLA-CS, s.k.o., Hradec Kralove, Czech Republic). Polydioxanone is a semicrystalline, biodegradable polymer belonging to the polyester family. It degrades by random hydrolysis of its molecule ester bonds. The degradation accelerates by low pH. None of the degradation products or intermediates is harmful. The stent is provided in unfolded form, and immediately before placement, it needs to be loaded into a dedicated applicator (28F) with an atraumatic dilator tip. The stent is designed to maintain the integrity and radial force for at least 8 weeks following implantation. Stent disintegration occurs 11–12 weeks after insertion. The stents are radio transparent and have radioopaque markers at both the proximal and distal ends. The diameter of the stent is 25 mm with lengths ranging from 60 to 135 mm. After releasing, the biodegradable stent, which is not removable, expands gradually and maintains its preformed diameter.

Poly-/-lactic acid monofilaments biodegradable esophageal stent (Tanaka-Marui stent; Marui Textile Machinery Co., Ltd., Osaka, Japan) is available in Japan.

In a Japanese case series, 13 patients with benign esophageal stenosis were treated with poly-/-lactic acid monofilaments biodegradable esophageal stent (Tanaka-Marui stent; Marui Textile Machinery Co., Ltd., Osaka, Japan). The stent was deployed successfully in all patients. In 10 of the 13 cases, spontaneous migration of stents occurred between 10 and 21 days after placement. In these cases, the migrated stents were excreted with feces, and no obstructive complication was experienced. In three cases, the stents remained at their proper position until 21 days after placement. The follow-up period of these patients was between seven month to 2 years, and no patient complained of symptoms of re-stenosis.

In recent European series, 21 patients received a treatment for refractory benign esophageal strictures with biodegradable stents (ELLA-CS, s.k.o., Hradec Kralove, Czech Republic).

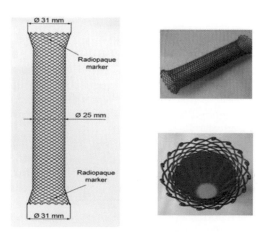
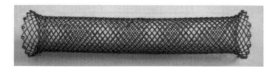

Figure 11.3 Biodegradable esophageal stent (ELLA-CS, s.k.o., Hradec Kralove, Czech Republic).

A 6 cm stent was inserted in eight patients and 9 cm stent was used in 13 patients. All procedures were performed without inter-procedure complications. Seven patients experienced chest pain and received medical therapy. One patient developed minor bleeding 6 weeks after stent placement. Stent migration was observed in 2 patients (9.5%).

Surveillance endoscopy 3 and 6 months after initial therapy revealed the presence of stent in 19 and zero patients respectively.

After a median follow-up of 53 weeks, nine patients (45%) remained free of dysphagia and received no additional therapy. The available data is encouraging but further studies are needed to refined the technique and prove the positive risk/benefit ratio.

Pediatric experience

The number of pediatric studies is limited. All reports are retrospective, mainly as case studies and lacking in uniform stenting techniques.

The initial experience with custom-made esophageal stent in children with corrosive esophagitis came from Turkey. The technique provided a much better outcome, leading to a healing in 68% of the patients compared to 33% with standard therapy (dilatations). Poor patient compliance and esophageal shortening during scar formation were the leading reasons for treatment failure. Another study from Turkey described a 10 year experience with a series of 11 children treated with esophageal stents. After stent removal, eight patients had a normal feeding pattern with a mean follow-up of 3.5 years. The results suggested esophageal stenting provided a good long-term outcome and decreased the need for surgical reconstruction.

A Chinese group advocated laparotomy for esophageal stent placement 2–3 weeks after caustic ingestion or even immediately in case of esophageal perforation. Eighteen children (1–4 years) were included. All custom-made stents were removed after 4–6 months. Eighty five percent of children remain asymptomatic 3 months after stent removal.

The first pediatric experience with SEPS (Polyflex/Rüsch) was reported in a series of 10 patients (aged 6 months to 23 years) with refractory esophageal stricture, mostly after corrosive ingestion. Deployment of SEPS required balloon dilatation before stent insertion. Stents remained in the esophagus for 20–133 days. Some children experienced nausea and vomiting several days after placement of the stent. The degree of dyspepsia was related to the length of the stent. Treatment with midazolam and ondansetron reduced the symptoms. All children received pain-relieving medication during the first days after stenting. Patients also required acid-blocking medication while the stent was in place. Five patients made a full recovery; others needed further treatment with additional stenting. During the entire treatment, children maintained oral feeding.

Fully covered tracheobronchial stents were endoscopically placed under general anesthesia in seven pediatric patients (6 months – 7 years old) with benign esophageal strictures. All patients had several unsuccessful dilatations before stent placement. Balloon dilatation preceded the stent deployment. Two factors determined the size of the stent: age appropriate esophageal diameter and the length of the stricture (plus 2 cm added to each side of the stricture). A few patients received more than one treatment with different sized stents. Stents remained within the esophagus for 3 and 15 days without complications. All of them were removed with biopsy forceps. The efficacy of treatment was directly related to the time of esophageal stenting. Six of seven children improved. There were no complications associated with esophageal stent therapy. Persistent gagging and respiratory distress led to early stent removal in two children.

Zhang and colleagues reported experience with covered retrievable expandable nitinol stents in 8 children with corrosive esophageal stenosis. The stents were placed in all patients without complications and were successfully removed 1 to 4 weeks later. After stent placement, all patients were able to eat solid food without dysphagia. Stent migration occurred in one patient; in this patient, the stent was repositioned successfully. During the 3-month follow-up period, all children could eat satisfactorily. After 6 months, two children required balloon dilatation (3 and 5 times respectively).

The first two cases of successful application of a biodegradable stent in children with caustic esophageal stricture were performed in Minsk, Byelorussia, in 2006. However, the case series was published in a local medical journal.

We reported a positive experience with the biodegradable esophageal stent (ELLA-CS, s.k.o., Hradec Kralove, Czech Repablic) in a child.

A 10-year-old healthy boy with normal psychomotor development ingested several full swallows of a drain cleaner by accident; a 15% NaOH solution with a pH of 12.5. He immediately vomited and started complaining of dysphagia and retrosternal pain.

An upper endoscopy was performed 15 hours after the ingestion. Major circumferential ulcerations over the whole length of the esophagus were present. There was no perforation, and the stomach was normal.

Initial therapy included: analgesics, parenteral nutrition, intravenous omperazole (2 mg kg^{-1} · day^{-1}), and high-dose intravenous corticosteroids (1 g/1.73 m^2), a large nasogastric tube for 16 days, antibiotics and antifungal medication. The endoscopic appearance of the esophagus had significantly improved, and the corticosteroids were switched to oral administration; after 3 weeks, they were decreased gradually.

A control endoscopy 2 weeks after discharge still showed ulcerations, sloughing, and granulomatous tissue, but also, and for the first time, a developing stenosis at the mid-esophagus. The length of stenosis in the middle esophagus was about 2 cm.

The patient complained at that time of dysphagia for solids.

After parental consent was obtained, a self-expandable biodegradable SX-ELLA esophageal stent was inserted under general anesthesia 6 weeks after the accidental ingestion. The stent had a body diameter of 25 mm and a length of 80 mm; insertion was uneventful (Figure 11.4).

During the first days after the insertion, he complained of retrosternal pain and dysphagia. He also had nausea and vomited several times per day, for which he was treated with alizapride. Two weeks after the insertion of the stent, he was discharged because he had been asymptomatic for several days. Oral omeprazole (20 mg/day) was continued.

The stent remained in place, although a control endoscopy after 3 weeks showed that the distal end had extended into the stomach (Figure 11.5). A control endoscopy was performed every 2 to 3 weeks. About 12 weeks after insertion, the stent had degraded about 50%. At that time, the esophageal mucosa had healed. Although the patient remained symptom-free during the 4 months, he developed a severe distal esophageal stenosis of more than 1 cm about 10 months after the initial ingestion and 6 months after the stent placement.

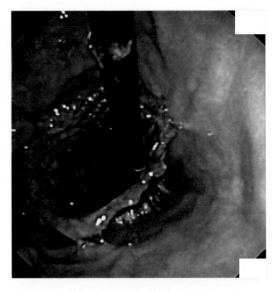

Figure 11.5 Retrograde view of the stent extended into the stomach.

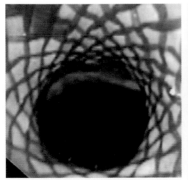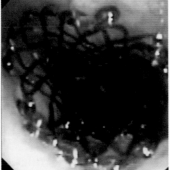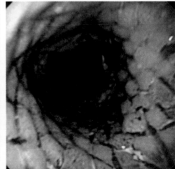

Figure 11.4 Endoscopic image of a biodegradable stent immediately after esophageal insertion.

The stenosis in the middle of the esophagus remained visible, but passage of the Olympus GIF-Q180, with external diameter of 8.8 mm, remained easy. Esophageal pH monitoring showed a reflux index of 15% in the lower esophagus; histology was compatible with a "reflux esophagitis." Repeated history and low gastrin levels confirmed noncompliance to the omeprazole treatment. After 4 balloon dilatations, and with careful control of the proton pump inhibitor intake (omeprazole 40 mg/day), the distal esophageal stenosis no longer relapsed. Histology of the distal esophageal biopsies is normal. Gastric pull-up or colonic interposition was avoided. The child now has normal eating habits.

A major advantage of biodegradable stents is that they can remain in place until full disintegration. As acid enhance stent dissolution, proton pump inhibitors must be administered to avoid premature disintegration. One drawback is that this stent is currently available in large-size only and cannot be used in small children.

Discussion and conclusion

There has been a recent trend for the treatment of benign esophageal disorders, such as refractory strictures, with stent technology. The results of SEMs and SEPs in the management of refractory benign esophageal strictures have been mixed. Until further improvement, these stents cannot be recommended as a standard therapy of refractory benign esophageal stricture. The use of self-expandable stents for the management of anastomic leaks and perforations appears promising. The development of a removable, fully-covered stent increases the potential application of this device in children with a wide range of congenital and acquired esophageal strictures. However, long-term prospective controlled trials with retrievable SEMS and biodegradable stents in the management of benign esophageal lesions are anticipated. In the meantime, stents may offer a temporary improvement for some children with refractory benign esophageal stricture. Since experience with esophageal stenting in children is very limited, we believe that it should be performed in referral centers.

The first line therapy of esophageal strictures remains endoscopic dilatation, followed by mitomycin application. If this fails, stenting of the stricture is a valuable option before the surgical option becomes inevitable. The timing of stenting is uncertain, but there are some indications that early stenting could be beneficial. It is likely that the patient tolerance to the initial placement of the stent without complication and remaining of the stent in proper position for an adequate time before removal are the two main contributing factors to success of the therapy.

In small children, large adult-size stents cannot be used due to risk of perforation and prolonged pain and nausea. The alternative options are tracheo-bronchial and custom-made stents. Tracheo-bronchial stents have a smaller diameter and double (proximal and distal) flanges, which makes displacement less likely. However, they are stiffer and have a higher radial force. The advantage is a relatively simple deployment technique. The disadvantage is that they may be more traumatic and less easy to remove due to stiffness. Custom-made stents are another option. These stents fit the specific diameter and the length appropriate to each patient. If necessary, anti-migration flaps can be added.

Another point of discussion is the duration of treatment. In general, covered stents remains in the esophagus for 1 to 4 weeks. It has been shown that results are better when stents are removed after more than 1 week. However, the longer a stent remains in place, the higher the risk of migration, the chance of tissue overgrowth, and difficult removal. A reasonable approach was proposed with replacement of the stent by a new one with incremental increased diameter of 2 mm every 2 weeks until the desired diameter is reached.

Removal of a fully covered stent is a relatively simple endoscopic procedure. Alligator or rat-tooth device or biopsy forceps allow grasping and pulling the purse-string suture into the endoscope channel, collapsing the top of the stent. An alternative approach is pulling the stent into the stomach before extraction. If the stent cannot be pulled into the biopsy channel, an overtube or endotracheal tube can be used. Complications after stent removal are infrequent, but it is safer to remove a stent under general anesthesia with endotracheal intubation.

We believe that esophageal stenting is a reasonable option for children with refractory esophageal stricture who failed dilatations and mitomycin application and facing surgical reconstruction. Knowledge of different stents specific properties and related complications is essential for proper choice of the optimal device. We believe that esophageal stent treatment should be performed in specialized centers under general anesthesia by experienced pediatric adult gastroenterologists. Currently, commercially available biodegradable stents, fully covered retrievable esophageal or perhaps smaller caliber (tracheobroncheal) SEMS can be used in carefully selected children with refractory esophageal strictures as the last non-surgical therapeutic option.

📖 FURTHER READING

Atabek C, Surer I, Demirbag S, *et al.* (2007) Increasing tendency in caustic esophageal burns and long-term polytetrafluorethylene stenting in severe cases: 10 years experience. *Journal of Pediatric Surgery*, **42,** 636–640.

Best C, Sudel B, Foker JE, *et al.* (2009) Esophageal stenting in children: indications, application, effectiveness, and complications. *Gastrointestinal Endoscopy*, **70,** 1248–1253.

Boukthir S, Fetni I, Mrad SM, *et al.* (2004) High doses of steroids in the management of caustic esophageal burns in children. *Archives of Pediatrics*, **11,** 13–17.

Broto J, Asensio M, Vernet JM. (2003) Results of a new technique in the treatment of severe esophageal stenosis in children: poliflex stents. *Journal of Pediatric Gastroenterology & Nutrition*, **37,** 203–206.

Burgos L, Barrena S, Andres AM, *et al.* (2010) Colonic interposition for esophageal replacement in children remains a good choice: 33-year median follow-up of 65 patients. *Journal of Pediatric Surgery*, **45,** 341–345.

Conigliaro R, Battaglia G, Repici A, *et al.* (2007) Polyflex stents for malignant oesophageal and oesophagogastric stricture: a prospective, multicentric study. *European Journal of Gastroenterology & Hepatology*, **19,** 195–203.

Conio M, Repici A, Battaglia G, *et al.* (2007) A randomized prospective comparison of self-expandable plastic stents and partially covered self-expandable metal stents in the palliation of malignant esophageal dysphagia. *American Journal of Gastroenterology*, **102,** 2667–2677.

Dua KS, Vleggaar FP, Santharam R, *et al.* (2008) Removable self-expanding plastic esophageal stent as a continuous, non-permanent dilator in treating refractory benign esophageal strictures: a prospective two-center study. *American Journal of Gastroenterology*, **103,** 2988–2994.

Evrard S, Le Moine O, Lazaraki G, *et al.* (2004) Self-expanding plastic stents for benign esophageal lesions. *Gastrointestinal Endoscopy*, **60,** 894–900.

Eickhoff A, Knoll M, Jakobs R, *et al.* (2005) Self-expanding metal stents versus plastic prostheses in the palliation of malignant dysphagia: long-term outcome of 153 consecutive patients. *Journal of Clinical Gastroenterology*, **39,** 877–885.

Elicevik M, Alim A, Tekant GT, *et al.* (2008) Management of esophageal perforation secondary to caustic esophageal injury in children. *Surgery Today*, **38,** 311–315.

Kramer RE, Quiros JA. (2010) Esophageal Stents for Severe Strictures in Young Children: Experience, Benefits, and Risk. *Current Gastroenterology Reports*, **12,** 203–210.

Knyrim K, Wagner HJ, Bethge N, *et al.* (1993) A controlled trial of an expansile metal stent for palliation of esophageal obstruction due to inoperable cancer. *New England Journal of Medicine*, **329,** 1302–1307.

Mrad SM, Boukthir S, Fetni I, *et al.* (2007) Severe corrosive oesophagitis : are high doses of methyl prednisolone efficient to prevent oesophageal caustic stricture in children? *Tunis Med*, **85,** 15–19.

Mutaf O. (1996) Treatment of corrosive esophageal strictures by long-term stenting. *Journal of Pediatric Surgery*, **31,** 681–685.

Oh YS, Kochman ML, Ahmad NA, *et al.* (2010) Clinical outcomes after self-expanding plastic stent placement for refractory benign esophageal strictures. *Digestive Diseases & Sciences*, **55,** 1344–1348.

Ott C, Ratiu N, Endlicher E, *et al.* (2007) Self-expanding Polyflex plastic stentts in esophageal disease: various indications, complications, and outcomes. *Surgical Endoscopy*, **21,** 889–96

Papachristou GI, Baron TH. (2007) Use of stents in benign and malignant esophageal disease. *Reviews in Gastroenterology Disorders*, **7,** 74–78.

Rahbar R, Jones DT, Nuss RC, *et al.* The role of mitomycin in the prevention and treatment of scar formation in the pediatric aerodigestive tract: friend or foe? *Archives of Otolaryngology Head & Neck Surgery*, **28,** 401–406.

Repici A, Conio M, De Angelis C, *et al.* (2004) Temporary placement of an expandable polyester silicone-covered stent for treatment of refractory benign esophageal strictures. *Gastrointestinal Endoscopy*, **60,** 513–519.

Repeci A, Vleggaar F.P, Hassn C, *et al.* (2010) Efficacy and safety of biodegradable stents for refractory benign esophageal strictures: the BEST (Biodegradable Esophageal Stent Study). *Gastrointest Endosc,* **72,** 927–934.

Riffat F, Cheng A. (2009) Pediatric caustic ingestion: 50 consecutive cases and a review of the literature. *Diseases of the Esophagus,* **22,** 89–94.

Repici A, Hassan C, Sharma P, *et al.* (2010) Systematic review: self-expanding plastic stent for benign oesophageal strictures. *Alimentary Pharmacology & Therapeutics,* **31,** 1268–75.

Saito Y, Tanaka T, Andoh A, *et al.* (2007) Usefulness of biodegradable stents constructed of poly-l-lactic acid monofilaments in patients with benign esophageal stenosis. *World Journal of Gastroenterology,* **13,** 3977–3980.

Saranovic D, Djuric-Stefanovic A, Ivanovic A, *et al.* (2005) Fluoroscopically guided insertion of self-expandable metal esophageal stents for palliative treatment of patients with malignant stenosis of esophagus and cardia: comparison of uncovered and covered stent types. *Diseases of the Esophagus,* **18,** 230–238.

Sharma P, Kozarek R. (2010) Role of esophageal stents in benign and malignant diseases. *American Journal of Gastroenterology,* **105,** 258–273.

Song HY, Park SI, Jung HY, *et al.* (1997) Benign and malignant esophageal strictures: treatment with a polyurethane-covered retrievable expandable metallic stent. *Radiology,* **203,** 747–752.

Song HY, Jung HY, Park SI, *et al.* (2000) Covered retrievable expandable nitinol stents in patients with benign esophageal strictures: initial experience. *Radiology,* **17,** 551–557.

Szegedi L, Gal I, Kosa I, *et al.* (2006) Palliative treatment of esophageal carcinoma with self-expanding plastic stents: a report on 69 cases. *European Journal of Gastroenterology & Hepatology,* **18,** 1197–1201.

Triester SL, Fleisher DE, Sharma VK. (2006) Failure of self-expanding plastic stents in treatment of refractory benign esophageal strictures. *Endoscopy,* **38,** 533–537

Uhlen S, Fayoux P, Vachin F, *et al.* (2006) Mitomycin C: an alternative conservative treatment for refractory esophageal stricture in children? *Endoscopy,* **38,** 404–407.

Vandenplas Y, Hauser B, Devreker T, *et al.* (2009) A biodegradable esophageal stent in the treatment of a corrosive esophageal stenosis in a child. *Journal of Pediatric Gastroenterology Nutrition,* **49,** 254–257.

Wang RW, Zhou JH, Jiang YG, *et al.* (2006) Prevention of stricture with intraluminal stenting through laparotomy after corrosive esophageal burns. *European Journal of Cardiothoracic Surgery,* **30,** 207–211.

Vakil N, Morris AI, Marcon N, *et al.* (2001) A prospective, randomized, controlled trial of covered expandable metal stents in the palliation of malignant esophageal obstruction at the gastro-esophageal junction. *American Journal of Gastroenterology,* **96,** 1791–1796.

Zhang C, Yu JM, Fan GP, *et al.* (2005) The use of a retrievable self-expanding stent in treating childhood benign esophageal strictures. *Journal of Pediatric Surgery,* **40,** 501–504.

12

Endoscopic application of Mitomycin C for intractable strictures

Mike Thomson

 KEY POINTS

- As fibrosis of a hollow organ causes stricture formation, it is logical to try to prevent this with topical application of an antifibrotic such as mitomycin C.
- Steroids are anti-inflammatory, are not appropriate, and do not work.
- Mitomycin C is effective post-balloon dilation for the prevention of re-stenosis in many conditions of various etiology in the esophagus, but this topical application is difficult in other parts of the GI tract.
- No adverse events have been encountered with its topical use, and it has been employed

  in many other areas of healthcare such as laryngeal reconstruction with no problems encountered.
- The protection of normal mucosa during topical application is standard although this may not strictly be necessary.
- The potential for primary prevention of post-caustic ingestion endoscopic application prior to esophageal stricture formation is interesting.

Esophateal dilation

Esophageal dilation is indicated in patients with symptomatic esophageal obstruction. The obstruction could be due to a wide range of anatomical and functional esophageal disorders.

The purpose of esophageal dilation is to alleviate symptoms, permit free intake of enteral nutrition, while reducing complications such as pulmonary aspiration. Esophageal perforation (2.6%) is a worrying complication of dilation therapy and is best managed in conjunction with pediatric surgeons. Readily available pediatric surgical support is vital while performing this procedure in children. Adult studies show that the risk

of perforation is 4 times higher if the endoscopist has performed fewer than 500 therapeutic endoscopies. In addition, it is higher in treatment of complex strictures particularly when weighted bougies are passed blindly. Perforation should be suspected in any child developing continued chest pain, breathlessness, fever or tachycardia. A chest X-ray is a useful first line investigation.

For dilation, two types of devices are available; one is the push bougie and the other the balloon dilator. Push dilators are made of rubber and may be weighted (tungsten/ mercury filled) or wire-guided (polyvinyl, metal or Celestin type). The weighted dilators may be used blindly and vary in size from 7–20 mm. The balloon dilators may also be wire-guided or they may be passed through the

---

endoscope. These vary from 6–40 mm with larger balloons used for treatment of achalasia. In most cases, fluoroscopy during the procedure is recommended, especially when using non-wire-guided dilators, during dilation of complex esophageal strictures, or in patients with a tortuous esophagus.

Bougie-type dilators exert both radial and longitudinal forces due to the shearing effect and balloon dilators exert a radial force. Because of this significant difference, it is recommended that radial balloon dilators are the tool of choice in children, with a lower rate of complications and equal efficacy. Adult literature supports that both bougie and balloon dilators are equally effective in relief of dysphagia in patients with esophageal strictures.

Dilation of a strictured esophageal lumen to 12–15 mm usually relieves symptoms of dysphagia in peptic strictures. To reduce the risk of perforation, it has been suggested that no more than 3 dilators of progressively increasing diameter should be passed in a single session. It is generally agreed that unguided passage of weighted bougies should only be used in treatment of simple strictures. In addition, dilators less than 10 mm are floppy and need screening. Again, with the guide wire technique it is suggested that these should preferably be placed under direct vision. The authors, in common with most endotherapeutic practitioners, prefer balloon dilation under direct vision with the balloon centered at the tightest point of the stricture. In adult practice, screening is more commonly used in cases with tortuous strictures. We, however, tend to take a more cautious approach in treatment of children and have a low threshold for screening, unless the stricture is simple and the anatomy extremely well known. Generally the 'rule of 3s' applies, in which, the dilation of a stricture should not be greater than 3 times the diameter of the stricture. This is particularly true if the stricture is man-made i.e. anastamotic, as perforation is more likely in such a situation.

Recurrent structuring, consequent to caustic ingestion, is a treatment nightmare. Circumferential or deep caustic burns have a poor outcome, with an increased risk of perforation and/or stricture formation, even with early steroid use (5% with second degree and 90–100% in 3rd degree burns). Holwell et al on the contrary, suggest some benefit with steroid use.

Historically, medical treatments, especially antifibrotic agents, have been successfully used in both manipulation of wound healing and scar formation in a number of disparate medical problems. These include; reduction of liver collagen, prevention of peritoneal fibrous adhesions to prevent mechanical intestinal obstruction, reduction in the amount of scar tissue on skin, restricting scar formation on gliding surfaces, and prevention of conduit stenosis after a circumferential internal injury. One such treatment mitomycin C, an anthracycline derived from Streptomyces bacteria, has been successfully used to prevent scar formation in childhood glaucoma, dacryocystorhinostomy and tracheal stenosis. It is an antibiotic, which interferes with DNA replication ('G2' stage RNA synthesis) and protein synthesis, in turn, inhibiting fibroblast proliferation. In an animal study, the vocal folds of dogs treated with mitomycin C showed fewer fibroblasts and less collagen in the superficial layer of lamina propria compared to controls, but no difference in the inflammatory infiltrate.

Use of mitomycin C

The author reported the first use of mitomycin C in a child with caustic stricture necessitating recurrent dilations. An eighteen-month-old girl developed two strictures after accidental ingestion of caustic soda. The first was 3 cm distal to the tracheo-esophageal bifurcation (1 mm in diameter and 3–5 mm in length), and a second 8 cm from the tracheo-esophageal bifurcation (3 mm wide and 1.5 cm long). (Figure 12.1) After the initial dilation, solid dysphagia resolved but returned within 5 days necessitating a second dilation, when dexamethasone (1 mg × 4) was injected circumferentially into the stricture. Subsequently, post-dilation symptom recurrence of solid dysphagia and drooling necessitated weekly dilations on a further 14

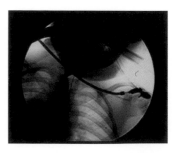

Figure 12.1 Videofluoroscopy picture of a proximal and a distal stricture in the same child.

occasions; size of the balloon progressively increased to 18 mm using a pressure of 35 psi for 2–7 minutes. Surgery and stent placement were not considered an option due to the proximity of the first stricture to the tracheo-esophageal bifurcation. The use of experimental topical mitomycin C was discussed and the first dose administered after consent of the parents. A cotton pledget soaked in a solution of mitomycin C (0.1 mg/ml) was applied topically under direct vision for 2 minutes at the strictured esophageal segment after dilation with the balloon. A second application was made one week later. After 3 months, for the first time without dilation, it was possible to pass a pediatric size endoscope (Fujinon EG 410PE, 8.4 mm diameter), showing very little residual stenosis. (Figure 12.2) Endoscopic views are seen in Figures 12.3, 12.4 and 12.5. At 5 years follow-up she has required one dilation, and continues to remain asymptomatic with good growth.

Presently, there is no known therapeutic dose of mitomycin C. Studies of intradermal mitomycin C (0.015 to 0.25 mg) in BALB/c mice showed formation of skin ulcers at clinically relevant mitomycin C dose levels of 0.05 and 0.075 mg (3.6 to 10.7 mg/m2). Filtering surgery in the eye, with 0.2 or 0.4 mg/ml of mitomycin C, showed no

difference in results between the use of two doses. In tracheal stenosis, an application of a dose of 0.1 mg/ml by cotton pledgets for 2 minutes at the site of lysed cicatrix, has been used in children. We used a similar concentration (0.1 mg/ml) for 2 minutes at the strictured esophageal segment following balloon dilation.

The available evidence suggests that short-term topical use of mitomycin C is safe. There were no reported complications in 15 patients with tracheal stenosis at 18 months follow-up. Adverse effects have been reported with high-dose, long-term topical use in bladder cancer. A 71-year-old man developed a self-resolving type III/IV hypersensitivity reaction with eczema, purpura,

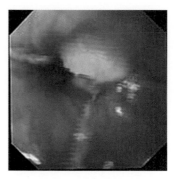

Figure 12.4 Application of cotton pledglet soaked in mitomycin C to post-dilation area, front-loaded onto grasping forceps through endoscope, and protecting normal mucosa with an EMR cap on the tip of the endoscope.

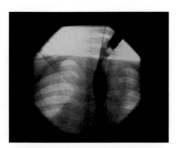

Figure 12.2 Resolution of strictures 3 months after application of mitomycin and dilation.

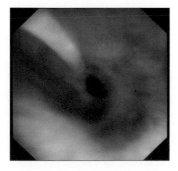

Figure 12.3 Pre-treatment stricture.

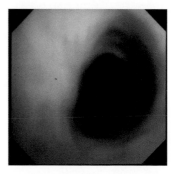

Figure 12.5 Post-treatment 12 months later with persistence of patency. Since publication of this first report, mitomycin C has been used worldwide and authors and colleagues are now reporting successful use of mitomycin C in a series of 16 children (caustic, post-surgical stenosis, epidermolysis bullosa strictures) jointly with colleagues from pediatric gastroenterology centers of the world.

and a positive patch test after intravesical instillation for bladder cancer. Eosinophilic cystitis has been reported with bladder instillation. Regular topical application of mitomycin C jelly may lead to urethral structuring.

It is not known if the early use of mitomycin C is more beneficial. Authors have used topical mitomycin C (uncontrolled) in a 2-year-old child presenting with acute burns at the angles of lips to prevent scarring. The child made an excellent recovery. There were no acute problems with its usage and no sequelae related to this.

FURTHER READING

Afzal NA, Albert D, Thomas AL, *et al.* (2002) A child with oesophageal strictures. *Lancet*, **359**, 1032.

Anderson KD, Rouse TM, Randolph JG. (1990) A controlled trial of corticosteroids in children with corrosive injury of the esophagus. *New England Journal of Medicine*, **323**, 637–640.

Camara JG, Bengzon AU, Henson RD. (2000) The safety and efficacy of mitomycin C in endonasal endoscopic laser-assisted dacryocystorhinostomy. *Ophthalmic Plastic & Reconstructive Surgery*, **16**, 114–118.

Cox JG, *et al.* (1994) Balloon or bougie for dilatation of benign esophageal stricture? *Digestive Diseases & Sciences*, **39**, 776–781.

Dorr RT, Soble MJ, Liddil JD, *et al.* (1986) Mitomycin C skin toxicity studies in mice: reduced ulceration and altered pharmacokinetics with topical dimethyl sulfoxide. *Journal of Clinical Oncology*, **4**, 1399–1404.

Inglis JA, Tolley DA, Grigor KM. (1987) Allergy to mitomycin C complicating topical administration for urothelial cancer. *British Journal of Urology*, **59**, 547–549.

Garrett CG, Soto J, Riddick J, *et al.* Effect of mitomycin C on vocal fold healing in a canine model. *Annals of Otology Rhinology & Laryngology*, **110**, 25–30.

Howell JM, Dalsey WC, Hartsell FW, *et al.* (1992) Steroids for the treatment of corrosive esophageal injury: a statistical analysis of past studies. *American Journal of Emergency Medicine*, **10**, 421–425.

Kirsh MM, Peterson A, Brown J.W, *et al.* (1978) Treatment of caustic injuries of the esophagus: a ten year experience. *Annals of Surgery*, **188**, 675–678.

Kunkeler L, Nieboer C, Bruynzeel DP. (2000) Type III and type IV hypersensitivity reactions due to mitomycin C. *Contact Dermatitis*, **42**, 74–76.

Langdon DE. (1997) The rule of three in esophageal dilation. *Gastrointestinal Endoscopy*, **45**, 111.

McClave SA, Brady PG, Wright RA, *et al.* (1996) Does fluoroscopic guidance for Maloney esophageal dilation impact on the clinical endpoint of therapy: relief of dysphagia and achievement of luminal patency. *Gastrointestinal Endoscopy*, **43**, 93–97.

McClave SA, Wright RA, Brady PG. (1990) Prospective randomized study of Maloney esophageal dilation–blinded versus fluoroscopic guidance. *Gastrointestinal Endoscopy*, **36**, 272–275.

Moazam F, Talbert JL, Miller D, *et al.* (1987) Caustic ingestion and its sequelae in children. *Southern Medical Journal*, **80**, 187–190.

Moore WR. (1986) Caustic ingestions. Pathophysiology, diagnosis, and treatment. *Clinical Pediatrics (Philadelphia)*, **25**, 192–196.

Peacock EE Jr. (1981) Control of wound healing and scar formation in surgical patients. *Archives of Surgery*, **116**, 1325–1329.

Quine, MA, Bell GD, McCloy RF, *et al.* (1995) Prospective audit of perforation rates following upper gastrointestinal endoscopy in two regions of England. *British Journal of Surgery*, **82**, 530–533.

Rahbar R, Shapshay SM, Healy GB. (2001) Mitomycin: effects on laryngeal and tracheal stenosis, benefits, and complications. *Annals of Otology Rhinology & Laryngology*, **110**, 1–6.

Riley SA, & Attwood SE. (2004) Guidelines on the use of oesophageal dilatation in clinical practice. *Gut*, **53(Suppl 1)**, i1–i6.

Rosseneu S, Afzal N, Yerushalmi B, *et al.* (2007) Topical application of Mitomycin C in oesophageal strictures. *Journal of Pediatric Gastroenterology & Nutrition*, Ref Type: In Press

Saeed ZA, Winchester CB, Ferro PS, *et al.* (1995) Prospective randomized comparison of polyvinyl bougies and through-the-scope balloons for dilation of peptic strictures of the esophagus. *Gastrointestinal Endoscopy*, **41**, 189–195.

Sanders SP, Cantor LB, Dobler AA, *et al.* (1999) Mitomycin C in higher risk trabeculectomy: a prospective comparison of 0.2 to 0.4 mg/cc doses. *Journal of Glaucoma*, **8**, 193–198.

Scolapio, JS, *et al.* (1999) A randomized prospective study comparing rigid to balloon dilators for benign esophageal strictures and rings. *Gastrointestinal Endoscopy*, **50**, 13–17.

Sidoti PA, Belmonte SJ, Liebmann JM, *et al.* (2000) Trabeculectomy with mitomycin C in the treatment of pediatric glaucomas. *Ophthalmology*, **107**, 422–429.

Stein GS, Rothstein H. (1968) Mitomycin C may inhibit mitosis by reducing "G2" RNA synthesis. *Current Modern Biology*, **2**, 254–263.

Ulman I, Mutaf O. (1998) A critique of systemic steroids in the management of caustic esophageal burns in children. *European Journal of Pediatric Surgery*, **8**, 71–74.

Ward RF, April MM. (1998) Mitomycin C in the treatment of tracheal cicatrix after tracheal reconstruction. *International Journal of Pediatric Otorhinolaryngology*, **44**, 221–226.

Yakubu A, Salanki PM, Cade M, *et al.* (1999) Extensive urethral stricture after using mitomycin in local anaesthetic jelly for urethral tumours. *British Journal of Urology International*, **83**, 873–874.

Yamamoto H, Hughes RW Jr, Schroeder KW, *et al.* (1992). Treatment of benign esophageal stricture by Eder-Puestow or balloon dilators: a comparison between randomized and prospective nonrandomized trials. *Mayo Clinic Proceedings*, **67**, 228–236.

13

Colonoscopic imaging and endoluminal treatment of intraepithelial neoplasia: clinical advances

Mike Thomson and David P. Hurlstone

 KEY POINTS

- Large sessile polyps or tumors can successfully and safely be removed in the upper and lower GI tract with EEMR.
- Use of endo-ultrasound can be helpful in identifying the margins and depth of any lesions prior to and during removal.
- Narrow band imaging, chromo-endoscopy, and magnification endoscopy can be used to identify lesions and margins of lesions aiding their successful removal by EEMR.

- Lesions straddling haustral folds can now be removed.
- Retroflexion in the colon using a gastroscope is a useful technique if a lesion is "hiding" behind a haustral fold.
- Significant morbidity associated with colectomy may be avoided using this minimalistic approach.

Introduction

Colonoscopy was first introduced as a means of directly visualizing the colon in the 1960s and the development of its therapeutic capabilities soon followed. Technological advancements and a greater understanding of the pathogenesis of colorectal diseases have allowed colonoscopy to evolve into the gold standard colorectal investigation with the endoluminal resection of early lesions also being possible. In adult gastroenter-

ology colonoscopy is at the heart of colorectal screening protocols aimed at the secondary prevention of colorectal cancer (CRC) in the West. The early detection of precancerous lesions:

- Allows targeted surveillance of an at-risk population.
- Facilitates early resection of the lesions therefore decreasing the incidence of CRC.
- Allows less radical resection procedures to be carried out resulting in decreased morbidity from CRC.

Practical Pediatric Gastrointestinal Endoscopy, Second Edition. George Gershman, Mike Thomson, Marvin Ament.
© 2012 Blackwell Publishing Ltd. Published 2012 by Blackwell Publishing Ltd.

- Is cost-effective in the long-term management of the at-risk population

The ideal goal is to detect and resect all potentially cancerous lesions via colonoscope. The aims outlined above have encouraged research into advanced colonoscopic imaging which, together with the discovery of new clinical carcinogenesis models, may change the way CRC is screened in the West.

The adenoma-carcinoma concept, which has formed the basis for current colonoscopic surveillance in the West over the past 30 years, only accounts for about two-thirds of CRCs. It is increasingly believed that the morphology of flat lesions and their pit patterns can suggest their propensity to develop into CRC. Japanese researchers reported flat and depressed colorectal lesions in the 1980s. Many depressed neoplasms arise through the *de novo* pathogenic sequence and demonstrate early invasive characteristics. Given the introduction of colorectal cancer screening programs in the West, it is essential to re-evaluate the significance of flat lesions as applicable to Western cohorts. All investigators report difficulties in identifying flat and depressed lesions using conventional colonoscopy. The development of new technology means that these lesions can be detected and assessed using various optical colonoscopic techniques *in vivo* and, furthermore, they allow targeted surgical and endoscopic resection.

Colonoscopic resection methods have traditionally aimed towards biopsy and polypectomy. Endoscopic mucosal resection (EMR) is in its infancy, but it allows early and effective treatment of selected superficial neoplasms, and obviates the need for major surgery in these patients. The safety and efficacy of new endoscopic interventional therapeutics in the form of EMR requires further evaluation.

New insights into CRC pathogenesis

Until recently, screening has been based on Morson's hypothesi that CRC develops from polypoid adenomata. It is also known that the likelihood of malignant change increases with the increasing size of a polyp. This morphological adenoma-carcinoma sequence is mirrored by genetic changes in the polypoid tissues. These morphological premises, combined with histological findings, form the rationale behind the management and subsequent surveillance of patients with colorectal polyps. It has been shown, however, that colonoscopic polypectomy of exophytic lesions (Paris class Ip/s, *see* Table 13.1) alone results in a higher incidence of colorectal cancer than expected. The UK National Polyp Study reported on the 6-year follow-up of 1418 patients after repeated colonoscopy to clear all polyps. While this study did not have a true control arm, the background, age and sex specific incidence of colorectal cancer was used as a control group. The findings demonstrated that the removal of all polyps seen, prevented the development of 75% of carcinomas. The Veterans Affairs Study found only 50% of cancers were prevented, but not all patients had received total colonoscopy. This makes it possible that the inability to prevent all subsequent CRC in these groups may be that flat and depressed colorectal lesions (Paris 0-II / 0-IIa/c / 0-IIc/a) were not detected or recognized. If they were, they may have been inadequately treated. Because this "flat adenoma" concept has not found widespread acceptance in the West, there is a paucity of data addressing the issues of atypical morphological, clinico-pathological features or validation of new colonoscopic technologies and therapeutics in Western cohorts. Although well-established in Japan, these concepts have currently failed to make a significant impact on colonoscopic practice in the UK, Europe and USA.

Recently, however, studies have been performed in the West corroborating Japanese findings. Our group prospectively studied the prevalence and clinico-pathological characteristics of flat and depressed colorectal lesions in a single UK-based cohort in patients at a high-risk of developing colorectal neoplasm. Thirty-eight per cent of all detected adenomas were flat lesions. This prevalence was similar to that reported by Rembacken, but was higher than that reported by Saito, and Wolber, in the USA and Canada respectively. Factors that may account for these differences may include case mix, inter-observer variation, endoscopic detection techniques (the use of high-magnification chromoscopic colonoscopy (HMCC)), and variation in histopathological reporting. It was also shown that these flat lesions have a predilection for the development of high-grade dysplasia (HGD). Twenty-five per cent of flat lesions in our series contained HGD or beyond. For lesions greater than 8 mm in diameter, a two-fold increase in the presence of HGD as compared to exophytic adenomatous lesions was observed. In addition, our data shows a significant prevalence of early invasive carcinoma in lesions smaller

Table 13.1 The Paris classification of endoscopic lesion morphology

Endoscopic appearance	Paris class		Description
Protruded lesions	Ip		Pedunculated polyps
	Ips		Subpedunculated polyps
	Is		Sessile polyps
Flat elevated lesions	IIa		Flat elevation of mucosa
	IIa / IIc		Flat elevation with central depression
Flat lesions	IIb		Flat mucosal change
	IIc		Mucosal depression
	IIc/IIa		Mucosal depression with raised edge

than conventional exophytic lesions, corroborating the observation of many Japanese groups. For example, in a study of 15 flat rectal cancer cases, Tada *et al.*, found that despite all the tumors being less than 2 cm in diameter, 9 had invaded the submucosa. The metastatic risk of flat and depressed lesions, however, is not clear. Shimoda *et al.*, showed that despite exophytic carcinomas being larger (mean 55 mm) than flat carcinomas (mean 43 mm) the rates of lymphovenous infiltration were 32% and 77% respectively. Also in this study, flat lesions were more likely to invade the submucosa. As CRC survival rates depend on the extent of local invasion and presence or absence of metastatic disease, if malignancy can be detected at an earlier stage in CRC, prognosis can improve significantly. In early colon cancer a 5-year survival in excess of 97% has been reported.

The anatomical location of these lesions is of clinical importance as it influences colonoscopic practice. In the Sheffield UK series, 82% of all flat lesions with HGD and 90% of all flat/depressed type adenocarcinomas clustered within the right hemi-colon, supporting the need for total colonoscopy in detecting such "high-risk" lesions.

The detection of aberrant crypt foci (ACF) in the rectum using high-magnification chromoscopic colonoscopy has also shown that such biomarkers are valid predictors of proximal right hemi-colonic flat and depressed neoplasia. Our group studied 1000 patients in whom the median number of ACF per patient in the endoscopically "normal", adenoma and cancer group was 1 (range 0–5), 9 (range 0–22) and 38 (range 14–64) respectively. The relative risk (RR) of dysplastic ACF when comparing the flat adenoma group with the endoscopically "normal" group was 4.68 and the RR for flat cancer versus the endoscopically "normal" group being 21.8. Patients with >5 adenomas also had higher ACF densities than those with <5 adenomas. These data may therefore provide the endoscopist with a novel tool to risk-stratify patients requiring total colonoscopy and help avoid interval cancers at the time of flexible sigmoidoscopy.

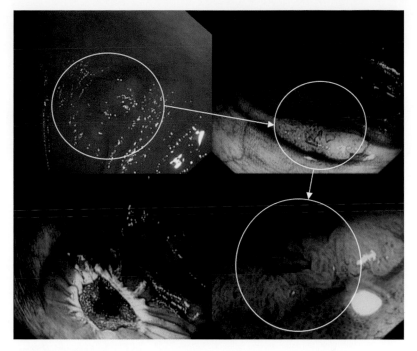

Figure 13.1 Top left: High-definition white light images of a proximal ascending colonic lesion. The lesion highlighted is distinguished by focal erythema and loss of vascular net architecture. Top right: High-definition indigo carmine 0.4% targeted chromoscopy imaging of the lesion. The lesion is now clearly circumscribed and can be classified as a Paris 0-IIa (flat elevated) lesion in the absence of a fixed type 0-IIc component (central depression). Bottom right: High magnification (100×) imaging shows a normal Kudo type I crypt pattern adjacent to the lesion with a predominant Kudo type IIIL pit pattern at the lesion's apex – i.e. intraepithelial neoplasia positive. Endoscopic excision is indicated. Bottom left: Post endoscopic mucosal resection *en bloc* resection imaging. The muscularis mucosa can be clearly visualized with no evident neoplastic crypt architecture at the horizontal or vertical resection margins. The lesions have been completely resected (R0 anticipated endoscopically).

It is important to remember that the inflammation-metaplasia-dysplasia-adenocarcinoma sequence is a concept not exclusive to adult patients and that children and adolescents have a part to play in this evolutionary pathology.

High magnification chromoscopic colonoscopy (HMCC)

High magnification colonoscopes enable the magnification of colonic mucosa up to 150 times and also offer higher resolution than older colonoscopes (Figure 13.1–3). Their use is maximized in conjunction with chromoscopy, and this represents the most common mode of visual enhancement used by endoscopists presently. Using this technique, clear lesion delineation and pit patterns (*see* Table 13.2) can be observed.

The technique involves initial visualization of the colon with conventional videocolonoscopy, looking out for the following mucosal signs, which may be subtle:

- Focal pallor or erythema.
- Hemorrhagic spots.
- Fold convergence.
- Disruption of mucosal vascular net pattern.
- Mucosal unevenness or discrete mucosal deformity.
- Air-induced deformation.

Once identified, the suspicious areas are washed down with the appropriate mucosal toilet and the dye applied. Lesions are then sized using an open biopsy forceps whose width is known. Morphological classification is then undertaken by activating the colonoscope's magnification lever and characterizing its appearances.

Table 13.2 The modified Kudo criteria for the classification of colorectal crypt architecture *in vivo* using high magnification chromoscopic colonoscopy

Pit Type	Characteristics	Appearance Using HMCC	Pit Size (mm)
I	Normal round pits		0.07 +/− 0.02 mm
II	Stella or papillary		0.09 +/− 0.02 mm
IIIs	Tubular / round pits Smaller than pit type I		0.03 +/− 0.01 mm
IIIL	Tubular / large		0.22 +/− 0.09 mm
IV	Sulcus / gyrus		0.93 +/− 0.32 mm
V(a)	Irregular arrangement and sizes of IIIL, IIIs, IV type pit		N/A

Pit patterns

Pit patterns were originally described by Kosaka in 1975 and were formally validated in Japanese studies by Kudo. Pit patterns have been shown to correlate strongly with their associated histopathological diagnoses and, as a result, this method of classification is widely used by authors. Types I and II are associated with normal and hyperplastic mucosa. Type IIIs are seen more often in depressed lesions and are associated with carcinomatous change. Type IIIL are associated with adenomas in protuberant lesions. Types IV and V are associated with adenomas with atypical cellularity whereas type V or non-pit patterns are indicative of adenocarcinoma.

Dyes

A summary of common dyes used in HMCC is shown in Table 13.3. Indigo carmine (IC) 0.2–1% is the most frequently used agent. It is a contrast enhancer that pools in recesses, aiding the visualization of abnormal mucosa. As there is no actual reaction with the tissues, it washes off easily which makes it unsuitable for prolonged procedures. IC has been shown to be sufficient in the visualization of Type I–IV pits but if further visualization is required, crystal violet (CV) can be used to stain the mucosa. This compound is a potentially toxic-reactive dye and should only be used sparingly when Type V pits are suspected. Methylene blue stains for a longer period of time and is commonly used in ulcerative colitis cancer surveillance.

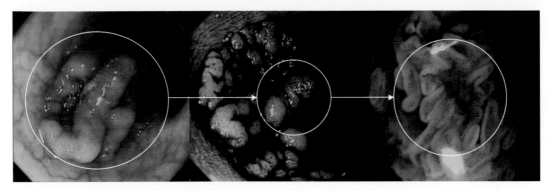

Figure 13.2 Left: Conventional high-definition white light views of a lateral spreading tumor (granular type) positioned at the recto-sigmoid junction. Middle: Indigo-carmine 0.4% chromoscopy has been applied to the recto-sigmoid segment. The peripheral neoplastic pit pattern can now be fully defined and the circumferential margins of the lesion identified. Right: High-magnification (100×) imaging of the largest nodule (highlighted) shows a Kudo type IV crypt pattern.

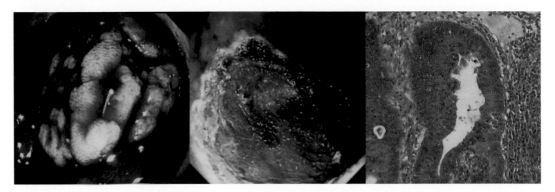

Figure 13.3 Left: Endoscopic mucosal resection of the lesion is indicated (neoplastic-non-invasive pit pattern). The lesions have been raised using a submucosal injection of 50% dextrose solution. The lesion has lifted in a symmetrical fashion with no tethering suggestive of submucosal deep invasion. Middle: Post endoscopic mucosal resection appearances shows the muscularis mucosa visible. There are some prominent vessels shown in the vertical dissection plane which have been prophylactically coagulated using argon plasma. Right: Hematoxylin and eosin stained fixed pathological specimen at high power. Features shown are of a high-grade villous adenoma without submucosal invasive characteristics. Curative resection endoscopically was achieved in this case.

In vivo optical biopsy using HMCC

Recent prospective studies have addressed the efficacy of HMCC at differentiating neoplastic from non-neoplastic colorectal lesions. Tung *et al.*, assessed 175 polyps from 141 consecutive patients. Although not described in the methodology, differentiation of the neoplastic type pit patterns (IIIs/V) can be enhanced by the use of CV staining post mucolysis. The use of CV in this study may have improved neoplastic sensitivity rates and

aided diagnosis in the 6 neoplastic lesions that were mis-classified. Kato *et al.*, found that diagnostic accuracy rates for non-neoplastic, adenomatous and cancerous lesions were 75%, 94% and 85% respectively. Tung *et al.*, found an overall diagnostic accuracy of 80.1% and Togashi et al., 88.4%. Our prospective study of 1 008 patients in the UK undergoing HMCC showed a 98% sensitivity rate in distinguishing neoplastic lesions from non-neoplastic ones with an overall accuracy of 95%. CV staining was used to aid diagnosis of the invasive crypt types, which may have influenced

Table 13.3 Classification of common chromoscopic dyes

Type of dye	Preparation	Application	Advantages	Side-effects
Contrast				
Indigo-Carmine Most commonly used Acetic acid	Standard mucosal toilet	Dye spraying via 'scope or diffusion catheter		None
Reactive				
Crystal Violet Kudo type V pit differentiation	Mucosal toilet with proteinase solution	Specialized catheter; 2–3 min wait for fixation		Possible long-term toxicity
Cresyl violet				
Absorptive				
Methylene Blue	Standard mucosal toilet	Dye spraying via 'scope or diffusion catheter	Longer staining pattern	Potentially mutagenic

the improved sensitivity and specificity when differentiating neoplastic from non-neoplastic lesions as compared to Tung (93.8% and 64.6% respectively). CV staining for diagnosis of the invasive pit patterns was used in Togashi's series of 923 lesions with a comparable sensitivity (92%) but improved specificity (73.3%) as compared to Tung's data. These studies illustrate that despite increased accuracy rates being widely shown, there is still conflicting data as to how sensitive, specific and accurate magnified chromoendoscopy is. This discrepancy may be caused by differences in operator experience, chromoscopic technique and histological interpretation. There are limited published data reporting on the learning curve required to fulfill the primary end-points of competence and sustained observer accuracy and inter/intra observer variability. It is clear from the above studies, however, that there is an increase in overall accuracy rates with more experience of the procedure. The colonoscopist in the Sheffield study had experience of over 800 lesions prior to commencing this study. For a widespread impact to be made in both Europe and the Unites States, further data is required to assess the learning curve and observer variability characteristics among endoscopists. Endoscopy training programs will need to evolve their curriculum should safe and effective practice of new techniques with sustainable standards be achieved.

In vivo staging of colorectal lesions using HMCC

Accurate *in vivo* staging is essential at colonoscopy as Paris class 0-II CRCs which are limited to the submucosal layer 1 can be managed by EMR as the risk of lympho-venous invasion and lymph node metastases (LNM) is <5%. Lesions with deeper vertical (Paris criteria >1000 microns) (i.e. stage T2) have an increased risk of LNM (10–15%). EMR in this group is therefore undesirable due to a higher risk of perforation, non-curative excision and untreated nodal disease. Surgical excision is recommended in this group.

The use of chromoscopic colonoscopy as an *in vivo* staging tool has been reported by Saitoh and colleagues. In their analysis of Paris 0-IIc CRCs, combined videoendoscopy and chromoscopy was used to characterize the essential endoscopic features favored by lesions with submucosal layer 1 and 2 invasion, which at the time of endoscopy may be used as a tool to guide the colonoscopists management. Using specific criteria (expansion appearance, present; surface depression, deep; irregularity of depressed surface, uneven; and converging folds toward the tumor), Saitoh found the sensitivity and specificity for determining submucosal layer 2 disease was 90%. However, when 21 lesions showing intramucosal carcinoma were excluded from the analysis, specificity rates fell to 70%. A recent prospective analysis of endoscopic morphological anticipation of submucosal invasion in Paris class 0-II lesions using the Nagata subtype analysis of the Kudo type V pit pattern showed a κ coefficient of agreement between pit type V and histologically confirmed sm2 invasion was 0.51 (95% CI). Using pit types Vn(B) and Vn(C) as clinical indicators of invasive disease, 97% of lesions were correctly anticipated to have sm2+ invasion, however specificity was low at 50% (overall accuracy 78%). The clinical implication of these data is that these lesions tend to be overstaged, which may deprive some patients the opportunity of curative local excision with EMR. Similar problems have been encountered using the 7.5 MHz ultrasound probe in the staging of rectal carcinoma, with variable

accuracy rates reported from 60–79% according to the T stage system. The introduction of high-frequency "mini probe" ultrasound has now been reported to have a high overall accuracy when used to determine submucosal invasion Paris class II lesions. However, ultrasound imaging requires further training, has significant expense and may prolong the procedure (Figure 13.4, 13.5).

HMCC in the detection of intraepithelial neoplasia and colitis associated cancer

Although many pediatric gastroenterologists will see this concept as a theoretical one for their patients, there is no doubt that knowledge of this

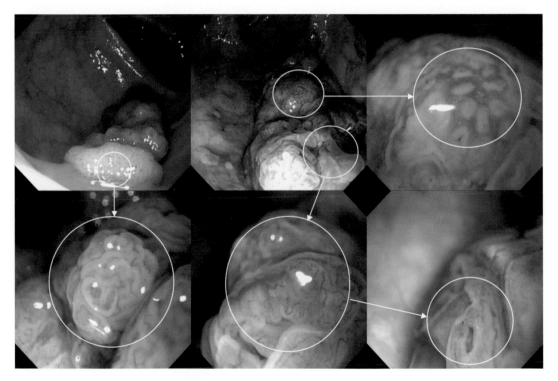

Figure 13.4 Top left: Conventional high-definition white light imaging of a descending colonic Paris class 0-Isp (sub-pendunculated) lesion. Bottom left: The basal polyp segment highlighted (top left) is shown at 100× magnification using 0.4% indigo carmine chromoscopy. The pit pattern is neoplastic-non-invasive (Kudo type IIIL). Top-middle: the lesion is shown at conventional non-magnified imaging following application of 0.4% indigo carmine chromoscopy. The highlighted areas show the lesion segments undergoing high magnification (100×) imaging.

Top-right: High magnification (100×) imaging of the highlighted segment shows a Kudo type II pit pattern (non-neoplastic non-invasive crypt). Bottom middle: High magnification (100×) imaging of the highlighted segment shows a tortuous vascular net architecture in combination with a IIL crypt pattern (bottom right) highly suggestive of a serrated adenoma component. Post-endoscopic mucosal resection showed complete excision (R0) of a "collision" lesion i.e. villous, tubular, serrated and hyperplastic component polyp.

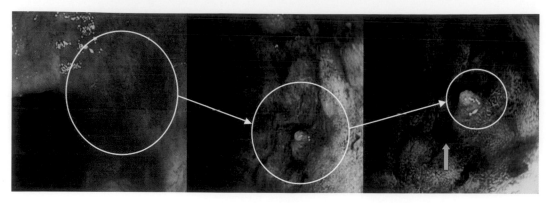

Figure 13.5 Left: conventional white light views of the distal descending colon in a patient with longstanding ulcerative colitis. There is focal erythema and subtle change in vascular net architecture as compared to the surrounding mucosa. Middle: Methylene blue 0.1% chromoscopy highlights an irregular raised nodule adjacent to a depressed mucosal area. Right: The adjacent mucosal depression is shown highlighted with the blue arrow.

area is an important corollary of our conception of IBD evolution – this is especially true when counseling adolescents not keen on following treatment regimes. For instance, azathioprine is now associated strongly with the diminution of CRC risk in long-term IBD. The management and clinical interpretation of dysplasia in the context of chronic ulcerative colitis is radically different to that of sporadic dysplastic lesions in the "normal" population. These patients have an increased risk of interval cancers, especially those with long-standing disease. The morphology of precancerous lesions may be flat and multifocal, making HMCC a useful adjunct in their detection. At the current time, dysplasia is the most reliable biomarker of malignant change, being present in >70% of ulcerative colitis patients with CRC. Recent published data suggest that using HMCC with targeted biopsies in the context of chronic ulcerative colitis (CUC) surveillance significantly increases the diagnostic yield for intraepithelial neoplasia (IN) as opposed to conventional colonoscopy and biopsy protocols by up to four times.

The ability to differentiate IN from hyperplastic or inflammatory mucosal change using HMCC in ulcerative colitis has also been shown to offer a sensitive and specific tool with a high overall diagnostic accuracy (96%). Data from two other groups confirm this. There are, however, indistinct mucosal appearances seen in the presence of acute inflammation which may result in equivocal histological diagnoses. It has therefore been recommended that HMCC targeted biopsies be used only when the disease is quiescent and even then, only in clearly demarcated lesions.

Summary of limitations of current imaging technology

- High sensitivity/specificity for the differentiation of non-neoplastic from neoplastic disease but low overall sensitivity for the anticipation of high-grade dysplasia.
- Effective over-staging of submucosal layer 3/T1 neoplasia.
- Operator-dependent error.
- Surface topographical imaging only.
- No ability to image surface/sub-surface lympho-vascular architecture, except with confocal endomicroscopy which is not widely available to date.

Emerging technologies – confocal endomicrosopy and histoendoscopy

Recently, the incorporation of a laser scanning microscope to a conventional video colonoscope (EC3870K; Pentax, Tokyo, Japan) has allowed the *in vivo* detection of neoplasia as well as estimation of depth invasion. Laser scanning confocal microscopy (LCM) is an adaptation of light microscopy whereby focal laser illumination is combined with "pinhole limited detection" to geometrically reject out of focus light. In single-point scanning confocal microscopes, the point is typically scanned in a raster pattern and measurements of light returning to the detector from successive points are digitized so an image of the scanned region can be constructed. It uses an argon-ion laser to transmit an excitation wavelength of 488 nm with a maximum laser output of <1 mW at the surface mucosa. Confocal images can then be collected at a scan rate of 0.8 frames/second (1024 × 1024 pixels) or 1.6 frames/second (1024 × 512 pixels). The optical slice thickness is 7 um with a lateral resolution of 0.7 um and z-axis range of 0–250 um below the surface layer. Optimized views are obtained with the use of fluorescein intravenously which is taken up by the cell to provide high-contrast image Acriflavine, tetracycline or cresyl violet can be used topically on the mucosa as image enhancers.

A German study in 2004 using fluorescein labeling found sensitivity rates of 97.4%, specificity rates of 99.4% and 99.2% accuracy comparing LCM to routine histology. Similar studies are underway in the UK to further validate the use of LCM in guiding subsequent diagnoses of colorectal neoplasia.

Clinical applicability of confocal endomicroscopy

- Early, improved tumor detection in a "curable" stage as a promising strategy for reduction of tumor mortality (applicable for both sporadic CRC and in the early detection of dysplasia in inflammatory bowel disease colorectal endoscopic screening).

- Fewer conventional biopsies if adequate sensitivity and specificity of CLM "optical biopsy" can be produced.
- Optimized work processes in endoscopy (e.g. immediate therapeutic decision).
- Incorporation of progress from field of immunology and genomics in endoscopy (molecular markers).
- Deep layer mucosal penetration for early CRC staging up to 250 microns.
- No substantial material consumption (stains)
- Currently, the only technology with potential for gastrointestinal molecular fluorescence marker imaging (Figure 13.6).

Auto-fluorescence colonoscopy

New endoscopic technology that is based on fluorescence is under evaluation by researchers. This concept utilizes either the "auto-fluorescence" of naturally occurring molecules such as collagen, NAD-H, flavins and porphyrins or fluorescence caused by exogenously administered fluorescent compounds.

The detection of neoplastic lesions using auto-fluorescence depends on subtle changes in the concentration or distribution in depth of endogenous fluorophores, changes in tissue micro-architecture and altered mucosal thickness or blood concentrations. These factors affect the

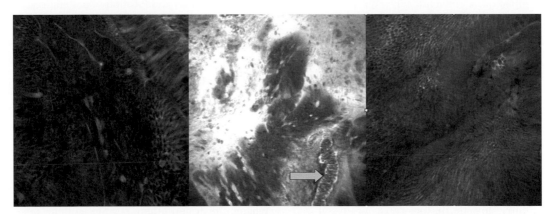

Figure 13.6 Left/right: confocal laser scanning endomicroscopic imaging using intravenous 10% fluorescence of the adjacent lesional mucosa. At 20 and 80 microns in the z axis (left figure/right figure respectively) there is clear crypt architectural distortion to imply adjacent flat dysplasia. There is mucin depletion, gross loss in regular crypt architecture and ridge lined epithelium present. Middle: The circumscribed lesion has been imaged at 50 microns in the z-axis using confocal endomicroscopy. There is gross extravasation of flurophore (white-out field) with a central dilated, tortuous capillary with red cells "stacked up" i.e. the red cell stack sign of neoplasia. The lesion can been characterized *in vivo* as a dysplasia-associated lesional mass. Urgent referral for pan-proctocolectomy should be considered in this clinical scenario.

fluorescence intensity or spectrum due to wavelength-specific light absorption. Using exogenous fluorophores, the detection of lesions is based on selective drug uptake or target tissue retention relative to uptake by normal tissue.

Kapadia *et al* using ultraviolet (UV) light in the colon were able to discriminate normal mucosa, adenomas and hyperplastic lesions with accuracies of 100%, 100% and 94% respectively. In the first *in vivo* human colonic spectroscopic study by Cothren *et al.*, differentiation between adenoma and non-adenomatous lesions was achieved in 97% of cases. Cotheran *et al.*, in the first blinded study, also identified colonic dysplasia with 90% sensitivity and 95% specificity. However, the clinical potential of spectroscopy in routine endoscopic practice is still unclear.

Endoscopic mucosal resection in Western practice

The benefits or early CRC detection are not exclusively those of increased survival as many patients can be curatively treated using novel resection techniques such as endoscopic mucosal resection (EMR). Such a procedure has a low cost and low associated morbidity and mortality when compared to conventional surgery. Data from Japan and our group in the UK now suggest that stage T1 disease can be curatively treated using novel colonoscopic resection techniques such as endoscopic mucosal resection (EMR) *see* Figure 13.7–9. As mentioned above, new endoscopic imaging techniques such as chromoscopic colonoscopy and high-magnification chromoscopic colonoscopy (HMCC) have highlighted the clinical importance of flat and depressed non-polypoid colorectal lesions. Data from centers outside Japan now suggest that novel endoscopic resection techniques such as EMR and endoscopic submucosal dissection are applicable to Western endoscopic practice.

EMR was originally described by Dehyle *et al.*, and has been developed by Japanese endoscopists for the resection of sessile and flat lesions of the stomach, oesophagus and colorectum. Simple snare resection is sufficient for pedunculated lesions. EMR permits the resection of flat and sessile lesions by longitudinal section through the submucosal layer. In the colorectum, EMR may provide curative resection for flat and sessile adenomas in addition to early colorectal cancer. EMR facilitates complete histological analysis of the resected lesion and makes it possible to determine precisely the completeness of excision in both the horizontal and vertical resection planes. This makes it advantageous compared to primary tissue ablative techniques such as argon plasma coagulation and electrocoagulation. Numerous EMR techniques have now been described using transparent caps fitted to the proximal aspect of the endoscope and that using an insulation tipped cutting knife. With the exception of submucosal posterior rectal tumors, these techniques are reserved for esophageal and gastric resection with the strip biopsy technique used routinely in the colorectum.

Basic EMR technique

The technique of EMR comprises 4 stages:

1. Diagnosis and localization of the lesion.
2. Evaluation of invasive depth to exclude lesions invading the deep submucosal layer 3 or beyond (i.e., T2 disease) using HMCC or ultrasound techniques.
3. Excision procedure.
4. Post resection evaluation.

Initial diagnosis and location of flat and sessile lesion of the colorectum is facilitated by the use of indigo carmine (IC) chromoscopy and allows the observation of detailed morphology. *In vivo* staging of identified lesions can then be achieved using high-magnification or through-the-scope mini-probe ultrasound techniques. Flat and sessile lesions up to 20 mm in diameter can be resected by *en block* or "single pass" resection with larger lesions requiring a piecemeal approach. A needle catheter is then inserted through the side-port of the colonoscope with sterile saline injected around the lesion and surrounding mucosa. A cleavage of the submucosa (having the effect of raising the lesion) then permits simple snare resection. A single cannulation can be used for small lesions (<10 mm) diameter with multiple cannulations usually required for lesions of 20 mm or larger. Some authors advocate the use of Adrenaline (1/100,000) mixed with saline or the use of twice-normal saline at submucosal injection. There are no randomized controlled trials proving the superiority of these methods with

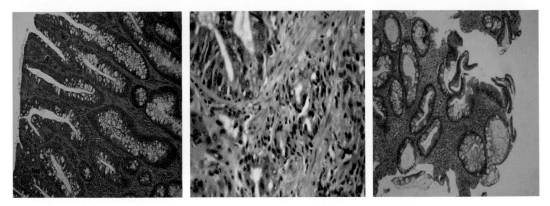

Figure 13.7 Left/right: High power Hematoxylin and eosin staining of the background mucosa shows abnormal crypt architecture compatible with chronic inflammatory bowel disease in addition to dysplastic crypt architecture. Middle: High power Hematoxylin and eosin staining of the circumscribed lesion shows high-grade dysplastic features with an invasive component. Histopathology confirms this lesion to be a dysplasia associated lesion mass where colectomy should be considered as the management of choice.

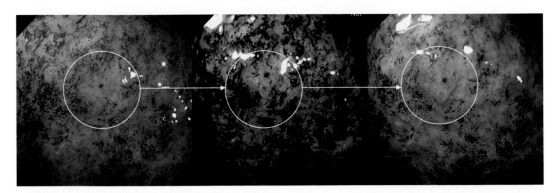

Figure 13.8 Left: high-definition white light imaging of the distal sigmoid colon in a patient with chronic pan-ulcerative colitis. There are florid neovascular changes but also a focus of focal pallor. Middle: Narrow band imaging of the segment shows the vascular architecture as brown tortuous streaks. The lesion is clearly defined as highlighted. Right: Indigo carmine 0.4% chromoscopy delineated the circumferential margin of the lesion according to SURFACE guidelines. The lesion was a flat *de novo* intraepithelial neoplastic lesion (Paris class 0-IIb).

regard to resection clearance, post EMR hemorrhage or perforation. Whatever injection medium is used, it is essential to maintain a sufficient mucosal lift or detachment throughout the EMR, which minimizes the risk of muscularis propria entrapment and subsequent perforation.

The Sheffield group advocates peripheral margin tattoos prior to saline submucosal injection that delineates the normal mucosal boundaries around the lesion prior to snaring. This is a helpful technique, as at submucosal lift, the lesion can become distorted and indistinct from the surrounding normal mucosa. If the lesion fails to lift (the non-lifting sign of Uno), or has an asymmetrical appearance, then the resection should be abandoned as this indicates tethering to the underlying muscularis mucosa. Perforation and risk of non-curative resection can occur in this scenario.

Following successful submucosal lift, a spiked or "barbed" snare is applied over the lesion and slowly closed under gentle suction. This permits the lesion to be retained within the snare boundaries before final resection. Prior to final cutting (usually using a 25W coagulation current) the

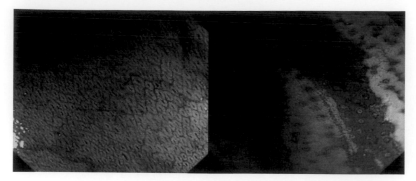

Figure 13.9 Left: High magnification (100×) chromoscopic colonoscopy (indigo carmine 0.4%) of a "normal" rectal mucosa. Note the regular ordered and "honeycomb" Kudo type I crypt pattern. Right: High magnification (100×) chromoscopic colonoscopy (indigo carmine 0.4%) of chronic ulcerative colitis. Note: there is gross fibrotic expansion of the inter-crypt spacing, a decrease in overall mucosal crypt density and prominent linear "tramline" fibrotic ridging characteristic of advanced fibrosis complicating long-standing ulcerative colitis.

snare should be relaxed slightly to allow any entrapped muscularis mucosa to retract. Following resection, the lesion is retrieved using a pronged grasping forcep or Roth net, followed by immediate fixation in 10% formalin solution. Japanese endoscopists "pin out" the lesion onto a solid cork or polystyrene plate prior to fixation that limits shrinkage of the resection specimen and permits easier and more accurate histopathological sectioning.

Post resection management

Following resection, it is important to re-evaluate the cut margin of the mucosa. High rates of adenoma recurrence, despite reported complete excision by the endoscopist have been reported. Performing EMR may, therefore, be considered a hazardous procedure if this is apparent, where remnant adenomatous tissue continues to assume a risk for carcinomatous transformation. The Sheffield group hypothesized that HMCC may provide a sensitive and specific tool to help guide the endoscopist as to whether resection was complete or not. By permitting the acquisition of this data *in vivo*, a key interventional point could be targeted to improve patient outcome (i.e. highlight patients at risk of incomplete resection and hence recurrent disease who require more intensive endoscopic follow-up or alternative management strategies). Hurlstone *et al.*, subsequently

demonstrated that for both *en bloc* and piecemeal resections, HMCC as an *in vivo* tool to predict remnant tissue post EMR, had an overall accuracy of 95%. Implications of these data may include, fewer follow-up procedures, improved therapeutic cure rates and the lowering of overall cost. All of these parameters are vitally important given the anticipated expansion in endoscopic requirements with the imminent introduction of CRC screening programs. On this basis, an extended EMR can therefore be performed at the same treatment session that limits the risk of recurrent disease at the resection site. Should a further EMR be unsuccessful argon plasma coagulation (APC) of any remnant tissue, including application to the entire circumference of the cut margin should be applied. All lesions should have an adjacent submucosal tattoo applied using Indian ink to facilitate localization at follow-up colonoscopy.

Complications of EMR

The main complications of EMR are hemorrhage, perforation and stenosis. The immediate and early complications (10% of cases) described in the first 12 hours post-resection are principally hemorrhage and rarely perforation. The Sheffield group reported bleeding complications in only 2% of patients undergoing EMR in their cohort of 599 lesions. This was significantly lower than that reported in Ahmed's retrospective analysis (22%). However, other Japanese authors have reported hemorrhage rates post-colonic EMR of 1.16%

(10/863), comparable to those observed in the Sheffield series. Okamoto's review of interventional colonoscopic resections also reports a perforation rate secondary to EMR of only 0.35% with Kaneko's multi-center analysis of endoscopic mortality showing rates of less than 0.0001% for this procedure. EMR may, therefore, be a safe and effective endoscopic therapy that may enhance our current strategies aimed at the secondary prevention of colorectal cancer.

Accurate *in vivo* staging is essential at colonoscopy prior to consideration of local endoluminal resection. Flat focal submucosal invasive CRCs which are limited to the submucosal layer 1 can be managed by EMR as the risk of lympho-venous invasion and nodal metastasis is rare (<5%). For lesions with deeper vertical invasion into the submucosal layer 3 or beyond (stage T2) the risk of nodal disease increases to 10–15%. EMR in this group is therefore undesirable due to a higher risk of perforation, non-curative excision and untreated nodal disease. Surgical excision is recommended in this group.

The Sheffield group aimed to prospectively assess the safety and efficacy of colorectal EMR for the endoscopic therapy of early lesions. Hemorrhage (immediate and delayed), perforation and mortality rates were all comparable to Okamoto's review of interventional colonoscopic resections and Kaneko's multi-center analysis of endoscopic mortality. These studies have now validated the use of these resection techniques in the West and may change the management of early colorectal neoplasia away from that of primary surgical resection to that of endoscopic based resection – a procedure that is usually ambulatory with minimal associated morbidity/mortality as compared to primary surgical resection. Furthermore, data supporting the efficacy of HMCC and high-frequency mini-probe ultrasound to distinguish invasive depth in early CRC were subsequently published, demonstrating their combined efficacy in early CRC staging – the largest cohort study within the literature. Given these data, the indications for EMR are again under review, with many authors suggesting extending the role of EMR further.

Given Moreaux's long-term survival and prognosis data for early CRC therefore (5-year survival >90%) EMR may represent an alternative therapeutic option from both a patient preference and health-economic perspective but further studies comparing conventional surgery to EMR with appropriate cost- effective modeling are now required. However, such favorable 5-year mortality is only applicable if early CRC is diagnosed more frequently and is treated by an endoscopist who has received the appropriate specialist endoscopic training and maintained an adequate skill level. Currently it would appear that Western endoscopists with conventional endoscopic training are less successful than Japanese endoscopists at diagnosing early stage cancer. This is not because the Japanese detect cancers by screening the complete asymptomatic population. Indeed, even in Japan, most cases of early cancer are incidental findings at endoscopy with only 10% of gastric cancers being diagnosed by formalized screening programs. At the National Cancer Centre in Tokyo, 20% of colonic cancers are now diagnosed in the intramucosal or T1 stage and hence numerous data regarding the efficacy of EMR exists due to therapeutic demand. Importantly, the data detailed above shows a similar prevalence and HGD rate amongst flat and depressed lesions to Japanese authors, which thus emphasizes the importance of a UK based study validating EMR techniques outside of Japanese endoscopic practice.

Clinical recommendations and conclusions

Colonic chromoscopy and HMCC have been shown to be useful in discriminating between neoplastic and non-neoplastic Paris 0-II colorectal lesions. The decision to target biopsies or progress to therapeutic intervention using EMR can be guided using this technology and avoid inappropriate biopsy or attempted endoscopic resection of lesions without a malignant potential or those which should be referred for surgical excision. We have, therefore, recommended the following endoscopic strategies based upon HMCC and pit pattern analysis.

1. Paris class 0-II lesions (<10 mm diameter without a type IIc component and demonstrable of a type I/II pit pattern can be left *in situ* without biopsy.
2. Paris 0-II lesions (excluding an associated type IIc component) with a type IIIL/IV pit pattern can be resected in a single-step procedure. A submucosal tattoo should be placed adjacent to the resection site to permit future

localization. Inclusion to a systematic surveillance programme of between 3–5 year intervals should then commence.

3. For lesions with a type IIc component and a type IIIs/V pit pattern either alone or in combination should receive cold biopsy only, even if small, and an adjacent mucosal tattoo placed for further localization. Further evaluation of such lesions using a 20 Mhz ultrasound mini-probe (USMP) may be helpful in assessing the invasive depth and possibility of LNM of the lesion and also improve safety if elective EMR is performed as tethering to the underlying muscularis mucosa can be clearly seen.

In conclusion, the techniques of colonic chromoscopy and HMCC have a high overall accuracy for the *in vivo* histopathological interpretation of sporadic Paris 0-II neoplasia and CUC IN detection, but are limited as they only provide surface topographical imaging. The techniques are not 100% sensitive or specific and although a useful diagnostic tool *in vivo*, are not currently a complete replacement for histopathology. It is important for this technology to be used and developed but also requirements for further education and colonoscopic training need to be addressed. In experienced hands, however, HMCC represents a significant advance in colonoscopic practice, which may improve diagnostic yield of significant lesions, lower the burden of insignificant biopsies interpreted by pathologists and enhance therapeutic safety. Finally, development of confocal endomicroscopy with chromoscopic assistance will potentially change the imaging paradigm again.

FURTHER READING

Ahmad NA, Kochman ML, Long WB, *et al.* (2002) Efficacy, safety, and clinical outcomes of endoscopic mucosal resection: a study of 101 cases. *Gastrointestinal Endoscopy*, **55**, 390–396.

Atkin WS, Morson BC, Cuzick J. (1992) Long-term risk of colorectal cancer after excision of rectosigmoid adenomas. *New England Journal of Medicine*, **326**, 658–662.

Bedenne L, Faivre J, Boutron MC, *et al.* (1992) Adenoma–carcinoma sequence or "de novo" carcinogenesis? A study of adenomatous remnants in a population-based series of large bowel cancers. *Cancer*, **69**, 883.

Brooker JC, Saunders BP, Shah SG, *et al.* (2002) Treatment with argon plasma coagulation reduces recurrence after piecemeal resection of large sessile colonic polyps: a randomised trial and recommendations. *Gastrointestinal Endoscopy*, **55**, 371–375.

Brostrom MO, Lofberg R, Ost A. (1986) Cancer surveillance of patients with longstanding ulcerative colitis: A clinical and endoscopical and histological study. *Gut*, **27**, 1408–1413.

Cothren RM, Richards-Koru R, Sivak MV, *et al.* (1990) Gastrointestinal tissue diagnosis by laser-induced fluorescence spectroscopy at endoscopy. *Gastrointestinal Endoscopy*, **36**, 105–111.

Cothren RM, Sivak MV, Van Dam J, *et al.* (1996) Detection of dysplasia at colonoscopy using laser-induced fluorescence: a blinded study. *Gastrointestinal Endoscopy*, **44**, 168–176.

Deyhle P, Largader F, Jenny S, *et al.* (1973) A method for endoscopic electroresection of sessile colonic polyps. *Endoscopy*, **5**, 38–40.

Fu KI, Sano Y, Kato S, *et al.* (2004) Chromoendoscopy using indigo carmine dye spraying with magnifying observation is the most reliable method for differential diagnosis between non-neoplastic and neoplastic colorectal lesions: a prospective study. *Endoscopy*, **36**, 1089–1093.

Goldmann H. (1996) Significance and detection of dysplasia in chronic colitis. *Cancer*, **78**, 2261–2263.

Haringsma J, Tytgat GNJ, Yano H, *et al.* (2001) Autofluorescence endoscopy: feasibility of detection of GI neoplasms unapparent to white light endoscopy with an evolving technology. *Gastrointestinal Endoscopy*, **53**, 642–650.

Hurlstone DP, Fujii T, Lobo AJ. (2002) Early detection of colorectal cancer using high-magnification chromoscopic colonoscopy. *British Journal of Surgery*, **89**, 272–282.

Hurlstone DP, Cross SS, Adam I, *et al.* (2003a) A prospective clinicopathological and endoscopic evaluation of flat and depressed colorectal lesions in the UK. *American Journal of Gastroenterology*, **98**, 2543–2549.

Hurlstone DP, Cross SS, Adam I, *et al.* (2003b) An evaluation of colorectal endoscopic mucosal resection using high-magnification chromoscopic colonoscopy: a prospective study of 1000 colonoscopies. *Endoscopy*, [in press].

Hurlstone DP, Lobo AJ. (2003c) Resection margin "thermal tattooing" for lateral spreading tumour resection using endoscopic mucosal resection: a new technique for assisting complete horizontal clearance. *World Journal of Surgery* (in press).

Hurlstone DP, Cross SS, Lobo AJ, *et al.* (2003) High magnification chromoscopic colonoscopy as a screening tool in acromegaly. *Gut,* **52,** 1797–1798.

Hurlstone DP, Cross SS, Adam I, *et al.* (2004a) Efficacy of high magnification chromoscopic colonoscopy for the diagnosis of neoplasia in flat and depressed lesions of the colorectum: a prospective analysis. *Gut,* **53,** 284–290.

Hurlstone DP, Sanders DS, Cross SS, *et al.* (2004b) Colonoscopic resection of lateral spreading tumours: a prospective analysis of endoscopic mucosal resection. *Gut,* **53,** 1334–1339.

Hurlstone DP, Cross SS, Drew K, *et al.* (2004c) An evaluation of colorectal endoscopic mucosal resection using high-magnification chromoscopic colonoscopy: a prospective study of 1000 colonoscopies. *Endoscopy,* **36,** 491–498.

Hurlstone DP, Cross SS, Adam I, *et al.* (2004d) Endoscopic morphological anticipation of submucosal invasion in flat and depressed colorectal lesions: clinical implications and subtype analysis of the Kudo type V pit pattern using high-magnification-chromoscopic colonoscopy. *Colorectal Disease,* **6,** 369–375.

Hurlstone DP, Cross SS, Adam I, *et al.* (2004e) Efficacy of high magnification chromoscopic colonoscopy for the diagnosis of neoplasia in flat and depressed lesions of the colorectum: a prospective analysis. *Gut,* **53,** 284–290.

Hurlstone DP, Karajeh MA, Shorthouse AJ. (2004f) Screening for colorectal cancer: implications for UK and European initiatives. *Techniques in Coloproctology,* **8,** 139–145.

Hurlstone DP, Cross SS. (2004g) Role of aberrant crypt foci detected using high-magnification chromoscopic colonoscopy in human colorectal carcinogenesis. *Journal of Gastroenterology and Hepatology,* (in press.)

Hurlstone DP, Brown S, Cross SS, *et al.* (2005a) High magnification chromoscopic colonoscopy or high frequency 20 MHz mini probe endoscopic ultrasound staging for early colorectal neoplasia: a comparative prospective analysis. *Gut,* **54,** 1585–1589.

Hurlstone DP, Brown S, Cross SS, *et al.* (2005b) Endoscopic ultrasound miniprobe staging of colorectal cancer: can management be modified? *Endoscopy,* **37,** 710–714.

Hurlstone DP, Fujii T. (2005c) Practical uses of chromoendoscopy and magnification at colon-oscopy. *Gastrointestinal Endoscopy Clinics of North America,* **15,** 687–702.

Hurlstone DP, Sanders DS, Lobo AJ, *et al.* (2005d) Indigo carmine-assisted high-magnification chromoscopic colonoscopy for the detection and characterisation of intraepithelial neoplasia in ulcerative colitis: a prospective evaluation. *Endoscopy,* **37,** 1186–1192.

Hurlstone DP, Karajeh M, Sanders DS, *et al.* (2005e) Rectal aberrant crypt foci identified using high-magnification-chromoscopic colonoscopy: biomarkers for flat and depressed neoplasia. *American Journal of Gastroenterology,* **100,** 1283–1289.

Inoue H, Takeshita K, Hori H, *et al.* (1993) Endoscopic mucosal resection with a cap-fitted panendoscope for esophagus, stomach, and colon mucosal lesions. *Gastrointestinal Endoscopy,* **39,** 58–62.

Kapadia CR, Cutruzzola FW, O'Brien KM, *et al.* Laser-induced fluorescence spectroscopy of human colonic mucosa. Detection of adenomatous transformation. *Gastroenterology,* **99,** 150–157.

Kitamura K, Taniguchi H, Yamaguchi T, *et al.* (1997) Clinical outcome of surgical treatment for invasive early colorectal cancer in Japan. *Hepatogastroenterology,* **44,** 108–115.

Kiesslich R, Fritsch J, Holtmann M, *et al.* (2003) Methylene Blue-Aided Chromoendoscopy for the Detection of Intraepithelial Neoplasia and Colon Cancer in Ulcerative Colitis. *Gastroenterology,* **124,** 880–888.

Kiesslich R, Neurath MF. (2004a) Chromoendoscopy: an evolving standard in surveillance for ulcerative colitis. *Inflammatory Bowel Disease,* **10,** 695–696.

Kiesslich R, Burg J, Vieth M, *et al.* (2004b) Confocal laser endoscopy for diagnosing intraepithelial neoplasias and colorectal cancer *in vivo.* *Gastroenterology,* **127,** 706–713.

Konishi K, Kaneko K, Kurahashi T, *et al.* (2003) A comparison of magnifying and nonmagnifying colonoscopy for diagnosis of colorectal polyps: A prospective study. *Gastrointestinal Endoscopy,* **57,** 48–53.

Kosaka T. (1975) Clinico-pathological study of the minute elevated lesion of the colorectal mucosa. *Journal of the Japanese Society of Coloproctology,* **28,** 218–226.

Kudo S, Hayashi S, Miura K, *et al.* (1989) The clinicopathological features of flat and depressed type of early colorectal cancer [in Japanese with English abstract]. *Stomach and Intestine,* **24,** 317–329.

Kudo S, Hirota S, Nakajima T, *et al.* (1994) Colorectal tumours and pit pattern. *Journal of Clinical Pathology*, **47,** 880–885.

Kudo S, Tamura S, Kashida H, *et al.* (1996) Endoscopic treatment in colorectal lesions –especially on endoscopic mucosal resection]. *Nippon Rinsho*, **54,** 1298–1306.

Kudo S, Kashida H, Nakajima T, *et al.* (1997) Endoscopic diagnosis and treatment of early colorectal cancer. *World Journal of Surgery*, **21,** 694–701.

Kudo S, Kashida H, Tamura T, *et al.* (2000) Colonoscopic diagnosis and management of nonpolypoid early colorectal cancer. *World Journal of Surgery*, **24,** 1081–1090.

Kudo S, Rubio CA, Teixeira CR, *et al.* (2001) Pit pattern in colorectal neoplasia: endoscopic magnifying view. *Endoscopy*, **33,** 367–373.

Lambert R, Provenzale D, Ectors N, *et al.* (2001) Early diagnosis and prevention of sporadic colorectal cancer. *Endoscopy*, **33,** 1042–1064.

Matsumoto T, Iida M, Yao T, *et al.* (1994) Role of nonpolypoid neoplastic lesions in the pathogenesis of colorectal cancer. *Diseases of the Colon and Rectum*, **37,** 450–455.

Medical Examinations for Digestive Cancer in 1995 Group. (1998) National Report. *Journal of Gastroenterology Mass*, **130,** 251–269.

Moreaux J, Catala M. (1987) Carcinoma of the colon: long-term survival and prognosis after surgical treatment in a series of 798 patients. *World Journal of Surgery*, **11,** 804–809.

Morson BC. (1968) Precancerous and early malignant lesions of the large intestine. *British Journal of Surgery*, **55,** 725–731.

Muller AD, Sonnenberg A. (1995) Prevention of colorectal cancer by flexible endoscopy and polypectomy. A case-control study of 32,702 veterans. *Annals of Internal Medicine*, **123,** 904–910.

Nagata S, Tanaka S, Haruma K, *et al.* (2000) Pit pattern diagnosis of early colorectal carcinoma by magnifying colonoscopy: clinical and histological implications. *International Journal of Oncology*, **16,** 927–934.

Nelson DB, Block KP, Bosco JJ, *et al.* (2000) High resolution and high-magnification endoscopy: September, *Gastrointestinal Endoscopy*, **52,** 864–866.

Newland RC, Chapuis PH, Pheils MT, *et al.* (1981) The relationship of survival to staging and grading of colorectal carcinoma: a prospective study of 503 cases. *Cancer*, **47,** 1424–1429.

Newland RC, Chapuis PH, Smyth EJ. (1987) The prognostic value of substaging colorectal carcinoma. A prospective study of 1117 cases with standardized pathology. *Cancer*, **60,** 852–857.

NHS-executive. (1997) Guidance on Commissioning Cancer Services. Improving Outcomes in Colorectal Cancer. Wetherby – UK. NHS Executive.

Okamoto H, Tanaka S, Haruma K. (1996) Japanese review of complications and measure by endoscopic treatment for colorectal tumor between 1989–1993 [in Japanese with English abstract]. *Hiroshimaigaku*, **49,** 585–591.

Palazzo MGL, Canard PJM. (2001) Guidelines of the French Society of Digestive Endoscopy: Endoscopic Mucosectomy. *Endoscopy*, **33,** 187–190.

Paris Workshop Participants. (2002) The Paris endoscopic classification of superficial neoplastic lesions: Esophagus, stomach and colon. *Gastrointestinal Endoscopy*, **58,** S3–43.

Ponchon T. (2001) Endoscopic mucosal resection. *Journal of Clinical Gastroenterology*, **32,** 6–10.

Rembacken BJ, Fujii T, Cairns A, *et al.* (2000) Flat and depressed colonic neoplasms: a prospective study of 1000 colonoscopies in the UK. *Lancet*, **355,** 1211–1214.

Riddell RH, Goldman H, Ransohoff DF, *et al.* (1983) Dysplasia in inflammatory bowel disease: standardized classification with provisional clinical implications. *Human Pathology*, **14,** 931–968.

Rutter MD, Saunders BP, Schofield G, *et al.* (2004) Pancolonic indigo carmine dye spraying for the detection of dysplasia in ulcerative colitis. *Gut*, **53,** 256–260.

Saitoh Y, Obara T, Einami K, *et al.* (1996) Efficacy of high-frequency ultrasound probes for the preoperative staging of invasion depth in flat and depressed colorectal tumors. *Gastrointestinal Endoscopy*, **44,** 34–39.

Saito Y, Waxman I, West AB, *et al.* (2001) Prevalence and Distinctive Biological Features of Flat Colorectal Adenomas in a North American Population. *Gastroenterology*, **120,** 1657–1665.

Shida H, Ban K, Matsumoto M, *et al.* (1992) Prognostic significance of location of lymph node metastases in colorectal cancer. *Diseases of the Colon and Rectum*, **35,** 1046–1050.

Shida H, Ban K, Matsumoto M, *et al.* (1996) Asymptomatic colorectal cancer detected by screening. *Diseases of the Colon and Rectum*, **39,** 1130–1135.

Tanaka S, Haruma K, Teixeira CR, *et al.* (1995) Endoscopic treatment of submucosal invasive colorectal carcinoma with special reference to risk factors for lymph node metastasis. *Journal of Gastroenterology*, **30,** 710–717.

Tung SY, Wu CS, Su MY. (2001) Magnifying colonoscopy in differentiating neoplastic from non-neoplastic colorectal lesions. *American Journal of Gastroenterology*, **96,** 2628–2632.

Wagnieres GA, Star WM, Wilson BC. (1998) *In vivo* fluorescence spectroscopy and imaging for oncological applications. *Photochemistry and Photobiology*, **68,** 603–632.

Willis J, Riddell RH. (2003) Biology versus terminology: East meets west in surgical pathology. *Gastrointestinal Endoscopy*, **57,** 369–376.

Winawer SJ, Zauber AG, Ho MN, *et al.* (1993) Prevention of colorectal cancer by colonoscopic polypectomy. The National Polyp Study Workgroup. *New England Journal of Medicine*, **329,** 1977–1981.

Wolber RA, Owen DA. (1991) Flat adenoma of the colon. *Human Pathology*, **22,** 70–74.

14

Endoscopic retrograde cholangio-pancreatography in children

Luigi Dall'Oglio, Paola De Angelis & Francesca Foschia

 KEY POINTS

- ERCP is a safe procedure even in infants with neonatal cholestasis.
- Proper equipment and technique minimizes the risk of ERCP related complications.
- MRCP is replacing ERCP as a preferred diagnostic procedure in infants and children with pancreatobiliary disorders.
- Besides the field of neonatal cholestasis and specific conditions requiring an endoscopic ultrasound or a fine needle aspiration

technique, ERCP is indicated primarily as a therapeutic procedure: sphincterotomy, stenting, naso-biliary drainage etc.
- ERCP plays an important role as a definitive treatment or a bridge therapy to surgery in children with acute post traumatic and chronic pancreatitis, choledochal cysts, complications after laparoscopic cholecystectomy and some form of intestinal duplications.

Introduction

ERCP represents a spectrum of techniques, each of which shares an initial step: retrograde opacification of bile and pancreatic ducts through the endoscopic cannulation of the major or minor papilla.

Each year thousands of ERCPs are performed in adult patients mainly due to a large spectrum of therapeutic applications.

However, a relatively low incidence of pancreatobiliary diseases in children and lack of experience among pediatric surgeons and gastro-

enterologists limited the application of ERCP in pediatric patients in the past.

In the last decade, significant progress has been made in the diagnosis of pancreatobiliary disorders in children, especially chronic pancreatitis. In addition, the rising incidence of cholelithiasis (particularly among obese children) has increased the demand for therapeutic ERCP.

Indications for ERCP in children vary from region to region. In Western countries, the main indication for ERCP is choledocolithiasis and biliary or chronic pancreatitis. In the Middle East, ERCP is commonly performed in children with choledocolithiasis due to sickle-cell anemia, and

---

Practical Pediatric Gastrointestinal Endoscopy, Second Edition. George Gershman, Mike Thomson, Marvin Ament.
© 2012 Blackwell Publishing Ltd. Published 2012 by Blackwell Publishing Ltd.

in Asian countries a choledocal cyst is the leading indication for ERCP.

In this chapter, our aim is to describe all the aspects of pediatric ERCP including indications, preparation, techniques, outcome and complications of diagnostic and therapeutic ERCP in infants and children.

Duodenoscopes and accessories

The smallest duodenoscope, the PJF 160 (Olympus), is only 7.5 mm wide. It has a 2 mm biopsy channel.

This instrument is designed for neonates and infants who weigh less than 10 Kg. The limitations are: difficulties passing a cannula through the distal portion of the scope, reduced capacity of the elevator to angle the cannula toward the major duodenal papilla, inadequate suction and application of 5 Fr wide accessories only. PJF 160 has a metal tip and, therefore, it is not routinely used for electrosurgical procedures due to risk of accidental thermal damage of the duodenal wall. However, successful sphincterotomy with a 5 Fr sphincterotome was reported. Some authors perform ERCP in infants and children less than 1.5 years of age using the PJF model, and standard adult diagnostic duodenoscope in older patients.

Other experts advocate an adult 11 mm wide therapeutic duodenoscope for children 7 years and older.

In our practice, we routinely use a standard adult therapeutic duodenoscope in children with a body mass more than 10–15 Kg. The list of commercially available endoscopes for pediatric ERCP is listed in Table 14.1.

The key to success and safety of pediatric ERCP is collaboration between a specially trained nurse and an experienced endoscopist and anesthesiologist. General anesthesia with intubation is mandatory for infants and children (except teenagers) avoiding compression of the trachea.

The list of commonly used accessories is summarized in Table 14.2.

Table 14.1 Duodenoscopes: specification

FUJINON	Insertion tube (mm)	Biopsy channel (mm)
ED450XL5	12.5	3.2
ED530XT	13. 4.2	4.2
OLYMPUS		
PJF	7.5	2.0
JF1T2	11.0	3.2
TJF160VR	12.5	4.2
PJF160	7.5	2.0
PENTAX		
ED3280K	10.8	3.2
PENTAX		
ED3480TK	11.6	4.2
ED3680TK	12.1	4.8

Table 14.2 List of commonly used accessories for ERCP

SPECIFIC ERCP ACCESSORIES
Cannulas: bolted and tapered catheters
Guidewires of different sizes and types: straight, "J", soft and stiff
Sphincterotomes
Precut needle sphincterotomes
Balloon hydrostatic dilators
Semirigid dilators
Stones extraction balloon
Stones retrieval basket (Dormia)
Catheter for naso-biliary and pancreatic drainage
Biliary and pancreatic stents
GENERAL ENDOSCOPIC ACCESSORIES
Foreign bodies forceps
Diatermic snares
Injection needles
Hemostatic metallic clip

The choice of particular accessories is dictated by specific indications, for example, narrowing or stricture of the common bile duct, the size of the papilla and the bile- or pancreatic ducts, and a matter of personal preference of the experienced endoscopist.

ERCP is a combined endoscopic and radiological technique and requires an optimal set up of fluoroscopy equipment and the participation of a well-trained radiologist capable of performing a percutaneous transhepatic cholangiography (PTC) to establish bile drainage in case of a failed ERCP. In addition, a PTC and ERCP *rendez vous* technique is an effective way to treat patients with cholestasis secondary to complex and difficult to approach biliary strictures. Different types of contrast media are available. The contrast is typically diluted in saline. Special endoscopes designed for endoscopic ultrasonography (EUS) are an important addition to the arsenal of instruments available for children with specific conditions (e.g. pancreatic cysts).

How to perform ERCP

ERCP is performed routinely with the patient in a prone position. Esophageal intubation with the side-view endoscope is different compared with frontal view instruments. It is almost a blind maneuver. It should be done properly to avoid trauma of the cervical esophagus or perforation of the piriform sinus. A duodenoscope is inserted into the mouth, along the middle line of the tongue, and advanced toward the pharynx then bent down toward the route of the tongue. Further insertion is combined with gradual deflection of the distal end of the scope upwards toward the posterior wall of the pharynx and advancement into the esophagus. The moment of esophageal intubation is associated with decreased resistance and appearance of gliding esophageal mucosa with a clear vascular pattern. Attempts to view the esophageal lumen are counterproductive and may lead to mucosal laceration. The endoscope is advanced without resistance until the vascular pattern disappears. It is usually associated with the entrance into the stomach and close contact of the lenses with gastric mucosa at the level of upper gastric body.

For proper orientation, a scope should be pulled back and rotated counterclockwise with simultaneous deflection of the distal end to the left. Once the panoramic view of the gastric body is estab-

lished, the duodenoscope is advanced forward and rotated clockwise. Care should be taken to avoid slipping back into the gastric body. During the transition between the gastric body and the antrum, the lumen of the stomach may disappear. Appearance of the sliding gastric mucosa is reassuring unless significant resistance occurs. The view of the gastric lumen is reestablished by elevating the tip of the scope and/or pulling the scope back gently. Longitudinal prepyloric folds are a good orienteer to follow. A transition through the pylorus is manifested by significant reduction of resistance and changes of the mucosal pattern from smooth to velvet types. The second portion of the duodenum is approached by upward deflection of the distal tip, clockwise rotation and advancement of the scope. It is the so-called "long" way technique. To convert it into the so-called "short" way position, which is more desirable for cannulation, the scope should be rotated clockwise and pulled back simultaneously.

In infants, it is quite difficult to navigate the instrument into the "short" position, leaving occasionally no alternative to the "long" way technique of ERCP despite some limitations: excessive stretching of the stomach and the duodenum, masking of the common bile duct by overlapping duodenoscope (leading to an obscure image), difficulties with control the distal tip of the scope, and positioning of the cannula or therapeutic accessories.

Indications and technique of endoscopic sphincterotomy (ES) are described in other sections of the chapter.

Complications

The incidence of ERCP related complications in adults is usually linked to therapeutic manipulation and fluctuates from 1% to 13%. Overall, the rate of complications associated with ERCP in children is under 5%. The most common complication is pancreatitis, which is usually resolved in one or two days. Isolated enzyme elevation in otherwise asymptomatic children should not be labeled as pancreatitis.

This complication can be prevented by precise and selective cannulation of the major papilla, avoidance of pancreatic parenchimography, and placement of a nasopancreatic drainage tube or pancreatic stent after pancreatic ES.

There is no consensus among pediatric and adult gastroenterologists regarding prophylactic use of sandostatine or serine protease inhibitors.

Bleeding after ES is rare and is well-controlled in most cases by injection of epinephrine 1:10 000 in saline during urgent endoscopy.

Few cases of retroperitoneal perforation of the duodenum after sphincterotomy have been described in children.

Important anatomical characteristics of bile ducts

Variations of normal anatomy of bile ducts and sphincter of Oddi are well known and should be considered for proper interpretation of cholangiogram. The diameter of a normal common bile duct just below the cystic duct in children 7 years and older varies from 2.1 to 4.9 mm. The confluence between cystic and common bile duct could be angled, parallel or spiral. For the most part, the sphincter of Oddi is located within the duodenal wall. The common bile and main pancreatic duct open into the ampula of major duodenal papilla or merge just above the duodenum.

Diagnostic and therapeutic biliary indication

Biliary indications for diagnostic and therapeutic ERCP are listed in Table 14.3.

Biliary atresia

Biliary atresia (BA) presents in the first months of life and is defined as segmental or diffuse obliteration of the extrahepatic bile ducts. The extent and the site of atresia are variable. Early diagnosis is critical for success of the Kasai portojejunostomy.

The main diagnostic dilemma in neonates with direct hyperbilirinemia is differentiation between BA and neonatal hepatitis. A combination of clinical signs such as jaundice, alcoholic stool, hepatomegaly, along with positive results of HIDA scan, liver ultrasound ("triangular-cord" sign) and liver biopsy, provide an accurate diagnosis of BA or neonatal hepatitis in 80–94%.

In the past, 10 to 20% of infants required a surgical exploration and intraoperative cholangiogram to establish a correct diagnosis.

Over the last decade, ERCP was proven safe and effective in the early diagnosis of BA in challenging

Table 14.3 Biliary indications for diagnostic and therapeutic ERCP

Diagnostic: clinical suspicion for	Therapeutic
Biliary atresia	Sphincterotomy
Choledocal cyst	Spincteroplasty
Choledocholithiasis	Stone extraction
Biliary obstruction due to parasitic infestation	Stricture dilation
Benign and malignant biliary strictures	Stent placement
Primary sclerosing cholangitis	Nasobiliary drainage
Pre-pos- operative evaluation	
Biliary neoplasia	
Hepatic injury and surgical complications	

cases. Three types of ERCP findings were described (Table 14.4).

Type 2 and type 3 findings are diagnostic. Type 1 findings are inconclusive and the diagnosis should be confirmed intraoperatively. Published data from King's College Hospital, London, UK showed that ERCP allowed avoidance of an exploratory laparotomy in about 42% of infants with cholestatic jaundice and suspected BA. A considerable proportion of these infants had no evidence of hepatic dysfunction during long-term follow up. The diagnosis established by ERCP was incorrect only in 1.6% of infants with neonatal cholestasis. Two novel approaches, laparoscopic cholangiography and magnetic resonance cholangiopancreatography (MRCP), are available but more data is necessary to validate their diagnostic accuracy.

Choledochal cysts

Choledochal cysts (CC) are anomalies of bile ducts frequently associated with anomalous pancreatobiliary junction (APJ), the so-called "common channel" (Figure 14.1) defined as a confluence of

Table 14.4 ERCP findings in infants with suspected biliary atresia	
Type 1	(35%): no visualization of biliary tree, absence of bile in the duodenum, normal pancreatogram
Type 2	35%): opacification of distal common bile duct and gallbladder, no bile in the duodenum, normal pancreatogram
Type 3	• 3a: visualization of the gallbladder and CBD. Presence of bile lakes in the porta hepatis • 3b (30%): visualization of both hepatic ducts and bile lakes

Table 14.5 Todani classification of choledochal cyst (based on the shape of the affected segments of bile ducts)

Type I (the most common type: 80–90%)

- IA: Segmental or diffuse saccular dilatation of extrahepatic biliary tree.
- IB: Segmental dilatation of CBD (more often in the distal portion), with normal bile duct between the cyst and the cystic duct
- IC: fusiform dilatation of CBD (Figure 14.2)

Type II (2%)

Choledochal diverticulum: isolated protrusion of the common bile duct wall

Type III (1.5–5%)

Choledococele: isolated involvement of the intraduodenal portion of CBD. The major duodenal papilla is bulging (Figure 14.3)

Type IV

- IVA (20%) Multiple dilatations of intra- and extrahepatic bile ducts
- IVB Multiple dilatations of the extrahepatic bile ducts

Type V

Caroli disease: multiple usually small dilatations of the intrahepatic bile ducts

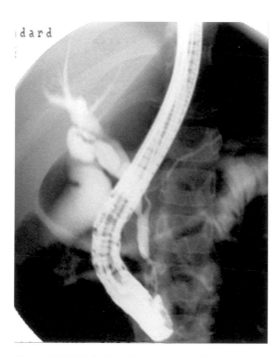

Figure 14.1 Choledochal cyst type 1 with a long common channel.

the common bile and main pancreatic ducts external to the duodenal wall. The association occurs in more than 80% of cases.

Choledochal cysts are usually found in infancy or childhood, although cases of delayed diagnosis in school age children and teenagers have been reported. The most accepted classification is listed in Table 14.5.

The common presentation includes abdominal pain, intermittent jaundice and recurrent acute pancreatitis. Associated complications include choledocolithiasis, cholelithiasis, biliary cirrhosis, intrahepatic abscess and biliary neoplasia. The treatment of choice of CC is hepaticojejunostomy in a Roux-en-Y fashion with complete cyst excision. The diagnostic role of ERCP is to define the anatomy of the pancreatobiliary junction. The information helps the surgeon estimate the distal level of CC resection, avoiding complications due to preservation of a long remnant of a choledochal cyst.

In many children with CC complicated by choledocholithiasis and biliary pancreatic, ERCP with sphincterotomy and biliary stent serves as a bridge therapy before definitive surgical correction.

In cases of small intramural choledococele (Figure 14.2), an endoscopic unroofing of the cyst

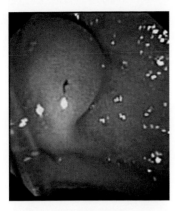

Figure 14.2 A bulging papilla in a 3-year-old girl with cholodochocele and recurrent pancreatitis.

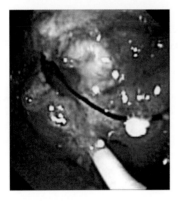

Figure 14.3 The endoscopic unroofing of the choledochocele.

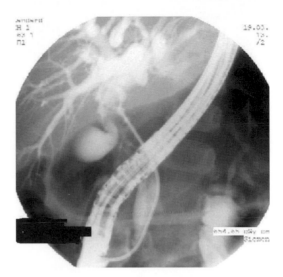

Figure 14.4 Endoscopic biopsy in 4-year-old boy with rhabdomiosarcoma of CBD. Markedly dilated common hepatic, right and left hepatic and intrahepatic bile ducts.

has been described (Figure 14.3) but there are no reports regarding the long-term follow-up of children managed by this method.

On rare occasions, biliary rhabdomiosarcoma can mimic clinical manifestation of CC. ERCP with endoscopic biopsies is an important method to avoid diagnostic laparotomy and tumour spreading related to percutaneous biopsy (Figure 14.4).

Choledocolithiasis

Cholelithiasis, although still rare, has become more frequently diagnosed in children. Recently, it was reported to occur in 0.15 to 0.22% of children. Choledocholithiasis was documented in 11% of children with cholelithisis. The incidence of choledocholithiasis increases from 3%, among children with acute or chronic calculus cholecystitis to almost 20% in children with gallstone

pancreatitis. Sickle cell disease (SCD) and other hemoglobinophathies are an additional risk factor. According to Issa *et al.*, stones in CBD were found in more than 37% of 125 children who underwent ERCP for obstructive jaundice or biliary colic. All cases were managed by ES and balloon stone extraction without laparoscopic or open CBD exploration.

Therapeutic ERCP with ES and stone extraction is the treatment of choice for children with retaining CBD stones after cholecystectomy. For children with cholelithiasis, there is no consensus whether suspicion of CBD stones warrants ERCP before laparascopic cholecystectomy or routine intraoperative cholangiogram to eliminate the needs for pre- or postoperative ERCP. In our practice, we perform ERCP prior to cholecystectomy in children with cholelithiasis, dilated CBD, and biliary pancreatitis or postoperatively in patients with persistently elevated or rising liver enzymes and escalating abdominal pain suggesting retaining CBD stones.

Primary sclerosing cholangitis (PSC)

PSC is a chronic progressive liver disorder, commonly associated with inflammatory bowel disease, characterized by ongoing inflammation, obliteration and fibrosis of both intra- and extrahepatic bile ducts with multiple strictures dividing bile ducts into short segments of normal

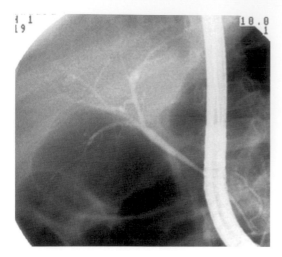

Figure 14.5 Early stage of PSC with narrowing of the right hepatic duct and of CBD.

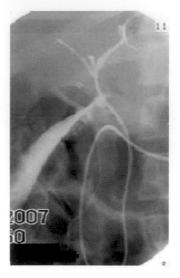

Figure 14.6 Post-cholecystectomy bile leak: extravasation of contrast into the peritoneal cavity. Bile leak completely resolved after sphincterotomy and naso-biliary drainage.

size or dilated bile ducts of a beaded or pearl necklace pattern (Figure. 14.5). The gallbladder and the cystic duct are involved in up to 15% of cases. PSC is a progressive disease wherein approximately 50% of the symptomatic patients will develop cirrhosis and liver failure and require liver transplantation. PSC carries an increased risk of malignancy, especially cholangiocarcinoma.

Diagnostic ERCP is indicated in children with suspected PSC, if the results of the MRCP are inconclusive. In some patients, cholestasis is due to dominant strictures defined as a discrete area of narrowing within the extrahepatic biliary tree. Dominant strictures of the extrahepatic bile duct occur in 7–20% of the patients with PSC and cholestasis. Patients with CBD stricture are candidates for therapeutic ERCP with ES with biliary stent placement. An alternative method is percutaneous balloon dilatation. Stenting is associated with more septic complications than balloon dilations. However, ERCP assisted treatment of dominant strictures can lower morbidity rates compared with percutaneous techniques.

Postsurgical and post-traumatic biliary disease

A bile leak after laparoscopic cholecystectomy, liver transplantation or traumatic injuries of bile ducts can be successfully treated by nasobiliary drainage (Figure 14.6) or ERCP with ES and biliary stent placement. A stricture of CBD after cholecystectomy can be treated by endoscopic placement of plastic stents.

Clinical manifestation of a bile leak after blind abdominal trauma is often insidious and nonspecific. It may delay the diagnosis by a few days despite utilization of radioisotope scintigraphy in all injuries carrying a high risk of a bile leak such as a laceration greater than 4 cm or extending into the porto hepatis. Early diagnosis reduces morbidity and hospitalization. ERCP with stent placement has been proven to contribute to prompt discovery of bile leak sources and dramatic recovery by effective reduction of the pressure in the bile ducts even if a stent does not bridge the gap between the damaged ducts.

Pancreatic indications for diagnostic and therapeutic ERCP

Acute recurrent and chronic pancreatitis are the most common pancreatic indications for ERCP in children. A complete list of pancreatic indications for diagnostic and therapeutic ERCP is listed in Table 14.6.

Acute pancreatitis

Non-invasive imaging studies such as an US (for non-obese children only), CT scan, and MRCP are the most important initial diagnostic steps in children with suspected acute pancreatitis. They allow for determining the extent and severity of the disease and complications of acute pancreatitis, e.g. pseudocysts. In fact, diagnostic ERCP is

Table 14.6 Diagnostic and Therapeutic ERCP in children with pancreatic disorders

Diagnostic ERCP
Recurrent pancreatitis
Chronic pancreatitis
Pancreatic mass
Therapeutic ERCP
Acute biliary pancreatitis
Papillary stenosis
Stenosis of the main pancreatic duct
Pancreas divisum
Pancrealitiasis
Pseudocyst
Duodenal duplication

now substituted for the most part by MRCP, which is less invasive and safer than ERCP (Table 14.7). A normal diameter of the major pancreatic duct ranges from 1.4 to 2.1 mm in the head of the pancreas and from 1.1 to 1.9 mm in the body.

During the acute phase of pancreatitis, ERCP is indicated only in children with biliary pancreatitis, or infants and children with CC or patients with acute cholangitis secondary to obstruction of CBD near the major duodenal papilla.

Therapeutic ERCP with biliary sphincterotomy is strongly indicated within 72 hours from the onset of symptoms in children with severe acute pancreatitis caused by choledocholithiasis with or without jaundice.

Recurrent pancreatitis

There are non-obstructive and obstructive forms of recurrent pancreatitis. ERCP can identify the causes of chronic pancreatitis in 40–75% of children. However, non-invasive methods such as MRCP should be used first because it has equal diagnostic value compared to ERCP in revealing anatomic abnormalities of the pancreatobiliary.

ERCP is indicated if additional diagnostic tests are considered: endoscopic biopsy or brush cytology.

Therapeutic ERCP embraces several techniques including pancreatic ES, pancreatic stone

Table 14.7 Role of MRCP and ERCP in children with pancreatic disorders

	Diagnostic Approach	Therapeutic Strategy
Acute Pancreatitis	MRCP or CT scan	Biliary pancreatitis with confirmed dilatation of CBD: sphincterotomy, stone extraction, occlusion cholangiogram
Recurrent Pancreatitis	MRCP ERCP reserved for children with unresolved diagnostic dilemmas and in cases when MRCP is not available	Biliary and pancreatic sphincterotomy, pancreatic stone extraction, dilation, pancreatic stent. • preoperative management: endoscopic sphinterotomy, dilations, stone removal for children with anomalous pancreatobiliary junction • Sphincterotomy of the major or minor duodenal papilla in children with pancreas divisum; • Endoscopic marsupialisation of the duplication into the duodenal lumen • pancreatic sphincterotomy for children with SOD.
Chronic Pancreatitis	Same	Endoscopic sphincterotomy, stone/sludge removal, drainage procedures

Table 14.8 Steps of biliary and pancreatic endoscopic sphyncterotomy (ES) technique

- Visualization of major papilla

- Cannulation and opacization of biliary and main pancreatic ducts

- Guidewire insertion

- Optimal direction of sphincterotome: 11–12 o'clock for biliary ES and 1–2 o'clock for pancreatic

- Pre-cut with needle-knife type sphincterotome for unsuccessful standard cannulation technique. Described immediate complication: bleeding; late complication papilla stenosis.

extraction, balloon dilations and pancreatic stent placement.

It is indicated for children with recurrent non-biliary pancreatitis and severe dilatation, strictures and stones of the main pancreatic duct and congenital anomalies such as pancreas divisum. A step by step technique of biliary and pancreatic ES is illustrated in Table 14.8.

Anomalous pancreatobiliary junction

Anomalous Pancreatobiliary Junction (APJ) is defined as a confluence of the common bile duct and the pancreatic duct outside the sphincter of Oddi, which allows mixing of pancreatic enzymes with bile; it is often associated with a choledochal cyst. It is considered an important contributing factor for development of choledocal cysts, cholangiocarcinoma and protein plugs. Common clinical manifestations of APJ anomalies are chronic abdominal pain, obstructive jaundice and/or recurrent pancreatitis. Endoscopic sphincterotomy is effective either as the definitive treatment or preoperative management of children with refractory pancreatitis.

Pancreas divisum

Pancreas divisum is considered the most common congenital anomaly of the pancreas. It occurs in approximately 6% of the general population. In most cases, it does not produce any symptoms. This malformation occurs due to lack of fusion between the ventral and dorsal embryologic part of the pancreas. The most reliable methods of diagnosis are ERCP or MRCP with secretin stimulation.

The main pancreatic duct appears short because it is not connected to the body of the pancreas. The Santorini duct drains the body and the tail of the pancreas. There is a complete form of the pancreas divisum (Figure 14.7) and an incomplete one (Figure 14.8), in which a partial communication between the ducts exists. Pancreatitis occurs when

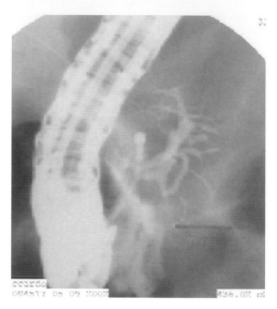

Figure 14.7 Complete pancreas divisum. A short main pancreatic duct that can only drain the pancreatic head.

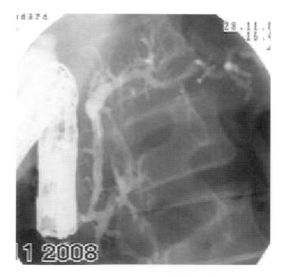

Figure 14.8 Incomplete pancreas divisum with dominant Santorini that appears dilated and tortuous in a 10-year-old girl with Crohn's disease and recurrent pancreatitis.

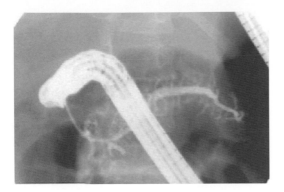

Figure 14.9 Duodenoscope is in a long position, which is often preferable for sphincterotomy of the minor duodenal papilla.

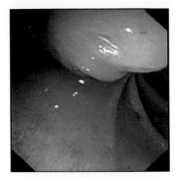

Figure 14.11 Endoscopic view of a duodenal duplication in a 2-year-old girl with recurrent acute pancreatitis. Major papilla in the center of the duplication.

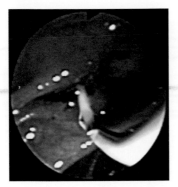

Figure 14.10 Pancreatic stent placed into the Santorini duct after successful sphincterotomy of minor duodenal papilla with complete resolution of chronic abdominal pain in patient with recurrent pancreatitis.

minor papilla become edematous or stenotic, preventing an adequate drainage of pancreatic fluid into the duodenum though the Santorini duct.

Therapeutic ERCP consists of ES of the minor and also major papilla (in the case of the incomplete form of pancreas divisum), allowing better pancreatic drainage (Figure 14.9). Temporary placement of a stent into the minor pancreatic duct may contribute to the resolution of abdominal pain in children with recurrent pancreatitis and pancreas divisum (Figure 14.10). One of the main concerns performing ES of the minor papilla is the length of the incision.

Two techniques of ES of the minor papilla are equally safe and effective: standard pull type of ES for patients with the naïve papilla or a needle-knife cut over existing plastic stent. The physician's choice of technique is based on his or her preference and specific endoscopic appearance of the papilla.

Duodenal duplications

A duodenal duplication cyst is a known but rare cause of recurrent acute pancreatitis. It represents 4–12% of all intestinal duplication. It is frequently located in the second portion of the duodenum. Duodenal duplications could be connected to or isolated from the biliary tree. Symptoms and signs are vomiting, chronic abdominal pain, and gastrointestinal bleeding due to ulceration of ectopic gastric mucosa.

Diagnosis of the duodenal duplication cyst is made by echo-tomography, MRCP and endoscopy (Figure 14.11). Treatment consists of surgical resection or endoscopic opening of the common wall (marsupialization into the duodenal lumen) (Figure 14.12) depending on the location of the duplication, its type, size and EUS findings (Figure 14.13).

EUS provides an essential information regarding relationship between duodenal duplication, CBD and pancreas. It helps with decision making for optimal treatment: surgery versus therapeutic endoscopy. Endoscopic therapy of duodenal duplication is summarized in Table 14.9.

Sphincter of Oddi dysfunction

Sphincter of Oddi dysfunction (SOD) is a rare cause of abdominal pain in children. It is related to an abnormal contractility of the sphincter without anatomic obstruction to bile flow or pancreatic fluid. SOD can manifest with chronic

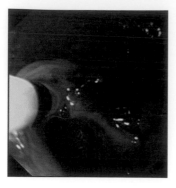

Figure 14.12 Complete dissection of the common wall complicated by bleeding, controlled with combination of 1:10000 epinephrine injection and coagulation.

Table 14.9 Steps of endoscopic marsupialisation of duodenal duplication

• Endoscopic visualization of cyst
• EUS: assessment of the common wall between the duplication cyst and the duodenum and involvement of the bile ducts
• ERCP: visualisation of the extrahepatic biliary tree
• Endoscopic dissection of duodenal duplication common wall with needle type or standard sphincterotome
• Haemostasis thorough verification.

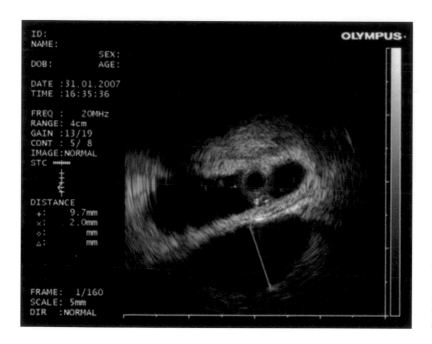

Figure 14.13
Endoscopic ultrasound, with 20 MhZ miniprobe in the duodenal lumen, shows the common wall (green markers) and the duplication.

abdominal pain and recurrent pancreatitis. The incidence of SOD in children is not established. In one study, SOD was diagnosed in 65 out of 245 paediatric patients who underwent ERCP. Dual sphincterotomy with pancreatic duct stent placement were recommended although the risk of postprocedure pancreatitis was significant. In such situations, the risks and benefits should be carefully weighed before intervention.

Chronic pancreatitis

There are three subgroups of chronic pancreatitis: chronic calcifying pancreatitis, chronic obstruc-

tive pancreatitis, and chronic inflammatory pancreatitis. A genetic testing (SPIN1 mutation) is essential for proper planning of the treatment and future prognosis. The current strategy consists of initial ERCP with pancreatic ES and pancreatic sludge or stone removal and stent placement with follow up sessions and stent replacements.

Pseudocyst and pancreatic trauma

Pseudocysts could be suspected on clinical grounds: persistent abdominal/epigastric pain, elevated pancreatic enzymes, or cholestasis due to distal CBD compression 3 to 6 weeks after an initial

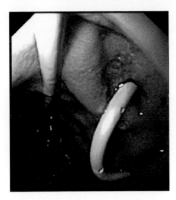

Figure 14.14 Post-traumatic pseudocysts in a 9-year-old boy treated with naso-pancreatic drainage and gastro-cystic double pig tail stent.

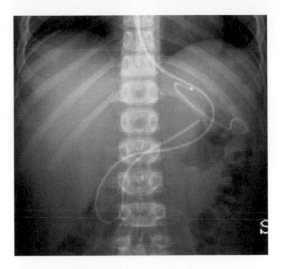

Figure 14.15 Radiogram of the pigtail stent and naso-pancreatic drainage tube.

attack of acute pancreatitis or trauma. Abdominal CT and MRCP are the best diagnostic options. Pseudocysts frequently resolve spontaneously.

Indications for intervention are trauma-related acute pancreatitis with increased risk of the main pancreatic duct disruption, presence of large, well organized pseudocysts 6 weeks since the onset of acute pancreatitis, and infected cysts.

The endoscopic approach for children with suspected pancreatic injury consists of ERCP and trans-ductal placement of a pancreatic stent over the guide wire, or transmural (usually trance gastric) passage of the guide wire followed by insertion of the pigtail drainage catheter into the cysts under EUS guidance to avoid accidental damage of the intramural vessels (Figures 14.14 & 14.15).

Steps of the EUS guided drainage technique of pancreatic pseudocysts are summarized in Table 14.10. The recurrence rate is about 15%. Surgery is indicated if pseudocysts persist.

EUS in pancreatitis

Multiple studies supported a high value of EUS as a source of valuable information contributing to the diagnosis and treatment of chronic pancreatitis, pancreatic pseudo-cysts, choledocholithiasis, pancreas divisum, and duodenal duplications. EUS improved the diagnostic and therapeutic outcome of ERCP in children with chronic and recurrent pancreatitis, and endoscopic treatment of pancreatic pseudo-cysts (EUS guided gastro-cystostomy) and duodenal duplication.

Table 14.10 Endoscopic steps of EUS guided drainage of pancreatic pseudocyst

- Endoscopic visualization and EUS confirmation*

- Diathermy needle puncture and section of the gastric wall toward the cyst's centre

- Opacification of cystic cavity

- Guidewire placement

- Hydrostatic balloon dilation of cystic opening

- Washing of cyst and removal of necrotic material

- Insertion of pigtail gastro-cystic stent or naso-gastro-cystic tube for drainage of cystic cavity

*according to our experience, radial mini probe is useful for marking the area for diathermy needle puncture of the gastric wall adjacent to the pseudo-cyst in small children or where small calibre linear EUS is not available.

Conclusion

ERCP is a very effective diagnostic and therapeutic procedure in children with pancreatobiliary disorders. It is safe in the hands of an experienced paediatric gastroenterologist. Therapeutic ERCP can be used as a definitive treatment for children with specific pancreatobiliary disorders and serves as a bridge therapy to surgery.

📖 FURTHER READING

Antaki F, Tringali A, Deprez P, *et al.* (2008) A case series of symptomatic intraluminal duodenal duplication cysts: presentation, endoscopic therapy, and long-term outcome. *Gastrointestinal Endoscopy*, Jan; **67(1)**, 163–168.

Attwell A, Borak G, Hawes R, *et al.* (2006) Endoscopic pancreatic sphincterotomy for pancreas divisum by using a needle-knife or standard pull-type technique: safety and reintervention rates. *Gastrointestinal Endoscopy*, **64(5)**, 705–711.

Barange K, Mas E, Railhac N, *et al.* (2009) Endoscopic management of biliary and pancreatic diseases in children. *Archives of Pediatrics* Jun; **16(6)**, 811–813.

Brown KO, Goldschmiedt M. (1994) Endoscopic therapy of biliary and pancreatic disorders in children. *Endoscopy*, **26**, 719–723.

Buscaglia JM, Kallo AN. (2007) Pancreatic sphincterotomy: technique, indications and complications. *World Journal of Gastroenterology*, **13(30)**, 4064–4071.

Canty TG Sr, Weinman D. (2001) Treatment of pancreatic duct disruption in children by endoscopically placed stent. *Journal of Pediatric Surgery*, **36**, 345–348.

Castagnetti M, Houben C, Patel S. (2006) Minimally invasive management of bile leaks after blunt liver trauma in children. *Journal of Pediatric Surgery*, **41**, 1539–1544.

Cheng CL, Fogel EL, Sherman S, *et al.* Diagnostic and therapeutic endoscopic retrograde cholangiopancreatography in children: a large series report. *Journal of Pediatric Gastroenterology & Nutrition*, **41**, 445–453.

Coehen S, Bacon BR, Berlin JA, *et al.* (2002) National Institutes of Health State-of-the-Science Conference Statement: ERCP for diagnosis and therapy. Jan 14–16, *Gastrointestinal Endoscopy*, **56**, 803–809.

Cohen S, Kalinin M, Yaron A, *et al.* (2008) Endoscopic ultrasonography in pediatric patients with gastrointestinal disorders. *Journal of Pediatric Gastroenterology & Nutrition*, May; **46(5)**, 551–554.

Consensus sulle patologie infiammatorie pancreatiche acute e croniche. Dicembre 2009 Area Qualità S.r.l.

Costamagna G, Shah SK, (2003) Tringali A. Current management of postoperative complications and benign biliary strictures. *Gastrointestinal Endoscopy Clinics of North America*, **13(4)**, 635–48).

Cotton PB, Laage NJ. (1982) Endoscopic retrograde cholangiopancreatography in children. *Archives of Disease in Childhood*, **57**, 131–136.

Etemad B, Whitcomb DC. (2001) Chronic pancreatitis: diagnosis, classification, and new genetic developments. *Gastroenterology*, **120(3)**, 682–707.

Guelrud M. (2001) Endoscopic retrograde cholangiopancreatography. *Gastrointestinal Endoscopy Clinics of North America*, **11**, 585–601.

Guerlud M, Jean D, Mendoza S, *et al.* (1991) ERCP in the diagnosis of extrahepatic biliary atresia. *Gastrointestinal Endoscopy*, **37**, 522–526.

Guerlund M. (1992) ERCP and endoscopic sphyncterotomy in infants and children with jaundice due to common bile ducts stones. *Gastrointestinal Endoscopy*, **38**, 450–453.

Hand BH. Anatomy and embriology of the biliary tract and pancreas. In: Sivak MV Jr, (ed), *Gastroenterologic endoscopy*, (2nd edn). 1995, pp. 862–77, WB Saunders, Philadelphia.

Holcomb GW III. Gallbladder disease. In: O'Neil JA Jr, Grosfeld JL, Fonkaslrud EW *et al*, (eds). *Principles of Pediatric Surgery*. 2003, pp. 645–646, Mosby Co, St Louis, Mo.

Issa H, Al Haddad A, Al Salem AH. (2007) Diagnostic and therapeutic ERCP in the pediatric age group. *Pediatric Surgery International*, **23**, 111–116.

Jang JY, Yoon CH, Kim KN. (2010) Endoscopic retrograde Cholangiopancreatography in pancreatic and biliary tract disease in Korean Children. *World Journal of Gastroenterology*, **16(4)**, 490–495.

Jeffrey GP. (1991) Histological and immunohistochemical study of the gallbladder lesion in primary sclerosing cholangitis. *Gut*, **32**, 424–429.

Keil R, Snajdauf J, *et al.* (2000) Endoscopic retrograde cholangiopancreatography in infants and children. *Indian Journal of Gastroenterology*, **19(4)**, 1757.

Lipsett PA, Segev DL, Colombani PM. (1997) Biliary atresia and biliary cyst. *Baillieres Clinical Gastroenterology*, **11**, 619–641.

Manfredi R, Lucidi V, Gui B, *et al.* (2002) Idiopathic chronic pancreatitis in children: MR cholangiopancreatography after secretin administration. *Radiology*, Sep; **224(3)**, 675–682.

Motte S. (1991) Risk factors for septicaemia following endoscopic biliary stenting. *Gastroenterology*, **101**, 1374–1381.

Mushin K. (2001) Balloon dilation compared to stenting of dominant strictures in primary sclerosing cholangitis. *The American Journal of Gastroenterology*, **96(4)**, 1059–1066.

Nathens AB, Curtis JR, Beale RJ, *et al.* (2004) Management of the critically ill patient with severe acute pancreatitis. *Critical Care Medicine*, **32(12)**, 2524–2536.

Newman KD, Powell DM, Holcom GW III. (1997) The management of cholidocholithiasis in children in era of laparoscopic cholecystectomy. *Journal of Pediatric Surgery*, **32**, 1116–1119.

Norton KI, Glass RB, Kogan D, *et al.* (2002) MR cholangiography in the evaluation of neonatal cholestasis: initial results. *Radiology*, **222**, 687–691.

Ostroff JW. (2001) Post transplant biliary problems. *Gastrointestinal Endoscopy Clinics of North America*, **11**, 163–183.

Perrelli L, Nanni L, Costamagna G, *et al.* (1996) Endoscopic treatment of chronic idiopathic pancreatitis in children. *Journal of Pediatric Surgery*, **31**, 1396–1400.

Pfau PR, Chelimsky GG, Kinnard MF, *et al.* (2002) Endoscopic Retrograde Cholangiopancreatography in children and adolescents. *Journal of Pediatric Gastroenterology Nutrition*, **35**, 619–623.

Rerknimitr R. (2002) Biliary tract complications after orthotopic liver transplantation with choledochocholedochostomy anastomosis: endoscopic findings and results of therapy. *Gastrointestinal Endoscopy*, **55**, 224–231.

Rocca R, Castellino F, Daperno M, *et al.* (2005) Therapeutic ERCP in pediatric patients. *Digestive Liver Disease*, **37**, 357–362.

Ryan WH, Raijman I, Finegold MJ. (2008) Diagnostic and therapeutic role of endoscopic retrograde cholangiopancreatography in biliary rhabdomiosarcoma. *World Journal of Gastroenterology*, **14(30)**, 4823–4825.

Saeky I, Takahashi Y, Matsuura T. (2009) Successful endoscopic unroofing for a pediatric choledochocele. *Journal of Pediatric Surgery*, **44**, 1643–1645.

Salemis NS, Liatsos C, Kolios M, *et al.* (2009) Recurrent acute pancreatitis secondary to a duodenal duplication cyst in an adult. A case report and literature review. *Canadian Journal of Gastroenterology*, **23(11)**, 749–752.

Saltzman JR. (2006) Endoscopic treatment of pancreas divisum: why, when, and how? *Gastrointestinal Endoscopy*, **64(5)**, 712–714.

Schaefer JF, Kirschner HJ, Lichy M, *et al.* (2006) Highly resolved free-breathing magnetic resonance cholangiopancreatography in the diagnostic workup of pancreaticobiliary diseases in infants and young children–initial experiences. *Journal of Pediatric Surgery*, **41(10)**, 1645–1651.

Screiber RA, Barker CC, Roberts EA. (2007) Biliary Atresia: The Canadian experience. *Journal of Pediatrics*, **151**, 659–665.

Shanmugam NP, Harrison PM, Devlin J, *et al.* (2009) Selective use of endoscopic retrograde cholangiopancreatography in the diagnosis of biliary atresia in infants younger than 100 days. *Journal of Pediatric Gastroenterology & Nutrition*, **49**, 435–441.

Sharma SS, Maharshi S. (2008) Endoscopic management of pancreatic pseudocyst in children; a long-term follow up. *Journal of Pediatric Surgery*, **43(9)**, 1636–1639.

Singham J, Yoshida EM, Scudamore C. (2010) Choledochal cysts. Part 3 of 3: Management. *Canadian Journal of Surgery*, **53(1)**, 51–56.

Suzuki M, Shimizu T, Kud T, *et al.* (2006) Non breath-hold MRCP in choledochal cyst in children. *Journal of Pediatric Gastroenterology & Nutrition*, **42**, 539–544.

Tagge EP, Hebra A, Goldberg A, *et al.* (1988) Pediatric laparoscopic biliary tract surgery. *Seminars in Pediatric Surgery*, **7**, 202–206.

Nose S, Hasegawa T, Soh H, *et al.* (2005) Laparoscopic cholecystocholangiography as an effective alternative exploratory laparotomy for differentiation of biliary atresia. *Surgery Today*, **35(11)**, 925–928.

Tarnasky PR, Palesch YY, Cunningham JT, *et al.* (1998) Minimally invasive therapy for choledocolithiasis in children. *Gastrointestinal Endoscopy*, **47**, 189–192.

Terui K, Hishiki T, Saito T, *et al.* (2010) Pancreas divisum in pancreaticobiliary malfunction in children. *Pediatric Surgery International*, **26(4)**, 419–422.

Terui K, Yoshida H, Kouchi K, *et al.* (2008) Endoscopic sphincterotomy is a useful preoperative management for refractory pancreatitis associated with pancreaticobiliary malfunction. *Journal of Pediatric Surgery*, **43**, 495–499.

Tipnis NA, Dua KS, Werlin SL. (2008) A retrospective assessment of magnetic resonance cholangiopancreatography in children. *Journal of Pediatric Gastroenterology & Nutrition*, **46**, 59–64.

Todani T, Watanabe Y, Narusue M, *et al.* (1977) Congenital bile duct cyst: classification, operative procedures and review of thirty-seven cases including cancer arising from choledocal cyst. *American Journal of Surgery*, **134,** 263–269.

Tröbs RB, Hemminghaus M, Cernaianu G, *et al.* (2009) Stone-containing periampullary duodenal duplication cyst with aberrant pancreatic duct. *Journal of Pediatric Surgery*, **44(1),** 33–35.

Varadarajulu S, Wilcox CM, Eloubeidi MA. (2005) Impact of EUS in the evaluation of pancreaticobiliary disorders in children. *Gastrointestinal Endoscopy*, **62(2),** 239–244.

Varadarajulu S, Wilcox CM, Hawes RH, *et al.* (2004) Technical outcomes and complications of ERCP in children. *Gastrointestinal Endoscopy*, **60,** 367–371.

Verting IL, Tabber MM, Taminiau JAJM, *et al.* (2009) Is endoscopic retrograde cholangiography valuable and safe in children all ages? *Journal of Pediatric Gastroenterology & Nutrition*, **48(1),** 66–71.

Waldhausen JHT. (2001) Routine intraoperative cholangiography during laparoscopic cholecistectomy minimized unnecessary endoscopic retrograde cholangiography in children. *Journal of Pediatric Surgery*, **36,** 881–884.

Waldhausen JHT, Benjamin DR. (1999) Cholecystectomy is becoming an increasingly common operation in children. *American Journal of Surgery*, **177,** 364–367.

Waters GS, Crist DW, Davoudi M, *et al.* (1996) Management of choledocholithiasis encountered during laparoscopic cholecystectomy. *American Journal of Surgery*, **62,** 256–258.

15

Endoscopic pancreatic cysto-gastrostomy

Mike Thomson

 KEY POINTS

- Endo-ultrasound is a useful adjunctive technique but is not mandatory.
- Initial incision preceded by sub-mucosal injection of epinephrine to prevent hemorrhage, occurs with an endo-knife.
- The incision can be enlarged with a sphincterotome.

- Pig-tailed or ERCP-type stents can be inserted.
- No adverse events have been encountered in the small pediatric series reported.
- Antibiotic prophylaxis may be required but this is not clear, and stents do not seem to need endoscopic removal as natural extrusion occurs.

Pancreatic pseudocysts are secondary to pancreatic damage, and maybe multi-etiological: traumatic; post-pancreatitis of idiopathic origin; following chemotherapy; or any other cause of acute pancreatitis. They should be differentiated from malignant cysts but this is unusual in childhood and is a distinction necessary predominantly in adult practice. Presentation may be with a persistently raised amylase, with chronic pain, as an abdominal mass, or with consistent nausea/vomiting. Treatment to date has either been conservative, surgical, with the use of (as yet unproven) anti-secretory agents such as octreotide or its longer-acting analogs (e.g. lanreotide), or via ERCP. More recently, trans-gastric cystostomies have been formed by endoscopy. These are either guided by endo-ultrasound which is a safer option avoiding gastric vessels (Figure 15.1), or blind with prior epinephrine injection into the bulge in the gastric wall from the luminal surface and then incision into the injected area. The former is preferable using linear endo-ultrasound ideally but radial endo-ultrasound may be sufficient at times, and

has been described in children. Indeed endosonography (EUS) has become the accepted procedure for drainage of pancreatic fluid collections over the past decade. EUS has been shown to be safe and effective and it has been the first-line therapy for uncomplicated pseudocysts. Where walled-off pancreatic necrosis was originally thought to be a contraindication for endoscopic treatment, multiple case series have now shown that these fluid collections can also be treated endoscopically with low morbidity and mortality. Usually the cyst can be indirectly identified abutting the lesser or greater curvature and is quite obvious as a mass effect into the gastric lumen. (Figure 15.2).

The initial incision may be made with an endo-knife (Figure 15.3), and once this is made, a sphincterotome may be inserted and employed to safely expand this incision. Subsequently, either straight ERCP plastic stents or pig-tailed stents can be inserted into the pseudocyst and left in situ. (Figure 15.4) Recently the temporary placement of self-expanding metal stents has been reported. Fluid will then follow the path of

Practical Pediatric Gastrointestinal Endoscopy, Second Edition. George Gershman, Mike Thomson, Marvin Ament.
© 2012 Blackwell Publishing Ltd. Published 2012 by Blackwell Publishing Ltd.

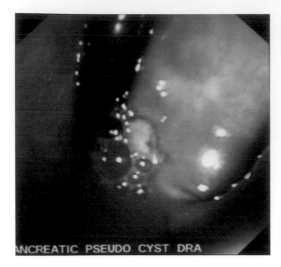

Figure 15.1 Trans-gastric endo-ultrasound of a pancreatic pseudocyst.

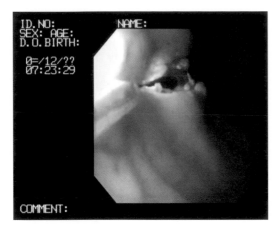

Figure 15.2 The indentation into the gastric wall can be seen easily identifying the position of the pseudocyst.

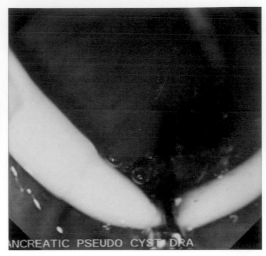

Figure 15.3 After endo-ultrasound has identified the cyst and a site which is free from gastric vessels, an endoknife or a sphincterotome (tapertome is best) is used to create a cauterised entry point from the stomach into the cyst. Adrenaline can be injected prior to the incision to further diminish the possibility of hemorrhage during incision.

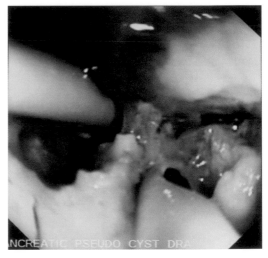

Figure 15.4 Grasping forceps are used to manipulate the stents (pig-tailed (blue) or straight (white)) through the gastro-cystostomy that was created.

least resistance and the presumed communication with the pancreatic duct will close preventing further accumulation of pancreatic fluid in the cyst. An endoscope may be inserted into the cyst, but this is not strictly necessary. (Figure 15.5) It is hoped that the gastric wall and the cyst will adhese and fibrose creating a channel so that, as the stents become unnecessary and as the cyst naturally deflates, the stents are extruded and the fistula closes. (Figure 15.6) This is the normal course of events. Patient symptom relief is acute and usually long-lasting. Complications are not common as long as gastric vessels are initially avoided. A combined approach involving drainage through the papilla and trans-mural endoscopic drainage can be useful in the larger and more loculated cysts.

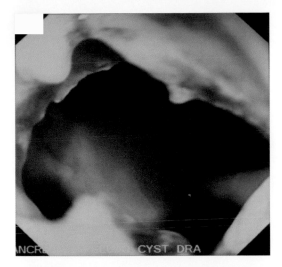

Figure 15.5 The stents are endoscopically observed in the pseudocyst.

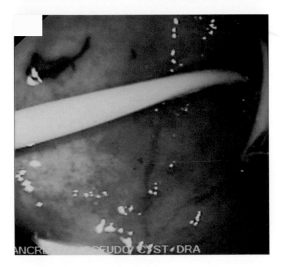

Figure 15.6 The endoscope is withdrawn from the stomach and the gastro-cystostomy is left in place.

 FURTHER READING

Al-Haddad M, El Hajj II, Eloubeidi MA. (2010) Endoscopic ultrasound for the evaluation of cystic lesions of the pancreas. *Journal of the Pancreas*, **11(4)**, 299–309.

Belle S, Collet P, Post S, *et al.* (2010) Temporary cystogastrostomy with self-expanding metallic stents for pancreatic necrosis. *Endoscopy*, **42(6)**, 493–495.

Bhasin DK, Rana SS. (2010) Combining transpapillary pancreatic duct stenting with endoscopic transmural drainage for pancreatic fluid collections: two heads are better than one! *Journal of Gastroenterology & Hepatology*, **25(3)**, 433–434.

Galasso D, Voermans RP, Fockens P. (2009) Role of endosonography in drainage of fluid collections and other NOTES procedures. *Best Practice & Research in Clinical Gastroenterology*, **23(5)**, 781–789.

Gumaste VV, Aron J. (2010) Pseudocyst management: endoscopic drainage and other emerging techniques. *Journal of Clinical Gastroenterology*, **44(5)**, 326–331.

Park DH, Lee SS, Moon SH, *et al.* (2009) Endoscopic ultrasound-guided versus conventional transmural drainage for pancreatic pseudocysts: a prospective randomized trial. *Endoscopy*, **41(10)**, 842–848.

Rossini CJ, Moriarty KP, Angelides AG. (2010) Hybrid notes: incisionless intragastric stapled cystogastrostomy of a pancreatic pseudocyst. *Journal of Pediatric Surgery*, **45(1)**, 80–83.

Theodoros D, Nikolaides P, Petousis G. (2010) Ultrasound-guided endoscopic transgastric drainage of a post-traumatic pancreatic pseudocyst in a child. *African Journal of Paediatric Surgery*, **7(3)**, 194–196.

16

Confocal laser endomicroscopy in the diagnosis of paediatric gastrointestinal disorders

Mike Thomson and Krishnappa Venkatesh

 KEY POINTS

- Confocal laser endo-microscopy (CLE) is feasible and safe in children as young as 18 months.
- Avoidance of biopsies in certain conditions such as graft-versus-host disease is desirable and CLE allows this.
- Targeting of biopsies is facilitated by CLE affording greater histological efficiency.
- Consequent cost savings on conventional histology are potentially large and a viable business case can be drawn around this

- premise for purchase and use of CLE in the pediatric setting.
- *In vivo* histology using CLE has revealed interesting new findings in situations such as celiac disease, which are lost in conventional histology due to fixing of tissue and associated artefact.
- CLE may prove particularly useful in situations such as the detection of polyp syndrome associated dysplasia.

Modern endoscopy has recently seen the development of technological advances with the aim of increasing and optimizing diagnostic yield from the procedure. These have included video and magnification endoscopes. Greater surface definition has been achieved with chromo-endoscopy, and recently, narrow-band imaging has allowed greater definition of vascular architecture. However, *in-vivo* sub-surface pathology remained obscure to the endoscopist until the advent of confocal endo-microscopy which affords magnification up to 1000×, and with sequentially deeper images from the epithelial surface to approximately 250 μm below the surface, producing histological

assessment of the *in-vivo* gastro-intestinal (GI) mucosal structure at the cellular and sub-cellular level. In addition, this technique avoids crush artefact from the grasp biopsy forceps and changes from histopathological processing.

The diagnosis of upper GI disorders in children depends, to a great extent, on endoscopy and subsequent histology of biopsy specimens. Pathologies such as: gastro-oesophageal reflux disease (GORD), eosinophilic oesophagitis (EO); *Helicobacter pylori* gastritis, and celiac disease (CD), in conjunction with various other investigative modalities have, as pivotal to their diagnosis, histological confirmation. Similarly, pediatric ileo-colonic conditions

---

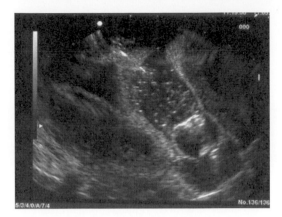

Figure 16.1 Confocal laser endomicroscopy.

such as inflammatory bowel disease (IBD), familial adenomatous polyposis (FAP), graft-versus-host disease (GVHD), and allergic colitis necessitate a tissue diagnosis.

CLE involves the use of a highly miniaturized confocal microscope which has been incorporated into the distal tip of a flexible endoscope to allow *in vivo* microscopic examination of the gut mucosa. The confocal microscope uses a single optical fiber to deliver 488 nm laser light to the distal tip of the endoscope where it is focused to a single diffraction limited point within the tissue. The laser light excites fluorescent molecules within the tissue. Fluorescent light emanating from the specific point of focus is collected into the same optical fiber of the confocal microscope and delivered to the photodetector. Light emanating from outside the focally illuminated spot is not focused into the optical fiber and, is therefore rejected from detection. The focused point of laser light is scanned in a raster pattern across the field of view, and the intensity of the fluorescent signal returning to the detector from successive points is measured (12-bit digitization) to produce two-dimensional images that are *en face* to the tissue surface. By moving the microscope optics within the confocal microscope, the operator can dynamically adjust the imaging depth to allow microscopic imaging at and below the surface of the mucosa; hence each image is an optical section representing one focal plane within the specimen, and collection of multiple optical sections at successive depths results in true volumetric sampling of the tissue. As a three-dimensional volume is thus sampled, this can be thought of as a "virtual biopsy".

The Pentax EC3870CILK endoscope (Figure 16.1) has a 5 mm diameter miniaturized confocal microscope integrated into the distal tip of the endoscope. The diameter of the distal tip and insertion tube of the endoscope is 12.8 mm. In addition to the integrated confocal microscope, the distal tip also contains a colour CCD camera which enables simultaneous confocal microscopy with standard video-endoscopy, air and water jet nozzles, two light guides, a 2.8 mm working channel and an auxiliary water jet channel. During CLE, the laser delivers an excitation wavelength of 488 nm at a maximum laser output of 1 mW to the tissue (typically 300–700 W). Confocal images can then be collected at either 1024×1024 pixels (0.8 frames/second) or 1024×512 pixels (1.6 frames second). The optical sections have a 475 m × 475 m field of view, with a lateral resolution of 0.7 m, axial resolution of 7.0 m, and the imaging depth (z axis) range of 0–250 m below the tissue surface in 4 m steps. The imaging depth below the tissue surface can be dynamically controlled by the operator. CLE magnifies images × 1000 fold and are visualized real-time on a monitor. A library of images is then collected and analyzed subsequently or contemporaneously.

Contrast agents

Fluorescein sodium (FS) 10% and acriflavine hydrochloride (AH) 0.05% are used as contrast agents. FS is highly water-soluble and, on intravenous administration, rapidly diffuses in seconds from the capillaries into the extra-vascular tissue. FS, when exposed to light of wavelength 465–490 nm (blue), emits light at longer wavelengths (520–650 nm, with the peak emission in the 520–530 nm green-yellow region). This enables visualization of micro-vessels, cells and connective tissue. However, FS is not enriched in the nuclei of intestinal epithelial cells and hence the nuclei are not readily visible in the confocal images. To circumvent this limitation, AF (0.05%) is used topically to enrich the superficial nuclei and to a lesser extent the cytoplasm.

To limit peristaltic artefacts, 10–20 mg Buscopan (hyoscine-N-butyl-bromide, Boehringer, Ingelheim, Germany) can be given intravenously. Following duodenal or ileal intubation, 0.05–0.1 ml/kg of 10% fluorescein sodium is administered intravenously and flushed adequately with normal saline. AF (0.05%) is applied to the mucosa using a spray catheter at all sites undergoing confocal imaging.

CLE image acquisition is performed by placing the tip of the colonoscope in direct contact with the target tissue site. Using gentle suction to stabilize the mucosa, image acquisition and focal plane z-axis scanning depth is actuated using two discrete hand-piece control buttons. Confocal images are sequentially obtained from third-part duodenum, gastric antrum and body, distal and proximal oesophagus in the upper GI tract, and ileum, cecum, ascending, transverse, descending, and sigmoid colon and rectum in the ileo-colon. Confocal images are acquired simultaneously with ongoing video endoscopic imaging. Same site mucosal specimens are obtained using standard biopsy forceps. The biopsy specimens are fixed in buffered formalin solution, embedded in paraffin wax, serial section obtained and stained with hematoxylin and eosin (H-E). The histologic specimens from each site are compared with same site confocal images jointly by the endoscopists and experienced pediatric and GI histopathologists, who are often in the endoscopy room. It is notable that the CLE images are cross-sectional in parallel with the mucosal surface, which is in contrast to standard histology in which a vertical section is made. Once this adjustment in perception is made by the observer, it is relatively easy to compare CLE images *in vivo* and post-fixed tissue sections by histology. Of course, no artefact due to fixing and staining occurs in the CLE images.

Recently in our centre, CLE occurred in 57 children intubating the duodenum at upper GI endoscopy, and the terminal ileum at ileo-colonoscopy. In all those in whom this occurred, the pylorus at upper GI CLE and the terminal ileum at lower GI CLE were intubated in all patients except one – the exception being a patient who weighed 10 kg and who was 8 months old in whom the pylorus and ileo-cecal valve were both too narrow to accept the confocal endomicroscope. The youngest and smallest patient to have full successful examinations up to third-part duodenum and terminal ileum was 18 months old and 11 kg. The procedure time for upper GI endoscopy ranged from 7–25 minutes (median 16.4 minutes), and for ileo-colonoscopy 15–45 minutes (median 27.9 minutes). A total of 132 pinch biopsies were taken from the upper GI tract from 33 procedures and 184 from the ileo-colon from 30 procedures i.e., not all patients had both upper and lower GI CLE.

No complications or adverse effects occurred except on one occasion when precipitation was observed in the peripheral venous line when fluorescein was injected immediately after neostigmine, but no patient morbidity occurred as the precipitant did not enter the patient.

Upper GI tract

In our unit, 33 patients underwent upper GI CLE, and duodenum was intubated in all but one. A total of 4 368 confocal images were obtained which included 1 835 from the duodenum, 1 451 from the stomach and 1 082 from the esophagus, which were compared with 44 biopsies from each site.

The esophagus is lined by non-keratinized squamous epithelium with polygonal epithelial cells. The nuclei of the epithelial cells are highlighted clearly following topical administration of acriflavine. Further, the capillary loops in the papillae are visible in deeper planes following subsurface optical sectioning, and surface to capillary distance can be measured as each level is deeper by 4 µm. This allows assessment of GORD-like histopathology given that papillary height is increased and epithelial surface to papillary tip (i.e. where capillary loops appear on confocal endomicroscopy) distance is thereby shorter. Recent *in-vivo* data indicate that the epithelium is thinner in GORD versus normal versus EoE and this is a very interesting phenomenon as it may allow real-time differentiation of esophageal pathologies.

The gastric pits or foveolae appear as invaginations on the surface epithelium. Each confocal image shows several evenly spaced such pits lined by columnar epithelium. The centers of the pits appear dark.

On confocal imaging, the duodenal villi have a long, slender and finger-like appearance similar to histologic specimens. The single layer of brush border columnar epithelial cells interspersed with intraepithelial lymphocytes and goblet cells is well-visualized. Crypts are not usually visible except in the presence of villous atrophy.

Celiac disease is particularly amenable to diagnosis by CLE. Comparative histological and CLE images are shown in Figure 16.2. On confocal imaging, in CD with subtotal villous atrophy (Marsh type 3a/b) (Figure 16.2A), the duodenal villi are broad with loss of the hexagonal pattern of the surface epithelium and a decrease in goblet

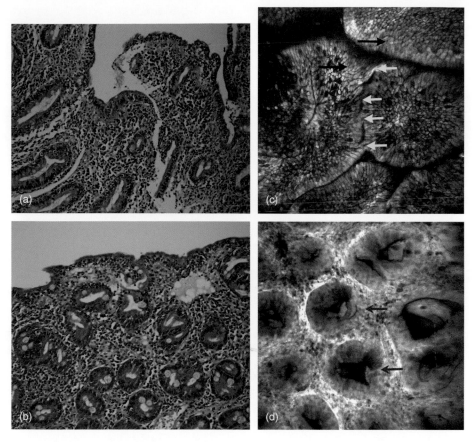

Figure 16.2 Comparison of confocal images with conventional histologic images in celiac disease. (a) Histologic image showing marked villous atrophy with increased intraepithelial lymphocytes and crypt hyperplasia. (b) Comparative confocal image. (c) Histologic image showing total villous atrophy of the duodenum. (d) Comparative confocal image.

cells. A characteristic feature observed was linking between adjacent villi giving an appearance of the villi being "sticky." (Figure 16.2B) Furthermore, the villi appear to be folded onto themselves. In contrast, in CD with total villous atrophy (Marsh type 3c on histology) (Figure 16.2C), on confocal imaging, villi are absent and crypts are visible with dense cellular infiltration in the surrounding stroma (Figure 16.2D) similar to histology.

Lower GI tract

The typical features of the colonic crypt pattern can be seen in Figure 16.3 with a polygonal appearance. Goblet cells show up as dark cells, whilst enterocytes are light grey.

Technological innovations have led to the development of chromo-endoscopy where dyes such as methylene blue and indigo carmine have been used to aid localization of lesions, and magnifying endoscopy has enabled visualization of surface structures at approximately ×100 fold magnification. In adults, several studies have validated these techniques in differentiating neoplastic from non-neoplastic lesions, diagnosis of neoplastic lesions in flat and depressed lesions in the colorectum, and in cancer surveillance in patients with long-standing ulcerative colitis. Differentiation of types of colitis is feasible although specificities such as presence of eosinophils are not observable. Typical features of ulcerative colitis are demonstrable, and CLE allows targeting of biopsy taking in order to allow such issues as dysplasia to be identified.

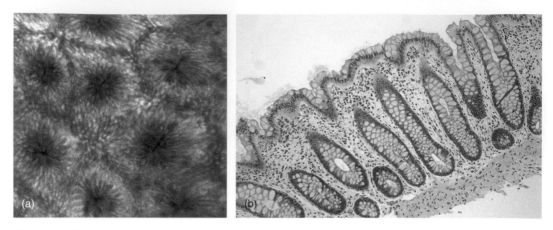

Figure 16.3 Comparison of confocal images with conventional histologic images of the lower GI tract. (a) Confocal image of normal colonic mucosa showing regularly spaced crypts with numerous goblet cells (arrow). (b) Comparative histologic image, note different plane.

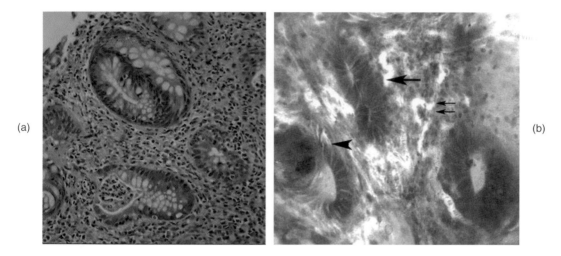

Figure 16.4 (a) Inflammatory bowel disease showing bifid crypt pattern, crypt distortion/destruction/abscess and cryptitis, goblet cell depletion, inflammatory cell infiltration prominence. (b) Comparative confocal image showing similar features plus tortuous vessel architecture suggesting inflammatory activity.

The following features are seen in inflammatory bowel disease on histology and on CLE (Figure 16.4).

1. Goblet cell depletion
2. Bifid crypt pattern
3. Crypt distortion
4. Crypt abscess/cryptitis
5. Crypt destruction
6. Tortuous vessels.

Granulomata cannot reliably be distinguished as yet in our experience, however ileal inflammatory features can be, and therefore distinction between UC and Crohn's disease is further aided. Other pathologies such as collagenous colitis are noted

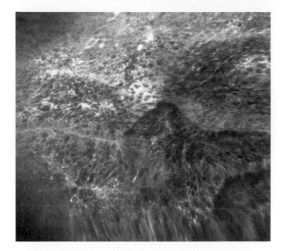

Figure 16.5 CLE of GVHD showing nuclear debris representing apoptotic bodies and obviating the need for taking of actual biopsies for histological confirmation.

easily with the typical increase in the thickness of the basement membrane. Graft- versus-host-disease (GVHD) may also be identified with nuclear debris representing apoptotic bodies in the rectal mucosa (Figure 16.5), and this would potentially negate the need for biopsy which, in immunocompromised children who may be at increased risk of mucosal infection and hemorrhage associated with biopsies being obtained, offers a cogent clinical benefit over standard endoscopy and biopsy.

Summary

The technology of CLE offers an insight into *in-vivo* histology and allows targeting of biopsies which not only allow more accurate diagnostics but may help in diminishing the number of biopsies and concurrent costs to an endoscopy service. Smaller endoscopes may be useful but we have shown this technology to be applicable practically in children as young as 18 months of age. The tantalising prospect of targeted biopsies or even a biopsy-free endoscopic procedure in the diagnosis of childhood GI disorders arises with obvious potential benefits in terms of avoidance of biopsy-associated complications, and diminution of the considerable histological burden that this patient cohort places on already over-stretched histopathological services with the prospect of considerable associated cost-savings.

FURTHER READING

Carvalho R, Hyams JS. (2007) Diagnosis and management of inflammatory bowel disease in children. *Seminars in Pediatric Surgery*, **16**, 164–171.

Delaney P & Harris M. (2006) Fiber-optics in scanning optical microscopy. In: Pawley JB, (ed) *Handbook of biological confocal microscopy* (3rd edn). pp. 501–515, New York Springer.

Fefferman DS, Farrell RJ. (2005) Endoscopy in inflammatory bowel disease: indications, surveillance, and use in clinical practice. *Clinical Gastroenterology & Hepatology*, **3**, 11–24.

Gono K, Obi T, Yamaguchi M, *et al.* (2004) Appearance of enhanced tissue features in narrow band endoscopic imaging. *Journal of Biomedical Optics*, **9**, 568–577.

Hoffman A, Goetz M, Vieth M, *et al.* (2006) Confocal laser endomicroscopy: technical status and current indications. *Endoscopy*, **38**, 1275–1283.

Jung M, Kiesslich R. (1999) Chromoendoscopy and intravital staining techniques. *Best Practice & Research in Clinical Gastroenterology*, **13**, 11–19.

Kiesslich R, Fritsch J, Holtman M, *et al.* (2003) Methylene blue-aided chromoendoscopy for the detection of intraepithelial neoplasia and colon cancer in ulcerative colitis. *Gastroenterology*, **124**, 880–888.

Kiesslich R, Burg J, Vieth M, *et al.* (2004) Confocal laser endoscopy for diagnosing intraepithelial neoplasias and colorectal cancer in vivo. *Gastroenterology*, **127**, 706–713.

Lipson BK and Yannuzzi L. (2006) Complications of intravenous fluorescein injections. *International Ophthalmology Clinics*, **29**, 200–205.

Polglase AL, McLaran WJ, Skinner SA, *et al.* (2005) A fluorescence confocal endomicroscope for in vivo microscopy of the upper- and the lower-GI tract. *Gastrointestinal Endoscopy Clinics of North America*, **62**, 686–695.

Thomson M, (2002) The pediatric esophagus comes of age. *Journal of Pediatric Gastroenterology & Nutrition*, **34(S1)**, 40–45.

Tung, SY, Wu CS, Su MY. (2001) Magnifying colonoscopy in differentiating neoplastic from non-neoplastic colorectal lesions. *American Journal of Gastroenterology*, **96**, 2628–2632.

Venkatesh K, Cohen M, Evans C, *et al.* (2009) Feasibility of confocal endomicroscopy in the diagnosis of paediatric gastrointestinal disorders. *World Journal of Gastroenterology*, **15(18),** 2214–2219.

Venkatesh K, Abou-Taleb A, Cohen M, *et al.* (2010) Role of confocal endomicroscopy in the diagnosis of celiac disease. *Journal of Pediatric Gastroenterology & Nutrition*, 2010; **51,** 274–279.

17

Enteroscopy

Mike Thomson

KEY POINTS

- The techniques of Sonde or push enteroscopy have now been superseded.
- Enteroscopy complements wireless capsule endoscopy and both should be available in any unit with pretensions towards becoming a small bowel investigation center.
- Single-balloon enteroscopy does not allow the operator to advance as far beyond the pylorus or in the retrograde manoeuver proximal to the ileo-cecal valve as double-balloon enteroscopy (DBE).
- DBE is the procedure of choice, is safe with CO_2 insufflation and has occurred many times in children to date with no adverse events reported, and allows endo-therapeutic procedures of any nature to occur throughout the small bowel.

- Tattooing lesions, or tattooing the most distal part of the small bowel reached in an antegrade fashion, allows subsequent identification of the lesion by a surgeon at laparoscopy, or identification of full small bowel visualization when the retrograde trans-anal procedure is performed, respectively.
- Spiral enteroscopy is an emerging technology that may be helpful in enteroscopy up to 150 cm beyond the pylorus and has the advantage of allowing the operator a static platform in the small bowel from which to perform endo-therapeutic procedures.

Introduction

The advent of flexible fiberoptic endoscopes transformed the diagnosis and management of gastrointestinal disorders in adults and children, allowing direct visualization with targeted mucosal biopsies. Furthermore endo-therapeutic procedures have now been possible throughout the upper GI tract and ileo-colon. However the small bowel, distal to the ligament of Trietz and proximal to the terminal ileum, has been to date inaccessible to conventional GI endoscopes.

The Sonde type enteroscope, developed in the 1970s, involved the introduction of a long thin fiberoscope with an inflatable balloon attached to its distal tip, through the nose into the stomach.

The fiberoscope was guided into the duodenum by a gastroscope and the balloon attached to the tip of the fiberoscope was inflated. Normal peristalsis ensured the movement of the fiberoscope down the small bowel and theoretical visualization of the entire small bowel. However, the procedure itself was cumbersome and limited by lack of therapeutic potential.

Push enteroscopy, introduced in the 1990s, allowed access of the proximal small bowel beyond the ligament of Trietz. This was improvised by the addition of a semi-rigid overtube which made it possible to reach up to 70–100 cm of small bowel beyond the pylorus. In addition to diagnosis, endotherapy became achievable with push enteroscopy, although limited to the jejunum. The indications in adults for push enteroscopy included overt and occult GI bleeding, iron deficiency anemia abdominal pain, Crohn's disease, PEJ placement and ERCP (Billroth type II). Push enteroscopy has been evaluated extensively in adults with a diagnostic yield ranging from 41–75%. There is one report of its use in children.

Nevertheless, the diagnosis of small bowel disease beyond the proximal jejunum still remained a challenge, never mind proximal to the distal ileum. Intra-operative enteroscopy technique was developed needing an operative colotomy or enterotomy through which the endoscope was passed to visualize the small bowel. This had a very good diagnostic yield but carried a high complication rat. This technique was further refined by performing an initial upper GI endoscopy, and a subsequent colonoscopy was performed and the surgeon manually threaded the small bowel over the tip of the endoscope thus avoiding an enterotomy, in subsequent years with the advent of laparoscopic assistance. Intra-operative laparoscopy-assisted push enteroscopy offers advantage in that the whole of the small bowel may be examined endo-luminally. However, of course, this involves handling of the bowel, and the need for both a surgeon and an endoscopist.

Wireless capsule endoscopy (WCE) was the next major advance in the diagnostic assessment of the mid-small bowel. WCE made it possible to visualize the entire small bowel. The main advantage has been the relative non-invasiveness of this procedure with good diagnostic yield. WCE has been found to be superior to push enteroscopy in the diagnosis of obscure GI bleeding in adults. However, the major limitations of WCE has been the inability to perform air insufflations, rinsing of tissue, taking biopsies or undertaking endotherapeutic procedures – and thus the major utility is limited to diagnostic input alone, at least so far. Complications although rare, exist and are mainly in the form of capsule retention that requires surgical intervention – however, the need for removal is extraordinarily rare.

In 2001, Yamamoto *et al* reported a new method where two balloons were used, one at the tip and the other at the distal end of an overtube, to perform total enteroscopy without the need for laparotomy. Double-balloon enteroscopy (DBE) was thus born. DBE enables high-resolution endoscopic imaging of the entire small bowel, with the advantage over WCE of potential for mucosal biopsies and interventional endo-therapy (e.g. non-variceal hemostasis, snare polypectomy and pneumatic balloon stricture dilatation).

DBE technique

The pediatric double-balloon enteroscopy system (Fujinon; Fujinon Inc., Japan) (Figure 17.1) consists of a high-resolution video enteroscope (EN-450P5/20) with a flexible overtube (TS-12140). The video enteroscope has a working length of 200 cm and an outer diameter of 8.5 mm while the flexible overtube has a length of 140 cm and outer diameter of 12 mm. The enteroscopes either have a 2.2 mm ("P" scope) or a 2.8 mm ("T" scope) forceps channel that enables routine biopsy, and the latter allows other common therapeutic interventions. The enteroscope, as well as the overtube, are fitted with a balloon each at the tip. The overtube and balloons are disposable. The balloons can be inflated and deflated with air from a pressure-controlled pump system with maximum inflatable pressure of 60 mmHg. Since the inflation of balloons is pressure-controlled they can be used safely, regardless of the diameter of the small bowel. The balloons help to anchor the scope and/or the overtube and stabilize the intestinal wall. This enables the further advance of the scope. The overtube prevents bending or looping of the intestine.

Both balloons are deflated at the start of the procedure. On reaching the distal duodenum or preferably jejunum the overtube balloon is inflated to fix and stabilize the overtube within the lumen. Subsequently, the enteroscope is advanced as far as possible. Then the enteroscope tip balloon is inflated and the overtube balloon is deflated. The overtube is now advanced to reach the

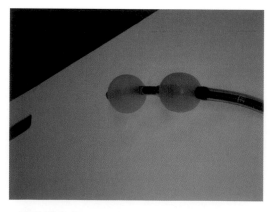

Figure 17.1 Double-balloon enteroscope system configuration.

enteroscope tip. The overtube is again inflated and both enteroscope and overtube are gently withdrawn together in order to "concertina" the small bowel over both. The whole procedure is repeated and each set of maneuvers (or "passes") can allow up to 40–60 cm of small bowel to be examined, until the terminal ileum (TI) is reached (Figure 17.2). If the TI is not reached then the most distal region reached is "tattooed" in the sub-mucosal plane with an endo-needle, using a bleb of normal saline then injected with methylene blue or indigo carmine (Figure 17.3). Alternatively 1 in 10 dyes in saline can be injected directly into the bowel wall, but there is a theoretical risk of intra-peritoneal leak with this one step technique. An approximate distance of post-pylorus small bowel negotiation can be calculated if one assumes that 5 cm of overtube insertion equates to approximately 40 cm of small bowel. The DBE can then be repeated via the trans-anal route and retrograde movement

from the TI proximally up the ileum allowing full examination of the whole small bowel. Colon negotiation can be facilitated with the overtube balloon in the colon itself. (Figure 17.4) Simultaneous fluoroscopy has not been found to allow further advancement of the DBE in recent studies.

On withdrawal in either procedure close examination of the mucosal surface occurs as with standard endoscopy, but lesions are dealt with as soon as they are found, whether this is on intubation or withdrawal. Bowel preparation is as for standard ileo-colonoscopy. The procedure is carried out under general anesthetic in children.

As noted above, there are two other Fujinon double-balloon enteroscopes used in adults, the EN450T5 with a diameter of 9.4 mm and an larger accessory channel of 2.8 mm allowing for the therapeutic enteroscopy and EN450B15 with a working

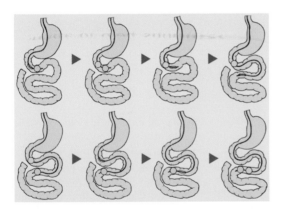

Figure 17.2 DBE technique.

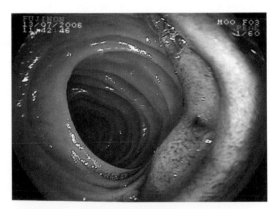

Figure 17.3 Double-balloon tattoo.

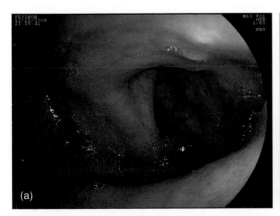

(a)

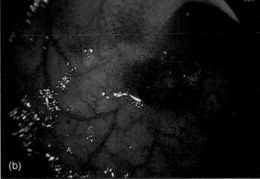

(b)

Figure 17.4 Polyp detected (a) and removed (b).

length of 152 cm useful in difficult colonoscopies and endoscopic retrograde cholangiography in patients with Roux-en-Y anastomosis. It is these scopes that allow endo-therapy as opposed to the smaller pediatric endo-diagnostic scope which we previously reserved for children under 3 years or 15 kg in weight. However, as experience has been gained it is clear that the more flexible smaller enteroscope has a greater chance of full small bowel examination than the stiffer "adult" enteroscope. We have attained full small bowel examination with the smaller scope. A newer smaller diameter enteroscope with a larger 2.8 mm working channel allowing more therapeutic procedures has been produced and is promising.

Indications for DBE

Obscure GI bleeding, polyps, and evaluation of Crohn's disease are by far the commonest indications for DBE in adult. DBE is also useful in the assessment of polyposis syndromes, ERCP in patients with Roux-en-Y anastomosis and suspected small intestinal tumors. A post-liver transplant child has benefited from DBE to identify and treat a bilio-enteric anastomotic stricture. DBE finds applications in the further evaluation of abnormal findings following WCE. Therapeutic roles include hemostasis, polypectomy, balloon dilation of strictures, and retrieval of foreign bodies. A summary of indications is listed in Table 17.1.

Pediatric experience

There are, to date, three papers including one from our center, in the pediatric literature reporting the use of DBE, all of them published in the last year.

Nishimura *et al* performed 92 procedures in 48 patients using four different double-balloon enteroscopes including a prototype. The mean duration of procedures was 96 minutes (range 30–220 minutes). The most common indication was stricture of biliary anastomosis following living donor liver transplantation (23 patients). Other indications included obscure GI bleeding (10 patients), surveillance and treatment of hereditary polyposis syndromes (5 patients), abdominal pain (4 patients), and inflammatory bowel disease

Table 17.1

Diagnostic	Therapeutic
Obscure GI bleeding	Haemostasis
evaluation of celiac disease	Polypectomy
malabsorption	Treatment of stenoses
Crohns disease	Retrieval of foreign bodies
Hereditary polyposis syndromes	ERCP in patients with Billroth type II stomach or Roux-en Y anastamosis
ERCP in patients with altered surgical anatomy	Gastrostomy placement in abnormal bowel anatomy
Suspected tumors	Treatment of early postoperative small-bowel obstruction

(2 patients). The overall diagnostic yield was 65%. Therapeutic interventions were performed in 40% of patients including balloon dilatation, biliary stenting, or removal of stones in 13 patients, polypectomy in 5 patients and argon plasma coagulation in 1 patient. Complications reported included self-limiting abdominal pain in 10 patients, mucosal injury of the small bowel in 1 patients and post-polypectomy bleeding in 1 patient.

Liu *et al* reported a retrospective case series of 31 patients. Oral approach was used in 18 patients and anal approach in 11 patients. Two patients underwent both oral and anal approaches and the entire small bowel was visualized. The procedure time ranged from 40 to 70 minutes. Twenty-seven patients of these were investigated for obscure GI bleeding. A source for the bleeding was found in 21 patients giving a diagnostic yield of 77%. Angiomata and Crohn's disease were the most common causes for bleeding. Four patients were investigated for chronic diarrhea; two were found to have lymphangiectasia, and one each had a diagnosis of IBD and celiac disease. The overall diagnostic yield was 80%.

In our own experience, initial description $n = 14$ (now $n = 40$), we have examined 40 patients, 8 for Peutz-Jeghers syndrome, 24 for obscure or occult GI bleeding, 2 for recurrent abdominal pain, 1 patient with Cowden's syndrome and persistent GI bleeding, and 5 for suspected but unproven (by conventional endoscopy) Crohn's disease. The median time was 118 minutes (range 95–195 minutes) for the whole procedure. The entire small bowel was examined in 6 patients and a length of 200–320 cm distal to pylorus in the remaining. Sixteen patients only had an oral approach; the remainder had oral and anal approaches. Polyps were detected and successfully removed (Figure 17.4a and b) in all 8 patients with PJ syndrome, in one patient with tubule-villous adenoma of the duodenum, in one patient with significant anemia and occult bleeding, and in a patient with Cowden's syndrome. A diagnosis was made in a patient with multiple angiomata (Figure 17.5) not amenable to endotherapy, and in one with a discrete angioma which was treated with argon plasma coagulation. The source of bleeding was identified in a further patient with varices. DBE was normal or revealed minor mucosal friability in the remaining patients. Hence, a diagnostic yield in the majority with therapeutic success in all but one in whom lesions requiring intervention was achieved. Incidentally, a Meckel's diverticulum was found (Figure 17.6) in one patient. Two patients with blue rubber bleb nevus syndrome had successful ablation of the lesions with argon plasma coagulation with no complications. (Figures 17.7a and 17.7b) No complications were encountered. All patients underwent general anesthesia and were allowed home on the same day. Part of the ability to perform

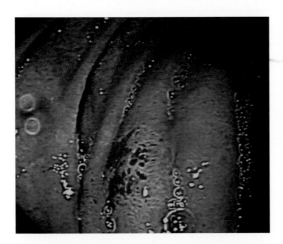

Figure 17.5 Multiple angiomas in small bowel.

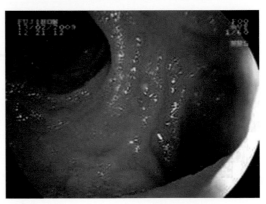

Figure 17.6 Meckel's diverticulum.

(a)

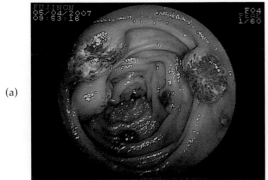

(b)

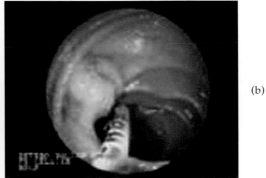

Figure 17.7 (a) Blue rubber bleb nevus syndrome lesions. (b) Blue rubber bleb nevus syndrome lesions after argon plasma coagulation

the procedure as a day case was allowed by the use of carbon dioxide insufflation – a much more rapid absorption led to a greater depth of intubation as the peritoneal cavity was thus less encumbered by gas-filled small bowel loops preventing advancement, and once woken the patients experienced minimal or no abdominal distension related pain. Interestingly the end expired CO_2 recorded during anesthesia rose, but not to any level that was considered compromising, nor higher than observed during CO_2-assisted laparoscopy. ERCP via a balloon enteroscope is now well-established in adult endoscopy, and is particularly useful when a Roux-en-Y loop is present.

Complications

From the three pediatric case series reported involving 107 children undergoing 186 procedures when oral and anal approaches are included, no major complications have been reported. Minor complications included abdominal pain, sore throat, minor aspiration, and bleeding following polypectomy. The lack of any significant complications reported reflects the small number of patients involved and the different indications for DBE in comparison to adults. In the adult literature, acute pancreatitis, perforation, and bleeding are known significant complications. Minor complications include pain, fever, vomiting. Single case reports of intraperitoneal bleeding and paralytic ileus have also been reported.

Several mechanisms have been proposed for the occurrence of acute pancreatitis. These include sphincter injury from direct compression by the balloons, duodenal pancreatic reflex, and direct pancreatic injury secondary to endoscopic compression of the pancreas against spine.

In one large international survey, 40 complications occurred from 2362 procedures (1.7%). The incidences of acute pancreatitis and perforations were similar at 0.3% each. Twelve bleeding complications were reported from 364 polypectomies, none of which were a major bleed. In another large pooled data from the German national register involving 3894 procedures, a complication rate of 1.2% was reported. Rates of acute pancreatitis were similar while perforations were higher at 3.4%. There were also six major bleeding episodes. Similar complication rates were reported in data from 9 US centers.

Training issues and learning curve

In view of the small number of cases requiring DBE in children, training remains an issue. In adults a step-by-step approach has been found to be useful. The first step is to be familiar with the pathological conditions in the small gut as well as the technique of DBE. The second step involves observation of live procedures in patients conducted by experienced endoscopists as well as hands on training using a fresh *ex vivo* model. Finally a one-to-one training with an experienced DBE endoscopist. Mehdizadeh *et al* found a significant decrease in the overall procedural time after the initial 10 DBE cases in a study involving 188 patients and 237 DBE procedures from 6 US centers. The mean duration decreased from 109 minutes for the first 10 cases to 92 minutes for subsequent cases. A close coordination with the adult GI units performing DBE may be beneficial. Further, with the low-case volume requiring DBE in children, it may be practicable and cost-effective to limit the use of DBE to specialized pediatric GI endoscopic units.

Single balloon enteroscopy

Using an Olympus platform and standard push enteroscope or pediatric-size colonoscope, this technique has its followers. (Figure 17.8) It has the advantage of a lack of requirement for a totally new endoscopic system, but suffers from certain

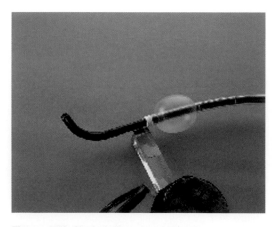

Figure 17.8 Single-balloon enteroscopy.

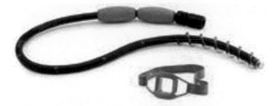

Figure 17.9 Spiral enteroscopy outside the patient.

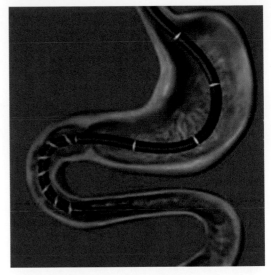

Figure 17.10 Spiral enteroscope advancing intra-luminally.

disadvantages that preclude deep small bowel intubation – this is identifed by most users. Hence, it is useful for proximal small bowel lesions, but rarely is full small bowel traverse observed or acquired. As there is only one balloon it relies (during the withdrawal to concertina the bowel over the scope, once the balloon has been deflated to facilitate this part of the enteroscopy) on the operator trying to hook the tip of the scope over one of the valvulae coneventes in the small bowel. However, inevitably during the withdrawal part of the procedure there is retrograde slippage, and a seesaw motion occurs during intubation and withdrawal, after only a few "passes". For deep small bowel intubation it is therefore **not** the procedure of choice, although it seems to be safe. Only one small series of seven patients exists in the pediatric literature to date. It has been used successfully in case reports in children, for example, for the treatment of small bowel varices with a child having a hepatico-jejunostomy.

Spiral enteroscopy

This is an exciting recent development as it exists due to the application of novel thinking to an enduring problem, that is, how to insert a flexible tube through a flexible tube. Then, instead of pushing this principle surrounds the screw and advance concept thus pulling the enteroscope through the small bowel. A mathematical relationship exists between the rotational force/movement, the acuteness of the spiral, and the resultant forward progression of the tip of the scope. A disposable overtube with an outer spiral is placed trans-orally over an endoscope (Figure 17.9) – typically, a Fujinon enteroscope at present – and after the pylorus is negotiated the operator simply rotates the handles of the overtube which remain outside the patient in a clockwise direction to produce forwards movement. (Figure 17.10) Remarkable forward movement with simultaneous "concertina"-ing of the small bowel over the

instrument occurs. When this motion is stopped, then stable non-movement of the tip of the scope can be observed. Simple reversal (counterclockwise) results in removal of the tip of the scope through the small bowel. With this degree of control lesions can be targeted accurately for endo-therapy without the distraction of intestinal peristalsis to inadvertently prevent accurate endo-therapy. Recent large adult studies are published, although some groups identify that the diagnostic yield may be less than that of DBE, although insertion depth seems to be greater than SBE.

Intraoperative or laparoscopy-assisted enteroscopy

It has to be said that this is an inferior technique to non-operative enteroscopy, Intraoperative or laparoscope-assisted enteroscopy starts with conventional enteroscopic jejunal intubation followed by surgical assistance. The endoscopist's role is relatively passive, deflecting the tip of the instrument while the surgeon, either with hands or laparoscopic instruments, concertinas examined parts of the small bowel over the enteroscope. Both the mucosal and serosal surfaces can be examined. Very little air is insufflated into the bowel to avoid hindering the surgeon. Dimmed lights in the operating field also help to identify the position of the tip of the instrument. In experienced hands, all the small bowel is examined in 60% of cases, taking up to 2 to 3 hours (Figure 17.11). An enterotomy may

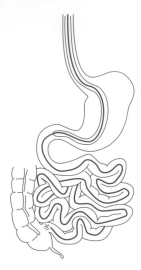

Figure 17.11 Extent of laparoscopic-assisted enteroscopy.

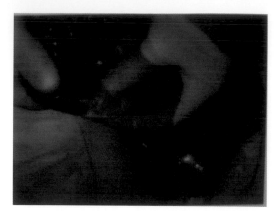

Figure 17.12 Intra-operative enteroscopy and trans-illumination of a discrete area of intestinal lymphangiectasia.

be used to insert a sterilized enteroscope in some situations. Lesions can be marked by injection of ink or placement of a suture. Intraoperative or laparoscopy-assisted enteroscopy is the most successful technique for identifying sites of obscure gastrointestinal bleeding with diagnostic yields of between 83 and 100%. Laser or bipolar coagulation can be used, and resection of lesions is recommended if intraoperative. This technique has demonstrable advantages in the assessment of the extent of polyposis syndromes. "On-table" enteroscopy has a better pick-up rate for polyps at laparotomy than external transillumination and palpation. It can be helpful to view both serosal and mucosal surfaces simultaneously, especially with trans-illumination, when trying to identify small isolated lesions such as isolated pockets of intestinal lymphangiectasia. (Figure 17.12) When attempted in Crohn's disease, up to 65% of patients have had lesions not previously identified in the small bowel by other investigations, including direct vision of the serosal surface of the bowel. As previously mentioned, occult Crohn's disease can be identified in children using enteroscopy. Partial intestinal obstruction and Meckel's diverticulum have also been identified at intraoperative enteroscopy. Small bowel neoplasia must not be forgotten as the second most common cause of obscure gastrointestinal bleeding in younger patients, accounting for 5 to 10% of cases in young adults. Exploratory laparoscopy and enteroscopy are important in preventing missed diagnoses. In essence intra-operative enteroscopy is likely to give way to DBE in the very near future.

Complications

Complications are not often encountered with simple push enteroscopy, but when the overtube is employed, significant patient discomfort has been described. Other, rare complications of the overtube include pharyngeal tear, Mallory-Weiss tear, gastric mucosal stripping, pancreatitis, and duodenal perforation. DBE may be associated with pancreatitis in some cases especially if the overtube balloon is first inflated too proximally, i.e. this needs to occur past the ligament of Treitz. Intraoperative enteroscopy has a 5% incidence of perforation and, in one series, a 50% incidence of mucosal laceration. Prolonged ileus has been occasionally described. None of these rare complications have been reported in the limited studies investigating children.

Conclusion

Flexible GI endoscopy is sufficient for diagnostic and therapeutic procedures in the vast majority of pediatric cases, and in adult patients with obscure gastrointestinal bleeding is known to determine the source in up to 90% of cases. However, in the small number of cases when the pathology is confined to the small bowel beyond the reach of conventional endoscopy, WCE and DBE have a role. DBE allows examination of the entire small bowel making it possible to diagnose small bowel Crohn's disease, obscure GI bleeding and tumors otherwise not attainable by conventional GI endoscopy and also to perform endotherapeutic procedures such as hemostasis, polypectomy, balloon dilatation of strictures, and retrieval of foreign bodies. DBE has a high diagnostic and therapeutic yield and has a low-risk of complications in 1–2% of cases. DBE is feasible and safe in children.

📖 FURTHER READING

Apelgren KN, Vargish T, Al-Kawas F. (1988) Principles for use of intraoperative enteroscopy for hemorrhage from the small bowel. *American Journal of Surgery*, **54,** 85–88.

Appleyard M, Fireman Z, Glukhovsky A, *et al.* (2000) A randomized trial comparing wireless capsule endoscopy with push enteroscopy for the detection of small-bowel lesions. *Gastroenterology*, **119,** 1431–1438.

Attar A, Maissiat E, Sebbagh V, *et al.* (2005) First case of paralytic intestinal ileus after double balloon enteroscopy. *Gut*, **54,** 1823–1824.

Barkin J, Lewis B, Reiner D, *et al.* (1996) Diagnostic and therapeutic jejunoscopy with a new, longer enteroscope. *Gastrointestinal Endoscopy*, **38,** 55–58.

Barth BA, Channabasappa N. (2010) Single-balloon enteroscopy in children: initial experience at a pediatric center. *Journal of Pediatric Gastroenterol ogy & Nutrition*, **51(5),** 680–684.

Bowden TA, Jr, Hooks VH, IIIrd, Teeslink CR, *et al.* (1980) Occult gastrointestinal bleeding: locating the cause. *American Journal of Surgery*, **46,** 80–87.

Chak A, Koehler MK, Sundaram SN, *et al.* (1998) Diagnostic and therapeutic impact of push enteroscopy: analysis of factors associated with positive findings. *Gastrointestinal Endoscopy*, **47,** 18–22.

Cheng DW, Han NJ, Mehdizadeh S, *et al.* Intraperitoneal bleeding after oral double-balloon enteroscopy: a case report and review of the literature. *Gastrointestinal Endoscopy*, **66,** 627–629.

Chong J, Tagle M, Barkin J, *et al.* (1994) Small bowel push-type fiberoptic enteroscopy for patients with occult gastrointestinal bleeding or suspected small bowel pathology. *American Journal of Gastroenterology*, **89,** 2143–2146.

Curcio G, Sciveres M, Mocciaro F, *et al.* (2010) Out-of-reach obscure bleeding: Single-balloon enteroscopy to diagnose and treat varices in hepaticojejunostomy after pediatric liver transplant. *Pediatric Transplantation*. doi: 10.1111/j.1399-3046.2010.01425.x

Darbari A, Kalloo AN, Cuffari C. (2006) Diagnostic yield, safety, and efficacy of push enteroscopy in pediatrics. *Gastrointestinal Endoscopy*, **64,** 224–228.

Di Caro S, May A, Heine DGN, *et al.* (2005) The European experience with double-balloon enteroscopy: indications, methodology, safety, and clinical impact. *Gastrointestinal Endoscopy*, **62,** 545–550.

Douard R, Wind P, Panis Y, *et al.* (2000) Intraoperative enteroscopy for diagnosis and management of unexplained gastrointestinal bleeding. *American Journal of Surgery*, **180,** 181–184.

Duggan C, Shamberger R, Antonioli D, *et al.* (1995) Intraoperative enteroscopy in the diagnosis of partial intestinal enteroscopy in infancy. *Digestive Diseases & Sciences*, **40,** 236–238.

Frieling T, Heise J, Sassenrath W, *et al.* (2010) Prospective comparison between double-balloon enteroscopy and spiral enteroscopy. *Endoscopy*, **42(11),** 885–888.

Foutch PG, Sawyer R, Sanowski RA. (1990) Push-enteroscopy for diagnosis of patients with gastrointestinal bleeding of obscure origin. *Gastrointestinal Endoscopy*, **36,** 337–341.

Gerson LB, Flodin JT, Miyabayashi K. (2008) Balloon-assisted enteroscopy: technology and troubleshooting. *Gastrointestinal Endoscopy*, **68,** 1158–1167.

Gerson LB, Tokar J, Chiorean M, *et al.* (2009) Complications associated with double balloon enteroscopy at nine US centers. *Clinical Gastroenterology & Hepatology*, **7,** 1177–1182, 1182, e1171–e1173.

Gong F, Swain P, Mills T. (2000) Wireless endoscopy. *Gastrointestinal Endoscopy*, **51,** 725–729.

Heine GD, Hadithi M, Groenen MJ, *et al.* (2006) Double-balloon enteroscopy: indications, diagnostic yield, and complications in a series of 275 patients with suspected small-bowel disease. *Endoscopy*, **38,** 42–48.

Hopkins H, Kapany YS. (1954). A flexible fiberoscope using static scanning. *Nature*, **173,** 39.

Hyer W, Neale K, Fell J, *et al.* (2000) At what age should routine screening start in children at risk of familial adenomatous polyposis? *Journal of Pediatric Gastroenterology & Nutrition*, **405**, 417.

Khashab MA, Lennon AM, Dunbar KB, *et al.* (2010) A comparative evaluation of single-balloon enteroscopy and spiral enteroscopy for patients with mid-gut disorders. *Gastrointestinal Endoscopy*, **72(4)**, 766–772.

Landi B, Cellier C, Fayemendy L, *et al.* (1996) Duodenal perforation occurring during push enteroscopy. *Gastrointestinal Endoscopy*, **43**, 631.

Lau WY. (1990) Intraoperative enteroscopy – indications and limitations. *Gastrointestinal Endoscopy*, **36**, 268–271.

Lewis B, Kornbluth A, Waye J. (1991) Small bowel tumors: the yield of enteroscopy. *Gut*, **32**, 763–765.

Lewis B, Wenger J, Waye J. (1991) Intraoperative enteroscopy versus small bowel enteroscopy in patients with obscure GI bleeding. *American Journal of Gastroenterology*, **86**, 171–174.

Lescut D, Vanco D, Bonniere P, *et al.* (1993) Perioperative endoscopy of the whole small bowel in Crohn's disease. *Gut*, **34**, 3647–3649.

Li XB, Dai J, Chen HM, *et al.* (2010) A novel modality for the estimation of the enteroscope insertion depth during double-balloon enteroscopy. *Gastrointestinal Endoscopy*, **72(5)**, 999–1005.

Liu W, Xu C, Zhong J. (2009) The diagnostic value of double-balloon enteroscopy in children with small bowel disease: report of 31 cases. *Canadian Journal of Gastroenterology*, **23**, 635–636.

Linder J, Cheruvattath R, Truss C, *et al.* (2002) Diagnostic yield and clinical implications of push enteroscopy: results from a nonspecialized center. *Journal of Clinical Gastroenterology*, **35**, 383–386.

Lo SK, Simpson PW. (2007). Pancreatitis associated with double-balloon enteroscopy: how common is it? *Gastrointestinal Endoscopy*, **66**, 1139–1141.

Manner H, May A, Pohl J, *et al.* (2010) Impact of fluoroscopy on oral double-balloon enteroscopy: results of a randomized trial in 156 patients. *Endoscopy*, **42(10)**, 820–826.

Manno M, Barbera C, Dabizzi E, *et al.* (2010) Safety of single-balloon enteroscopy: our experience of 72 procedures. *Endoscopy*, **42(9)**, 773, author reply, 774.

Mata A, Bordas JM, Feu F, *et al.* (2004) Wireless capsule endoscopy in patients with obscure gastrointestinal bleeding: a comparative study with push enteroscopy. *Alimentary Pharmacology & Therapeutics*, **20**, 189–194.

Mathus-Vliegen E. (1989) Laser treatment of intestinal vascular abnormalities. *International Journal of Colorectal Disease* **4**, 20–25.

May A, Nachbar L, Wardak A, *et al.* (2003) Double-balloon enteroscopy: preliminary experience in patients with obscure gastrointestinal bleeding or chronic abdominal pain. *Endoscopy*, **35**, 985–991.

May A. (2008) Performing Double-Balloon Enteroscopy: The Utility of the Erlangen EndoTrainer. *Techniques in Gastrointestinal Endoscopy*, **10**, 54–58.

Mehdizadeh S, Ross A, Gerson L, *et al.* (2006) What is the learning curve associated with double-balloon enteroscopy? Technical details and early experience in 6 U.S. tertiary care centers. *Gastrointestinal Endoscopy*, **64**, 740–750.

Mensink PBF. (2008) Complications of Double Balloon Enteroscopy. *Techniques in Gastrointestnal Endoscopy*, **10**, 66–69.

Monkemuller K, Bellutti M, Fry LC, Malfertheiner P. (2008) Enteroscopy. *Best Practice & Research in Clinical Gastroenterology*, **22**, 789–811.

Morgan D, Upchurch B, Draganov, P *et al.* Spiral enteroscopy: prospective U.S. multicenter study in patients with small-bowel disorders. *Gastrointestinal Endoscopy*, **72(5)**, 992–998.

Mylonaki M, Fritscher-Ravens A, Swain P. (2003) Wireless capsule endoscopy: a comparison with push enteroscopy in patients with gastroscopy and colonoscopy negative gastrointestinal bleeding. *Gut*, **52**, 1122–1126.

Nishimura N, Yamamoto H, Yano T, *et al.* (2009) Safety and efficacy of double-balloon enteroscopy in pediatric patients. *Gastrointestinal Endoscopy*, **71**, 287–294.

O'Mahony S, Morris AJ, Straiton M, et al. (1996) Push enteroscopy in the investigation of small-intestinal disease. *Quarterly Journal in Medicine*, **89**, 685.

Pennazio M, Arrigoni A, Risio M, *et al.* (1995) Clinical evaluation of push-type enteroscopy. *Endoscopy*, **27**, 164–170.

Sanada Y, Mizuta K, Yano T, *et al.*(1995) Double-balloon enteroscopy for bilioenteric anastomotic stricture after pediatric living donor liver transplantation. *Transplant International.* Jan, **24(1)**, 85–90.

Schnoll-Sussman F, Kulkarni K. (2008) Risks of Capsule Endoscopy. *Techniques in Gastrointestinal Endoscopy*, **10**, 25–30.

Shimizu S, Tada M, Kawai K. (1987) Development of a new insertion technique in push-type enteroscopy. *American Journal of Gastroenterology*, **82,** 844–847.

Sunada K, Yamamoto H. (2008) Double Balloon Enterosocopy: Techniques. *Techniques in Gastrointestinal Endoscopy*, **10,** 46–53.

Tada M, Akasaka Y, Misaki F, *et al.* (1977) Clinical evaluation of a sonde-type small intestinal fiberscope. *Endoscopy*, **9,** 33–38.

Thomson M, Venkatesh K, Elmalik K, *et al.* (2010) Double balloon enteroscopy in children: diagnosis, treatment and safety. *World Journal of Gastroenterology*, **16,** 56–62.

Turck D, Bonnevalle M, Gottrand F, *et al.* (1990) Intraoperative endoscopic diagnosis of heterotopic gastric mucosa in the ileum causing recurrent acute intussusception. *Journal of Pediatric Gastroenterology & Nutrition*, **11,** 275–278.

Turck, D, Bonnevalle M, Gottrand F, *et al.* (1990) Intraoperative endoscopic diagnosis of heterotopic gastric mucosa in the ileum causing recurrent acute intussusception. *Journal of Pediatric Gastroenterology & Nutrition*, **11,** 275–278.

Whelan R, Buls J, Goldberg S, *et al.* 1989, Intraoperative enteroscopy: University of Minnesota experience. *American Journal of Surgery*, **55,** 281–286.

Yamamoto H, Sekine Y, Sato Y, *et al.* (2001) Total enteroscopy with a nonsurgical steerable double-balloon method. *Gastrointestinal Endoscopy*, **53,** 216–220.

Yamamoto H, Kita H, Sunada K, *et al.* (2004) Clinical outcomes of double-balloon endoscopy for the diagnosis and treatment of small-intestinal diseases. *Clinical Gastroenterology & Hepatology*, **2,** 1010–1016.

Yang R, Laine L. (1995) Mucosal stripping: a complication of push enteroscopy. *Gastrointestinal Endoscopy*, **41,** 156–158.

Zaman A, Katon RM. (1998) Push enteroscopy for obscure gastrointestinal bleeding yields a high incidence of proximal lesions within reach of a standard endoscope. *Gastrointestinal Endoscopy*, **47,** 372–376.

18

Endoscopic approaches to the treatment of GERD

Mike Thomson

 KEY POINTS

- Evolution of this approach has occurred over the last 10 years and the present generation (trans-oral incisionless fundoplication (TIF)) is safe and effective in adults and, in a small series, in children.
- With CO_2 insufflation, no adverse events have occurred. Air insufflation should not be used.
- One year objective efficacy with pH studies, and quality-of-life with standardized validated scoring systems, has shown medium-term success in children.

- In the UK in day case procedures this approach compares favorably with laparoscopic, and even more so with open, fundoplication.
- The technique at present is limited by the size of the patient to approximately 25 kg body weight.
- Clearly, this technique requires further evaluation but initial studies are encouraging.

Gastroesophageal reflux disease (GERD) is symptomatic reflux associated with sequelae. These include failing to thrive, refractory wheezing, coughing aspiration, acute life-threatening events, apnoea, chronic otitis media, sinusitis, hematemesis, anemia, esophageal strictures and Barrett's esophagus. A follow-up of 126 children with gastroesophageal reflux disease in infancy showed 55% were symptom-free by 10 months and 81% by 18 months of age. However, those with frequent symptoms (>90 days) in the first two years of life are more likely to have symptoms by 9 years of age.

Gastroesophageal reflux treatment aims to achieve symptom relief while preventing complications. Patients who fail to achieve control with

medical therapy, may have persisten, severe esophagitis or become long-term dependent on anti-reflux treatments. In such cases, an anti-reflux procedure may be indicated. The principle of surgery in gastroesophageal reflux disease is to form some kind of reconstruction of the anti-reflux barrier, although exactly how efficacy is achieved is not fully understood. Open Nissen's fundoplication has been the treatment of choice to date, but is invasive and associated with morbidity and mortality. In recent years, laparoscopic fundoplication has become popular, and in general, has replaced the open Nissen's procedure, although superior efficacy and safety has yet to be demonstrated. With the laparoscopic procedure cosmesis is clearly superior, and in adult studies complications appear

Practical Pediatric Gastrointestinal Endoscopy, Second Edition. George Gershman, Mike Thomson, Marvin Ament.
© 2012 Blackwell Publishing Ltd. Published 2012 by Blackwell Publishing Ltd.

less common, with good success rates. It could be argued, therefore, that there remains little or no place for open anti-reflux procedures in pediatrics.

Three endoscopic techniques have been devised and used for treatment of pediatric GERD. These are described below.

Endoscopic suturing devices

Endoluminal gastroplication makes use of an EndoCinch® sewing machine attached to the endoscope (gastroscope) placing three pairs of stitches below the gastroesophageal junction to create three internal plications of the stomach. Plications may be applied in any manner dependent on operator preference. These may be applied circumferentially or longitudinally. The authors have a preference for placing two plications circumferentially 1.5 cm below the gastroesophageal junction and one 0.5 cm below the gastroesophageal junction, which we believe anatomically may be superior to other formations. (Figures 18.1–4)

Endoluminal gastroplication is now routinely carried out as a day-case procedure in adults. Preliminary studies have shown it to be quick, non-invasive, effective and safe. Results are comparable to the laparoscopic fundoplication in adults, which has been studied as a preferable alternative choice to an open Nissen's fundoplication.

Recently, the authors have reported use of Endocinch® (endoscopic gastroplication using a flexible endoscopic sewing device) in the treatment of 17 children (8 males, median age 12.9 years – range 6.1–17.7, median weight 45 kg – range 16.5–75) with gastroesophageal reflux disease refractory to, or dependent on (>12 months) proton pump inhibitors. All patients showed post-treatment improvement in symptom severity, frequency, and validated reflux-related quality of life scores (p < 0.0001) (Figure 18.5). At 36 months

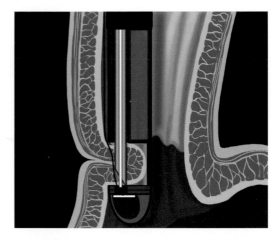

Figure 18.2 Suction applied and full-thickness tissue capture followed by needle and pusher wire placement of stitch.

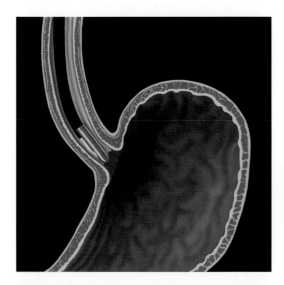

Figure 18.1 Endocinch front-mounted on endoscope.

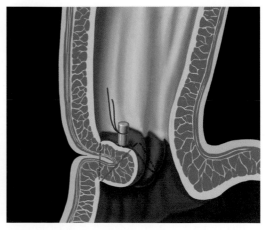

Figure 18.3 Endoscopic gastroplication. This figure shows the pattern of a zig-zag stich when applied with an Endocinch® sewing machine.

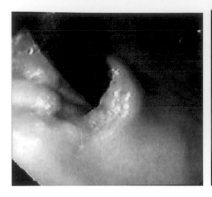
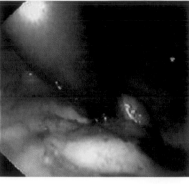

Figure 18.4 View (J manoeuver) of a lax GE junction in a child with major reflux after application of stitch with the EndoCinch®.

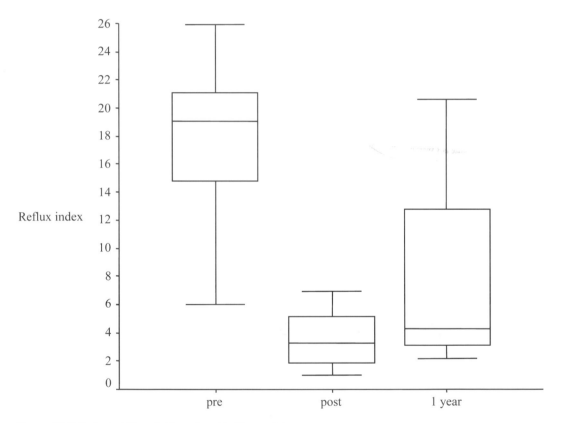

Figure 18.5 Endocinch® pediatric series pH efficacy at 1 year.

median follow-up 11 out of 17 patients were asymptomatic and no longer taking any anti-reflux medications. At 12 months follow-up, all pH parameters improved and had returned to normal in 8 out of 9 patients who underwent pH studies (reflux index fell from 16.6% (0.9–67%) to 2.5% (0.7–15.7%) ($p < 0.0001$)) (Figure 18.5).

The duration of action is open to ongoing assessment and debate, and has not been particu-larly impressive in adult studies. The reasons for superior efficacy and duration in children may be conjectured and due to some or all of the follow-ing: 3 pairs versus 2 pairs of sutures; greater time and care taken by the operator allowed by general anesthetic with the added advantage of absence of movement or retching during the procedure; and lastly the relatively deeper suture depth in the thinner pediatric esophagus compared to the

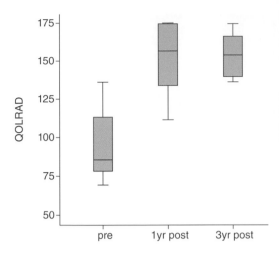

Figure 18.6 Significant improvement in the total QOLRAD score 1 and 3 years after gastroplication with the Endocinch®.

larger adult one. Data are now available indicating medium-term success in terms of reflux related quality-of-life scoring at 3 years post-Endocinch and in terms of avoidance of PPI need in the majority of patients. This is a small study but worthy of mention (Figure 18.6).

Despite the loss of sutures on observational follow-up studies some efficacy has been maintained, and the human and porcine endo-ultrasound studies of Liu *et al*, along with cadaveric analysis of the porcine model post-Endocinch® may throw some light on this observation. They suggest that the tissue remodeling in response to the foreign body, which is the suture, resulting in significant hypertrophy of the circular muscle layer of the esophagus may be the reason.

Nevertheless, Endocinch® has not maintained its initial enthusiastic uptake, and has been recently superseded by the next generation of full-thickness gastroplication trans-oral endoscopic techniques.

The next to appear was the Full Thickness Plicator® (Ndo-Surgical). This is placed under direct vision with a neonatal size endoscope passed through a specially designed endoscopic delivery system with an outer diameter of more than 20 mm. The retroflexion of both allows observation firstly of the opening of the jaws of the device, followed by the insertion of the corkscrew into the fundal tissue, allowing capture of the fundus and withdrawal into the jaws which are then closed. A pre-tied full thickness plication is then applied by the mechanism of shutting the

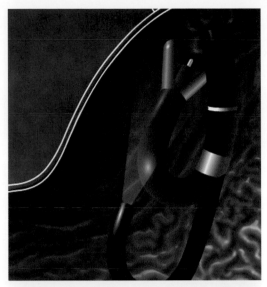

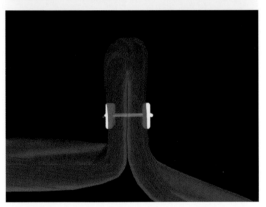

Figures 18.7 and 18.8 Application of the Full Thickness Plicator® (Ndo-Surgical).

jaws and a serosa to serosa plication is made. (Figures 18.7–9) A multicenter adult study has shown acceptable efficacy and a reduction of PPI requirement in a small adult cohort, and further study is necessary before this should be applied to children – the device is size and age-constrained due to its large outer diameter.

Esophyx

This device is representative of an alternative to the Plicator technology along a similar theme, although not identical.

The novel Transoral Incisionless Fundoplication (TIF)® procedure using EsophyX®

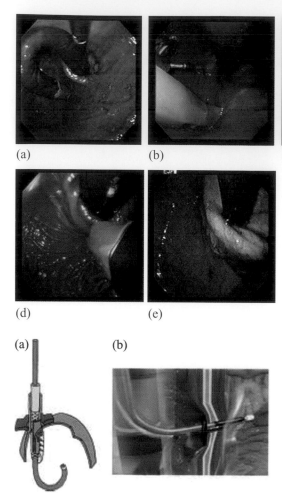

(a)

(b)

(c)

(d)

(e)

Figure 18.9 Retroverted views of stages of application of Full Thickness Plicator® (Ndo-Surgical) (a) Plicator and gastroscope retroflexed to GEJ. (b) Arms opened, tissue retractor advanced to serosa. (c) Gastric wall retracted. (d) Resulting full-thickness plication. (e) Arms closed, single pre-tied implant deployed.

(a)

(b)

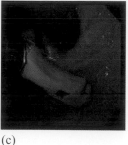

Figure 18.10 Distal end of the EsophyX® device (a) and SerosaFuse fastener (b). The valve is constructed by drawing tissue into the device with the aid of a helical retractor. The tissue mold is then closed over the retracted tissue and the fasteners are deployed. The fastener is delivered by a pusher that slides over a stylet. (From: Jobe BA, O'Rourke RW, McMahon BP, et al. (2008) Transoral endoscopic fundoplication in the treatment of gastroesophageal reflux disease: the anatomic and physiologic basis for reconstruction of the esophagogastric junction using a novel device. *Annals of Surgery*, 248, 69–76, with permission.)

mimics anti-reflux surgery in constructing an anterior partial fundoplication with tailored delivery of multiple fasteners during a single-device insertion (Figures 18.10 and 18.11). The TIF procedure was designed to restore the anti-reflux competency of the gastroesophageal junction by reducing small hiatal hernias, increasing LES resting pressure, narrowing cardia and recreation of acute angle of His.

Clinical results with TIF at 1, 2 and 3 years support its efficacy in eliminating heartburn and regurgitation, reducing the daily use of PPIs, normalizing esophageal acid exposure and reducing proximal extent of refluxate. Based on one-year results FDA cleared EsophyX in September 2007 for the treatment of GERD and small (<2 cm) hiatal hernia.

The TIF procedure has been demonstrated to be safe in adults. Post-TIF adverse events are mild and transient and include musculoskeletal and epigastric pain, nausea, and dysphagia up to one week secondary to sore throat. Only three esophageal perforations have been reported to date for 3000 cases performed world-wide. None of the subjects experienced chronic dysphagia, gas bloating, or diarrhea at long-term follow-up.

A feasibility study was started in December 2008 after obtaining appropriate training in the use of the EsophyX® device in its second iteration – the so-called TIF2.procedure. The feasibility study was conducted with 12 children (8 male) with a median age of 12.25 years (8–18) years and weight of 38.2 kg (26–91). The median duration of GERD symptoms was 45 months (24–70) and all subjects were on GERD medication for more than 6 months. The median pre-TIF2 reflux index off treatment was 11.4% (6–48). Hiatus hernia was present in 17% (2/12). Median operative time was 42 minutes (range 25–94). Adverse events were experienced by three subjects and consisted of mild or moderate pharyngeal irritation and epigastric pain. Two of the three subjects also had retrosternal chest pain

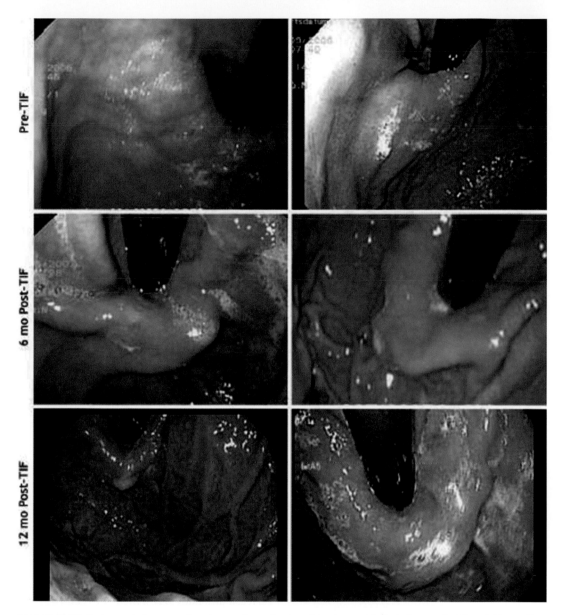

Figure 18.11 Endoscopic images of gastroesophageal valves from two subjects before and at 6 and 12 months following TIF1 (From: Cadiere GB, Buset M, Muls V, Rajan A, *et al* (2008). Antireflux transoral incisionless fundoplication using EsophyX: 12-month results of a prospective multicenter study. *World J Surg* 32:1676–88; with kind permission from Springer Science+Business Media B.V.)

and were subsequently found to have pneumomediastinum on CT chest but no leak on barium swallow. One of these two patients had pyrexia accompanying chest pain and was treated for possible mediastinitis and discharged home after 5 days of intravenous antibiotics. Subsequently, CO_2 insufflation was employed and more rapid absorption resulted in no further peri-procedure mediastinal gas leak.

At 6-month follow-up, all subjects ($n = 10$) discontinued PPIs, 80% were asymptomatic and 70% had normalized or clinically significantly reduced reflux index (10% time pH < 4). The results of this feasibility study showed that the TIF procedure was feasible, safe (with CO_2 insufflation) and clinically effective in treating GERD in children. Ongoing studies are occurring. Furthermore, the speed of the procedure, the days

Operation times

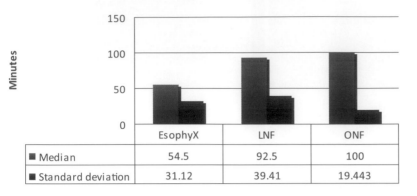

	EsophyX	LNF	ONF
■ Median	54.5	92.5	100
■ Standard deviation	31.12	39.41	19.443

Figure 18.12 Operation times comparing endoscopic, laparoscopic and open fundoplication.

Hospital Stay

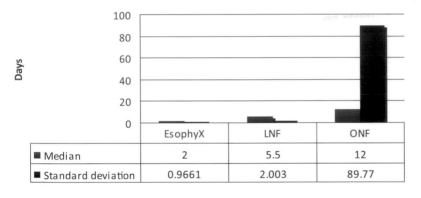

	EsophyX	LNF	ONF
■ Median	2	5.5	12
■ Standard deviation	0.9661	2.003	89.77

Figure 18.13 Hospital stay (days) comparing endoscopic, laparoscopic, and open fundoplication.

Total costs including HDU/NSU/ITU

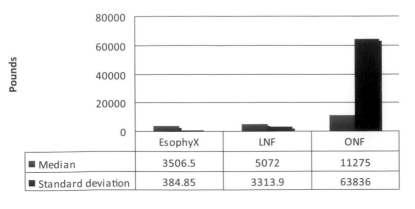

	EsophyX	LNF	ONF
■ Median	3506.5	5072	11275
■ Standard deviation	384.85	3313.9	63836

Figure 18.14 Total cost comparing endoscopic, laparoscopic and open fundoplication (British pounds).

of hospitalization, the relative cost-efficacy, and cost-benefit are identified in Figures 18.12–18.14.

Delivery of radiofrequency energy (the STRETTA® system)

The STRETTA® system has two parts; one a Stretta® catheter and the other Stretta® control module. The Stretta® catheter is a flexible, hand-held, single patient-use device that delivers radiofrequency energy generated by the control module (Figure 18.15). It is inserted into the patient's mouth and advanced to the gastro-esophageal junction. A balloon is inflated and needle electrodes are deployed into the tissue. Radiofrequency energy is delivered through the electrodes to create thermal lesions in the muscle of the lower esophageal sphincter and gastric cardia. As these lesions heal, the tissue contracts, resulting in a reduction of reflux episodes with improvement in symptoms. The Stretta® control module delivers this radiofrequency, while, at the same time, providing feedback to the physician regarding treatment temperatures, tissue impedance values, elapsed time, catheter position measurement and irrigation rate.

This treatment has been used in adults since 1999. Complications are rare but among those reported are ulcerative esophagitis with gas-troparesis, esophageal perforation and a case of aspiration following the procedure. Short-term (1 year) success was reported in an open-label trial. In a prospective study (non-randomized controlled trial) of 75 patients (age 49 +/– 14 years, 44% male, 56% female) undergoing laparoscopic fundoplication and 65 (age 46 +/– 12 years, 42%, 58% female) the Stretta® procedure, at 6 months, 58% of Stretta® patients were off proton pump inhibitors, and an additional 31% had reduced their dose significantly. In comparison, 97% of laparoscopic fundoplication patients were off PPIs. With long-term follow-up of these patients receiving the Stretta® treatment, beyond two years, 56% had discontinued use of all anti-secretory drugs.

This treatment has been reported in an uncontroled study of a group of eight children with a variable follow up period of 5–15 months. It was reported that 6 out of 8 children improved, and the cohort included 3 neurologically impaired children who also had concomitant PEG placement. One of this group had a post-procedure aspiration which was successfully treated. Of the two failures, one remained dependent on PPI and the other had a successful Nissen's fundoplication.

Pediatric gastroenterologists may be guarded in using this form of treatment as clearly using thermal energy treatment in a 70-year-old is different to a child who may have unknown consequences in the long-term. Hence this is not recommended.

Gastroesophageal biopolymer injection

In the Enteryx® procedure, a liquid polymer is injected into the lower esophageal sphincter (LES) with a needle catheter via an endoscope. After the injection, the polymer solidifies into a sponge-like permanent implant. This improves the gastroesophageal junction, by supporting and improving its elasticity and therefore reducing the degree of gastroesophageal reflux (Figure 18.16).

Cohen, in an international open-label clinical trial on 144 patients, showed a greater than 50% reduction in PPI in 84% at end of one year and 72% by two years with elimination in 67% patients. In a prospective, randomized trial, endoluminal gastroplasty (EndoCinch®) was compared with Enteryx® in 51 consecutive patients dependent on proton pump inhibitor therapy. At 6 months, proton pump inhibitor therapy could be stopped or dosage was reduced by more than 50% in 20 of

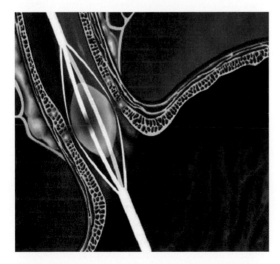

Figure 18.15 The Stretta® system. Use of a balloon to deliver radiofrequency energy via needle electrodes to the mucosa.

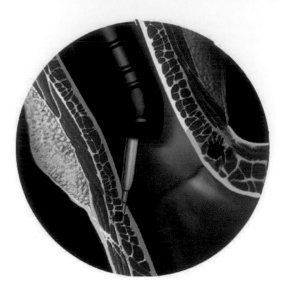

Figure 18.16 Injection of liquid polymer into the oesophageal mucosa. The Enteryx® procedure.

26 (77%) EndoCinch®-treated patients and in 20 of 23 patients treated by Enteryx® (87%, $p = 0.365$). Approximately 25% of the patients in both groups required retreatment in an attempt to achieve symptom control. To date, an estimated 3800 patients have been treated with the Enteryx® device, which was approved in 2003 by the FDA. To date, there are no published records of its use in pediatrics.

However, the FDA & Boston Scientific notified healthcare professionals and patients about serious adverse events, including death, occurring in patients treated with the Enteryx® device. Based upon reports filed with the FDA, patients suffered leakage, swelling, and ulcers in the esophagus. One elderly patient died after some of the polymer had been injected into the woman's aorta, which ruptured, causing her to bleed to death.

On September 23, 2005, Boston Scientific ordered a recall of all Enteryx® Procedure Kits and Enteryx® Injector Single Packs from commercial distribution. The company's recall notice stated some doctors accidentally punctured the wall of the esophagus while injecting the substance, causing adverse events. Additionally, Boston Scientific Corp. recently suspended sales of its Enteryx® device after more than two dozen reports of problems. The notice was posted on the company's Website, during the week of September 19, 2005.

Summary

The most promising results seem to accrue in the mid-term with the suturing devices which attain full-thickness plications, increase the intra-abdominal portion of the esophagus (most likely by plication tags inserting through the diaphragmatic crura as well as the full thickness of the oesophageal wall i.e., actual change in anatomy), and raised intra-sphincteric length and resting pressure. Endo-ultrasound may provide a more controled and sophisticated approach to this technology in the future.

FURTHER READING

Cadiere GB, Rajan A, Germay O, *et al.* (2008) Endoluminal fundoplication by a transoral device for the treatment of GERD: A feasibility study. *Surgical Endoscopy*, **22**, 333–342.

Cadiere GB, Van Sante N, Graves JE, *et al.* (2009) Two-year results of a feasibility study on antire-flux transoral incisionless fundoplication (TIF) using EsophyX. *Surgical Endoscopy*, **23**, 957–964.

Cohen LB, Johnson DA, Ganz RA, *et al.* (2005) Enteryx implantation for GERD: expanded multicenter trial results and interim postapproval follow-up to 24 months. *Gastrointestinal Endoscopy*, **61**, 650–658.

FDA. (2005) FDA preliminary public health notification. Internet Communication.

Festen C. (1981) Paraesophageal hernia: a major complication of Nissen's fundoplication. *Journal of Pediatric Surgery*, **16**, 496–499.

Filipi CJ, Lehman GA, Rothstein RI, *et al.* (2001) Transoral, flexible endoscopic suturing for treatment of GERD: a multicenter trial. *Gastrointestinal Endoscopy*, **53**, 416–422.

Gotley DC, Smithers BM, Rhodes M, *et al.* (1996) Laparoscopic Nissen fundoplication – 200 consecutive cases. *Gut*, **38**, 487–491.

Hyams JS, Ricci A Jr, Leichtner AM. (1988) Clinical and laboratory correlates of esophagitis in young children. *Journal of Pediatric Gastroenterology & Nutrition*, **7**, 52–56.

Islam S, Geiger JD, Coran AG, *et al.* (2004) Use of radiofrequency ablation of the lower esophageal sphincter to treat recurrent gastroesophageal reflux disease. *Journal of Pediatric Surgery*, **39**, 282–286.

Jobe BA, O'Rourke RW, McMahon BP, *et al.* (2008) Transoral endoscopic fundoplication in the treatment of gastroesophageal reflux disease: the anatomic and physiologic basis for reconstruction of the esophagogastric junction using a novel device. *Annals of Surgery*, **248**, 69–76.

Liu DC, Somme S, Mavrelis PG, *et al.* (2005) Stretta as the initial antireflux procedure in children. *Journal of Pediatric Surgery*, **40**, 148–151.

Liu JJ, Glickman JN, Carr-Locke DL, *et al.* (2004) Gastroesophageal junction smooth muscle remodeling after endoluminal gastroplication. *American Journal of Gastroenterology*, **99,** 1895–1901.

Mahmood Z, McMahon BP, Arfin Q, *et al.* (2003) Endocinch therapy for gastro-oesophageal reflux disease: a one- year prospective follow-up. *Gut*, **52,** 34–39.

Mahmood, Z. Byrne PJ, McMahon BP, *et al.* (2006) Comparison of transesophageal endoscopic plication (TEP) with laparoscopic Nissen fundoplication (LNF) in the treatment of uncomplicated reflux disease. *American Journal of Gastroenterology*, **101,** 431–436.

Martin AJ, Pratt N, Kennedy JD, *et al.* (2002) Natural history and familial relationships of infant spilling to 9 years of age. *Pediatrics*, **109,** 1061–1067.

Mattioli G, Repetto P, Carlini C, *et al.* (2002) Laparoscopic vs open approach for the treatment of gastroesophageal reflux in children. *Surgical Endoscopy*, **16,** 750–752.

Park P, Kjellin T, Kadirkamanathan S. (2001) Results of endoscopic gastroplasty for gastro-oesophageal reflux disease. *Gastrointestinal Endoscopy*, [Abstract].

Pleskow D, Rothstein R, Lo S, *et al.* (2004) Endoscopic full-thickness plication for the treatment of GERD: a multicenter trial. *Gastrointestinal Endoscopy*, **59,** 163–171.

Raijman I, Ben-Menachem T, Reddy G. (2001) Symptomatic response to endoluminal gastroplication (ELGP) in patients with gastroesophageal reflux disease (GERD): a multicentre experience. *Gastrointestinal Endoscopy*, [Abstract].

Repici A, Fumagalli U, Malesci A, *et al.* (2009) Endoluminal fundoplication (ELF) for GERD using EsophyX: a 12-month follow-up in a single-center experience. *J Gastrointestinal Surgery*, (ePub ahead of print).

Richards WO, Scholz S, Khaitan L, *et al.* (2001) Initial experience with the stretta procedure for the treatment of gastroesophageal reflux disease. *Journal of Laparoendoscopic & Advanced Surgical Techniques*, **11,** 267–273.

Richards WO, Houston HL, Torquati A, *et al.* Paradigm shift in the management of gastroesophageal reflux disease. *Annals of Surgery*, **237,** 638–647.

Rudolph CD, Mazur LA, Liptak GP, *et al.* (2001) Guidelines for evaluation and treatment of gastroesophageal reflux in infants and children: recommendations of the North American Society for Pediatric Gastroenterology and Nutrition. *Journal of Pediatric Gastroenterology & Nutrition*, **32(Suppl 2),** S1–S31.

Shepherd RW, Wren J, Evans S, *et al.* (1987) Gastroesophageal reflux in children. Clinical profile, course and outcome with active therapy in 126 cases. *Clinical Pediatrics (Philadelphia)*, **26,** 55–60.

Swain CP, Kadirkamanathan SS, Gong F, *et al.* (1994) Knot tying at flexible endoscopy. *Gastrointestinal Endoscopy*, **40,** 722–729.

Swain P, Park PO, Mills T. (2003) Bard EndoCinch: the device, the technique, and pre-clinical studies. *Gastrointestinal Endoscopy Clinics of North America*, **13,** 75–88.

Swain P, Park PO. (2004) Endoscopic suturing. *Best Practice and Research in Clinical Gastroenterology*, **18,** 37–47.

Thiny MT, Shaheen NJ. (2002) Is Stretta ready for primetime? *Gastroenterology*, **123,** 643–644.

Thomson, M. (1997) Disorders of the oesophagus and stomach in infants. *Baillieres Clinical Gastroenterology*, **11,** 547–571.

Thomson M, Frischer-Ravens A, Hall S, *et al.* (2004) Endoluminal gastroplication in children with significant gastro-oesophageal reflux disease. *Gut*, **53,** 1745–1750.

Thomson M, Antao B, Hall S, *et al.* (2008) Medium-term outcome of endoluminal gastroplication with the Endocinch device in children. *Journal of Pediatric Gastroenterology & Nutrition*, **46,** 172–177.

Thomson M, Lobontiu A, Stewart R, *et al.* Transoral incisionless fundoplication for the treatment of pediatric gastroesophageal reflux disease: a feasibility study. *(in preparation)*.

Torquati A, Houston HL, Kaiser J, *et al.* (2004) Long-term follow-up study of the Stretta procedure for the treatment of gastroesophageal reflux disease. *Surgical Endoscopy*, **18,** 1475–1479.

Veit F, Schwagten K, Auldist AW, *et al.* (1995) Trends in the use of fundoplication in children with gastro-oesophageal reflux. *Journal of Paediatric Child Health*, **31,** 121–126.

Velanovich V, Ben-Menachem T, Goel S. (2002) Case-control comparison of endoscopic gastroplication with laparoscopic fundoplication in the management of gastroesophageal reflux disease: early symptomatic outcomes. *Surgical Laparoscopy Endoscopy & Percutaneous Techniques*, **12,** 219–223.

Watson DI. (2008) Endoscopic antireflux surgery: are we there yet? *World Journal of Surgery*, **32,** 1578–1580.

Youd P, Emmanuel A, Sivanesan S, *et al.* Cessation of proton pump inhibitors following transoral incisionless fundoplication is associated with reduced proximal extent of refluxate. *Endoscopy* (submitted).

Index

Notes: Pages numbers in *italics* refer to Figures; those in **bold** to Tables